D1428661

Commissioning Editor: Oliver Walter
Development Editor: Kate Newell

Pediatric Cardiology

The Essential Pocket Guide

Walter H. Johnson, Jr., M.D.
Associate Professor of Pediatrics
Department of Pediatrics
Division of Pediatric Cardiology
University of Alabama at Birmingham
H 320
620 South 20th Street
Birmingham AL 35233
USA

James H. Moller, M.D.
University of Minnesota Medical School
MMC 288, Room 203 VCRC
420 Delaware St SE
Minneapolis MN 55455-0374
USA

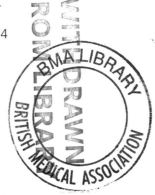

WILEY-BLACKWELL

A John Wiley & Sons, Ltd., Publication

This edition first published 2008 © by Blackwell Publishing Ltd

Blackwell Publishing was acquired by John Wiley & Sons in February 2007. Blackwell's publishing program has been merged with Wiley's global Scientific, Technical and Medical business to form Wiley-Blackwell.

Registered office: John Wiley & Sons Ltd, The Atrium, Southern Gate, Chichester, West Sussex, PO19 8SQ, UK

Editorial offices: 9600 Garsington Road, Oxford, OX4 2DQ, UK
        The Atrium, Southern Gate, Chichester, West Sussex, PO19 8SQ, UK
        111 River Street, Hoboken, NJ 07030-5774, USA

For details of our global editorial offices, for customer services and for information about how to apply for permission to reuse the copyright material in this book please see our website at www.wiley.com/wiley-blackwell

Library of Congress Cataloging-in-Publication Data

Johnson, Walter H., Jr.
Pediatric cardiology : the essential pocket guide / Walter H. Johnson Jr., James H. Moller. – 2nd ed.
    p. ; cm.
Includes bibliographical references and index.
ISBN 978-1-4051-7818-1 (pbk. : alk. paper)
1. Pediatric cardiology–Handbooks, manuals, etc. I. Moller, James H., 1933-   II. Title.
[DNLM: 1. Heart Diseases–Handbooks. 2. Child. WS 39 J71pa 2008]

RJ421.J64 2008
618.92′12–dc22

                                   2008023443 ISBN:

978-1-4051-7818-1

A catalogue record for this book is available from the British Library.

Set in 8/10 pt Frutiger Light by Aptara® Inc., New Delhi, India
Printed in Singapore by Utopia Press Pte Ltd

1 2008

Contents

Preface

Since the development of pediatric cardiac catheterization, echocardiography, and magnetic resonance imaging, less emphasis has been placed on the more traditional methods of evaluating a cardiac patient. Most practitioners, however, do not have these refined diagnostic techniques available to them or the training to apply them. To evaluate a cardiac patient, the practitioner therefore depends upon either the combination of physical examination, electrocardiogram, and chest X-ray, or the referral of the patient to a cardiac diagnostic center.

The purpose of this book is to formulate guidelines by which the practitioner, medical student, and house officer can approach the diagnostic problem presented by an infant or child with a cardiac finding. Through proper assessment and integration of the history, physical examination, electrocardiogram, and chest X-ray, the type of problem can be diagnosed correctly in 80% of patients, and the severity and hemodynamics can be correctly estimated.

Even though a patient may require referral to a cardiac center, the practitioner will appreciate and understand better the specific type of specialized diagnostic studies performed, and the approach, timing, and results of operation or management. This book will help in the selection of patients for referral and offer guidelines for the timing of referrals.

This book is divided into 12 chapters:

Diagnostic Methods includes sections on history, physical examination, electrocardiography, and chest radiography, and discusses functional murmurs. A brief overview of special procedures, such as echocardiography and cardiac catheterization, is included.

Heart Disease in Special Populations presents syndromes, genetic disorders, and maternal conditions commonly associated with congenital heart disease.

The chapters entitled Classification and Pathophysiology, Acyanotic Lesions, Obstructive Lesions, Cyanotic Lesions, and Other Cardiac Malformations discuss specific congenital cardiac malformations. The hemodynamics of the malformations are presented as a basis for understanding the physical findings, electrocardiogram, and chest radiographs. Emphasis is placed on features that permit differential diagnosis.

Cardiac Conditions in the Neonate describes the cardiac malformations leading to symptoms in the neonatal period and in the transition from the fetal to the adult circulation.

Acquired Cardiac Conditions includes common cardiac problems affecting children, such as Kawasaki disease, rheumatic fever, and the cardiac manifestations of systemic diseases.

Arrhythmias presents the practical basics of diagnosis and management of rhythm disorders in children.

Congestive Cardiac Failure presents the pathophysiology and management of cardiac failure in children. Medical and surgical (including transplantation) management is discussed.

Preventive Cardiology and Health Promotion discusses preventive issues for children with normal hearts (the vast majority) including smoking, hypertension, lipids, exercise, and other risk factors for adult-manifest cardiovascular disease. Prevention and health maintenance issues particular to children with heart disease are also discussed.

This book is not a substitute for the many excellent and encyclopedic texts of pediatric cardiology, or for the expanding number of electronic resources. Appendix G and the Additional Reading and References sections accompanying some chapters include both traditional and online resources chosen to be of greatest value to the practitioner. The Appendices deal with other issues such as management of tachycardia, outpatient drug therapy of heart failure, and tetralogy spells.

Certain generalizations are made. In pediatric cardiology, as in all fields, exceptions occur. Therefore, not all instances of cardiac abnormality will be correctly diagnosed on the basis of the criteria set forth here.

Chapter 1
Diagnostic methods

The history and physical examination are the keystones for diagnosis of cardiac problems. A variety of other diagnostic techniques can be employed beyond the history and physical examination. With each technique, different aspects of the cardiovascular system are viewed, and by combining the data derived, an accurate assessment of the patient's condition can be obtained.

HISTORY

General principles of the cardiovascular history
The suspicion of a cardiovascular abnormality may be raised initially by specific symptoms, but more commonly the presenting feature is the discovery of a cardiac murmur. Many children with a cardiac abnormality are asymptomatic

Pediatric Cardiology, by W Johnson, J Moller © 2008 Blackwell Publishing,
ISBN: 978-1-4051-7818-1.

because the malformation does not result in major hemodynamic alterations. Even with a significant cardiac problem, the child may be asymptomatic because the myocardium is capable of responding normally to the stresses placed upon it by the altered hemodynamics. A comparable lesion in an adult might produce symptoms because of coexistent coronary arterial disease or myocardial fibrosis.

In obtaining the history of a child suspected of cardiac disease, the physician seeks three types of data.

Diagnostic clues
Diagnostic clues (e.g., cyanosis or squatting) and other more general factors include the following.

Gender. Certain cardiac malformations have a definite gender predominance. Atrial septal defect (ASD) and patent ductus arteriosus are two to three times more likely in female than in male children. Coarctation of the aorta, aortic stenosis, and transposition of the great vessels more commonly occur in male children.

Age. The age at which a cardiac murmur or a symptom develops may give a diagnostic clue. The murmurs of congenital aortic stenosis and pulmonary stenosis are often heard in the neonatal period. Ventricular septal defect (VSD) is usually first recognized because of symptoms and murmur, at 4–6 weeks. The murmur of an ASD may not be discovered until the preschool examination. Among school age children, a functional (innocent) murmur is found in half.

Severity of the cardiac condition
The physician seeks information that suggests the condition's severity (e.g., dyspnea).

Etiology
The physician seeks information that suggests an etiology of cardiac disease (e.g., maternal lupus).

Chief complaint and/or presenting sign
Certain presenting complaints and signs are more common in certain cardiac disorders and the "index of suspicion" aids the physician in organizing the data to make a differential diagnosis. For many of the signs and symptoms discussed later, *noncardiac causes are often more likely than cardiac causes* (e.g., acute dyspnea in a previously healthy 4-month-old infant with no murmur is more likely a result of bronchiolitis than of congestive heart failure). Therefore, a complete history must be integrated with the physical examination and other diagnostic studies to arrive at the correct cardiac diagnosis.

Murmur

Murmur is the most common presenting finding because virtually all children and adults with a normal heart have an innocent (normal) murmur heard sometime during their lifetime. Certain historical features are associated with an innocent murmur; the child is asymptomatic and murmurs appearing after infancy tend to be innocent. The murmur of atrial septal defect is one important exception.

Chest pain

Chest pain is a common and benign symptom in older children and adolescents, estimated to occur at some time in 70% of school-aged children. About 1 in 200 visits to a pediatric emergency room is for chest pain.

Chest pain rarely occurs with cardiovascular disease in this age group. Myocardial ischemic syndromes (e.g., Kawasaki disease with aneurysms; hypertrophic cardiomyopathy) may lead to true angina. Patients with connective tissue disorders (e.g., Marfan syndrome) may have chest (or back) pain from arterial dissection. Although pericarditis may cause chest pain, it is almost always associated with fever and other signs of inflammation. Occasionally, chest pain accompanies supraventricular tachycardia. The vast majority of children with congenital cardiac malformations, including those who are fully recovered from surgery, do not have chest pain, and the majority of children and adolescents who do present with chest pain as their chief complaint do not have cardiac malformations or disease.

Benign chest pain is usually transient, appearing abruptly, lasting 30 seconds to 5 minutes and localized to the parasternal area. It can be distinguished from angina by the absence of diaphoresis, nausea, emesis, and paresthesias in an ulnar distribution. Benign chest pain is "sharp," not "crushing" like angina. Chest pain may occur as a result of chest wall tenderness, which is typically well localized, sharp in character, short (seconds to minutes) in duration, often aggravated by certain positions or movements, and can be induced by palpation over the area. These findings tend to be good evidence against cardiac cause for the pain. Some other noncardiac conditions (e.g., asthma) may be associated with childhood chest pain. However, benign pain is often described as "functional" because an organic cause cannot be found.

Palpitations

Palpitations, the sensation of irregular heartbeats, "skipped beats," or more commonly, rapid beats, are also common in the school-aged child and adolescent. They frequently occur in patients with other symptoms, such as chest pain, but often not simultaneously with the other symptoms. Palpitations are often found to be associated with normal sinus rhythm when the electrocardiogram is monitored during the symptom. Palpitations are not usually present in patients with known premature beats. Palpitations of sudden onset (approximately the time span of a single beat) and termination suggest tachyarrhythmia.

Near-syncope

Near-syncope is a complex of symptoms that includes vertigo and weakness. It is often induced by a postural change (orthostatic), is found commonly in older children and adolescents, and is almost always benign. The history often reveals little fluid and caloric intake beforehand. *True syncope*, characterized by complete loss of consciousness and loss of skeletal muscle tone, rarely results from a cardiac abnormality. It is often autonomic (vasovagal) in origin. Benign syncope is usually very brief in duration, often lasting only seconds. Benign syncope may follow a period of physical activity by several minutes; however, *syncope during exercise* often indicates a serious cardiac problem, such as aortic stenosis, arrhythmia, or myocardial abnormality. Because some life-threatening conditions (e.g., long QT syndrome) may result in syncope after a patient has been startled or has experienced an emotionally stressful situation, similar to benign syncope, an electrocardiogram is advisable for any child with a history of syncope. The family history should be explored for sudden death, syncope, seizures, SIDS, swimming deaths, and single-occupant motor vehicle fatalities.

Dyspnea

Dyspnea (labored breathing) is a symptom present in patients with pulmonary congestion from either left-sided cardiac failure or other conditions raising pulmonary venous pressure or from marked hypoxia. Dyspnea is manifested in infants by rapid, grunting respirations associated with retractions. Older children complain of shortness of breath. The most common causes in children are asthma and bronchitis.

Fatigue

Fatigue on exercise must be distinguished from dyspnea as it has a different physiologic basis.

Exercise intolerance of cardiac origin indicates an inability of the heart to meet the increased metabolic demands for oxygen delivery to the tissues during this state. This can occur in three situations:

Cyanotic congenital heart disease (arterial oxygen desaturation).

Congestive cardiac failure (inadequate myocardial function).

Severe outflow obstructive conditions or those causing cardiac filling impairment (inadequate cardiac output).

Fatigue on exercise or exercise intolerance is a difficult symptom to interpret because other factors, such as motivation or amount of training, influence the amount of exercise an individual can perform. To assess exercise intolerance, compare the child's response to physical activity with that of peers and siblings or to their previous level of activity.

Growth retardation

Growth retardation is common in many children who present with other cardiac symptoms within the first year of life.

Infants with cardiac failure or cyanosis. Infants with cardiac failure or cyanosis show retarded growth, which is more marked if they both are present. Usually, the rate of weight increase is more delayed than that of height. The cause of growth retardation is unknown, but it is probably related to inadequate caloric intake due to dyspnea during feeding and to the excessive energy requirements of congestive cardiac failure.

Growth. Growth may also be retarded in children with a cardiac anomaly associated with a syndrome, such as Down syndrome, which in itself causes growth retardation.

Developmental milestones. Developmental milestones requiring muscle strength may be delayed, but usually mental development is normal. In assessing growth and development, obtaining growth development data for siblings as well as for the parents and grandparents is helpful.

Congestive cardiac failure

Congestive cardiac failure leads to the most frequently described symptom complex in infants and children with cardiac disease. In infants and children, 80% of instances of heart failure occur during the first year of life; these are usually associated with a cardiac malformation. The remaining 20% occurring during childhood are usually related to acquired conditions. Infants with cardiac failure are described as slow feeders who tire when feeding, this symptom indicating dyspnea on exertion (the act of sucking a bottle). The infant perspires excessively, presumably from increased catecholamine release. Rapid respiration, particularly when the infant is asleep, is an invaluable clue for cardiac failure in the absence of pulmonary disease. The ultimate diagnosis of cardiac failure rests on a compilation of information from the history, the physical examination, and laboratory studies such as chest X-ray.

Respiratory infections

Respiratory infections, particularly pneumonia, are frequently present in infants and, less commonly, in older children with cardiac anomalies, especially those associated with increased pulmonary blood flow (left-to-right shunt) or with a greatly enlarged heart. The factors leading to the increased incidence of pneumonia are largely unknown but may be related to compression of the major bronchi by either enlarged pulmonary arteries, an enlarged left atrium, or distended pulmonary lymphatics.

Atelectasis may also occur, particularly in the right upper or middle lobe, in children with greatly increased pulmonary blood flow; or in the left lower lobe in children with cardiomyopathies and massively dilated left hearts.

Cyanosis

Cyanosis is a bluish or purplish color of the skin caused by the presence of at least 5 g/dL of reduced hemoglobin in capillary beds. The desaturated blood imparts a bluish color to the appearance, particularly in areas with a rich capillary network, such as the lips or oral mucosa. The degree of cyanosis reflects the magnitude of unsaturated blood. Mild degrees of arterial desaturation may be present without cyanosis being noted. Usually, if the systemic arterial oxygen saturation is less than 88%, cyanosis can be recognized—this varies with skin pigmentation, adequacy of lighting, and experience of the observer. A minimal degree of cyanosis may appear as a mottled complexion, darkened lips, or plethoric fingertips. Clubbing develops with more significant degrees of cyanosis.

Cyanosis is classified as either peripheral or central.

Peripheral cyanosis. Peripheral cyanosis, also called *acrocyanosis*, is associated with normal cardiac and pulmonary function. Related to sluggish blood flow through capillaries, the continued oxygen extraction eventually leads to increased amounts of desaturated blood in the capillary beds. It typically involves the extremities and usually spares the trunk and mucous membranes. Exposure to cold is the most frequent cause of acrocyanosis, leading to blue hands and feet in neonates and circumoral cyanosis in older children. The cyanosis disappears upon warming. The normal polycythemia of neonates may contribute to the appearance of acrocyanosis.

Central cyanosis. Central cyanosis is related to any abnormality of the lungs, heart, or hemoglobin that interferes with oxygen transport from the atmosphere to systemic capillaries. Cyanosis of this type involves the trunk and mucous membranes as well as the extremities. A variety of pulmonary conditions, such as atelectasis, pneumothorax, and respiratory distress syndrome, can cause cyanosis. Areas of the lungs, though not ventilated, are perfused, and blood flowing through that portion of the lung is unoxygenated. Thus, desaturated blood returns to the left atrium and mixes with fully saturated blood from the ventilated portions of the lungs. Rarely, dysfunctional hemoglobin disorders, such as excessive levels of methemoglobin, result in cyanosis because hemoglobin is unable to bind normal quantities of oxygen.

Cardiac conditions cause central cyanosis by either of two mechanisms.
(1) *Structural abnormalities*. Structural abnormalities which divert portions of the systemic venous return (desaturated blood) away from the lungs can be caused by two categories of cardiac anomalies:
   (a) *Conditions with obstruction to pulmonary blood flow and an intracardiac septal defect* (e.g., tetralogy of Fallot).
   (b) *Conditions in which the systemic venous and pulmonary venous returns are mixed in a common chamber before being ejected* (e.g., single ventricle).
(2) *Pulmonary edema of cardiac origin*. Mitral stenosis and similar conditions raise pulmonary capillary pressure. When capillary pressure exceeds oncotic pressure, fluid crosses the capillary wall into alveoli. The fluid accumulation interferes with oxygen transport from the alveolus to the capillary so that hemoglobin leaving the capillaries remains desaturated.
  Cyanosis resulting from pulmonary edema may be strikingly improved by oxygen administration, whereas cyanosis occurring with structural cardiovascular anomalies may show little change with this maneuver.

Squatting

Squatting is a relatively specific symptom, occurring almost exclusively in patients with tetralogy of Fallot. When experiencing a hypercyanotic or "tet" spell, cyanotic infants assume a knee/chest position, whereas older children squat in order to rest. In this position the systemic arterial resistance rises, the right-to-left shunt decreases, and the patient becomes less desaturated.

Neurologic symptoms

Neurologic symptoms may occur in children with cardiac disease, particularly those with cyanosis but are seldom the presenting symptoms. Rarely, in otherwise normal children, *seizures* stem from arrhythmias, such as the ventricular tachycardia seen in the long QT syndrome, and are the sole presenting symptom.

Prenatal history

A prenatal history may also suggest an etiology of the cardiac malformation if it yields information, such as maternal rubella, drug ingestion, or other teratogen.

Family history

The physician should obtain a complete family history and pedigree to disclose the presence of congenital cardiac malformations, syndromes, or other disorders, such as hypertrophic cardiomyopathy (associated with sudden death in young persons) or long QT syndrome (associated with a family history of seizures, syncope, and sudden death).

Other historical facts that may be diagnostically significant will be discussed in relation to specific cardiac anomalies.

PHYSICAL EXAMINATION

When examining a child with suspected cardiac abnormalities, the physician may focus too quickly on the auscultatory findings, overlooking the general physical characteristics of the child. In some patients, these findings equal the diagnostic value of the cardiovascular findings.

Cardiac abnormalities are often an integral part of generalized diseases and syndromes: recognition of the syndrome can often provide a clinician with either an answer or a clue as to the nature of the associated cardiac disease. These syndromes are discussed in Chapter 2.

Vital signs
Blood pressure

In all patients suspected of cardiac disease, examiners should record accurately the blood pressure in both arms and one leg. Doing this aids in diagnosis of conditions causing obstruction, such as coarctation of the aorta: recognition of conditions with "aortic runoff," such as patent ductus arteriosus, and identification of reduced cardiac output.

Many errors can be made in obtaining the blood pressure recording. The patient should be in a quiet, resting state, and the extremity in which blood pressure is being recorded should be at the same level as the heart. A properly sized blood pressure cuff must be used because an undersized cuff causes false elevation of the blood pressure reading. A slightly oversized cuff is unlikely to greatly affect readings. Therefore, blood pressure cuffs of various sizes should be available. A guide to the appropriate size for each age group is given in Table 1.1. Generally, the width of the inflatable bladder within the cuff should be at least 40% of the circumference of the limb, and the bladder length should encompass 80–100% of the circumference of the limb at the point of measurement. In infants, placing the cuff around the forearm and leg rather than around the arm and thigh is easier.

Although a 1-inch-wide cuff is available, it should never be used because it leads uniformly to a falsely elevated pressure except in the tiniest prematures. A 2-inch-wide cuff can be used for almost all infants.

Failure to pause between readings does not allow adequate time for return of venous blood trapped during the inflation and may falsely elevate the next reading.

Table 1.1 Recommended Dimensions for Blood Pressure Cuff Bladders.

Age Range	Width (cm)	Length (cm)	Maximum Arm Circumference (cm)*
Newborn	4	8	10
Infant	6	12	15
Child	9	18	22
Small adult	10	24	26
Adult	13	30	34
Large adult	16	38	44
Thigh	20	42	52

*Calculated so that the largest arm would still allow bladder to encircle arm by at least 80%. Adapted from National High Blood Pressure Education Program Working Group on High Blood Pressure in Children and Adolescents. The fourth report on the diagnosis, evaluation, and treatment of high blood pressure in children and adolescents. Pediatrics 2004; 114:555–576.

This is a work of the US government, published in the public domain by the American Academy of Pediatrics, available online at http://pediatrics.aappublications. org/cgi/content/full/114/2/S2/555 and http://www.nhlbi.nih.gov/health/prof/heart/hbp/ hbp_ped.pdf.

Methods. Four methods of obtaining blood pressure can be used in infants and children—three manual methods (flush, palpatory, and auscultatory) and an automated method (oscillometric).

For manual methods, the cuff should be applied snugly and the manometer pressure quickly elevated. The pressure should then be released at a rate of 1–3 mm Hg/s and allowed to fall to zero. After a pause, the cuff can be reinflated. Pressure recordings should be repeated at least once.

Flush method. In this method used in infants, a blood pressure cuff is placed about the infant's extremity, and the hand or foot is tightly squeezed by the physician's hand. The cuff is rapidly inflated, and the infant's hand or foot is released. As the pressure slowly falls, the pressure value at which the blanched hand or foot flushes reflects the mean arterial pressure. In infants, blood pressure should be taken simultaneously in an upper and lower extremity because fussiness and crying lead to falsely elevated, rapidly changing values. The practitioner can accomplish this by connecting two blood pressure cuffs by a Y-tubing to a manometer and placing one cuff on the arm and the other cuff on the leg, thereby obtaining the pressure simultaneously by the flush method.

Palpation. Palpation can also be used in infants. During release of the pressure from the cuff, the pressure reading at which the pulse appears distal to the cuff indicates the systolic blood pressure. A more precise but similar method uses an ultrasonic Doppler probe to register the arterial pulse in lieu of palpating it.

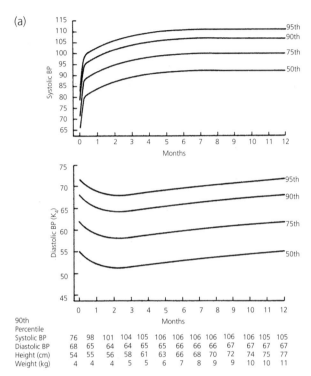

90th Percentile													
Systolic BP	76	98	101	104	105	106	106	106	106	106	106	105	105
Diastolic BP	68	65	64	64	65	66	66	66	67	67	67	67
Height (cm)	54	55	56	58	61	63	66	68	70	72	74	75	77
Weight (kg)	4	4	4	5	5	6	7	8	9	9	10	10	11

Figure 1.1 Blood pressure upper limits for boys and girls from birth to 1 year of age. (a) Girls; (b) boys. (Adapted from Report of the second task force on blood pressure control in children. Pediatrics 1987;79:1–25.)

Auscultation. In the older child, blood pressure can be obtained by the auscultatory method: in the arm, by listening over the brachial artery in the antecubital space, or in the leg and in the thigh, by listening to the popliteal artery. The pressure at which the first Korotkoff sound (K_1) is heard represents the systolic pressure. As the cuff pressure is released, the pressure at which the sound muffles (K_4) and the pressure at which the sound disappears (K_5) should also be recorded. The diastolic blood pressure is located between these two values.

Automated. Oscillometric methods utilize a machine that automatically inflates and deflates the cuff while monitoring pulse-related air pressure fluctuations within the cuff. Deflation is performed in stepwise fashion, and at each step the machine pauses for 2 seconds or less while the cuff pressure oscillations

(b)

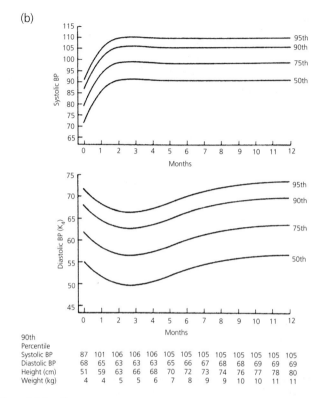

90th Percentile													
Systolic BP	87	101	106	106	106	105	105	105	105	105	105	105	105
Diastolic BP	68	65	63	63	63	65	66	67	68	68	69	69	69
Height (cm)	51	59	63	66	68	70	72	73	74	76	77	78	80
Weight (kg)	4	4	5	5	6	7	8	9	9	10	10	11	11

Figure 1.1 (*cont.*)

are recorded. The amplitude of these pulsatile oscillations begins to increase as the cuff pressure falls to the level of the systolic blood pressure, reaches a maximum amplitude at a cuff pressure equal to mean blood pressure, and diminishes as cuff pressure falls to diastolic levels. Because the method depends on measurement of faint pulsatile pressure oscillations, irregular heart rhythm (e.g., atrial fibrillation), conditions with beat-to-beat variability in pulse pressure (e.g., the pulsus alternans of heart failure or mechanical ventilator-induced changes), and patient movement may lead to inaccurate or absent readings.

Normal values. The normal blood pressure values for different age groups are given in Fig. 1.1 and Tables 1.2 and 1.3. The blood pressure in the leg should be the same as that in the arm. Leg blood pressure should also be taken with an

Table 1.2 Blood Pressure Levels for Boys by Age (1–17 years) and Height Percentile.

Age (year)	BP Percentile	Systolic BP (mm Hg) ←Percentile of Height→							Diastolic BP (mm Hg) ←Percentile of Height→						
		5th	10th	25th	50th	75th	90th	95th	5th	10th	25th	50th	75th	90th	95th
1	50th	80	81	83	85	87	88	89	34	35	36	37	38	39	39
	90th	94	95	97	99	100	102	103	49	50	51	52	53	53	54
	95th	98	99	101	103	104	106	106	54	54	55	56	57	58	58
	99th	105	106	108	110	112	113	114	61	62	63	64	65	66	66
2	50th	84	85	87	88	90	92	92	39	40	41	42	43	44	44
	90th	97	99	100	102	04	105	106	54	55	56	57	58	58	59
	95th	101	102	104	106	108	109	110	59	59	60	61	62	63	63
	99th	109	110	111	113	115	117	117	66	67	68	69	70	71	71
3	50th	86	87	89	91	93	94	95	44	44	45	46	47	48	48
	90th	100	101	103	105	107	108	109	59	59	60	61	62	63	63
	95th	104	105	107	109	110	112	113	63	63	64	65	66	67	67
	99th	111	112	114	116	118	119	120	71	71	72	73	74	75	75
4	50th	88	89	91	93	95	96	97	47	48	49	50	51	51	52
	90th	102	103	105	107	109	110	111	62	63	64	65	66	66	67
	95th	106	107	109	111	112	114	115	66	67	68	69	70	71	71
	99th	113	114	116	118	120	121	122	74	75	76	77	78	78	79
5	50th	90	91	93	95	96	98	98	50	51	52	53	54	55	55
	90th	104	105	106	108	110	111	112	65	66	67	68	69	69	70
	95th	108	109	110	112	114	115	116	69	70	71	72	73	74	74
	99th	115	116	118	120	121	123	123	77	78	79	80	81	81	82

Age	BP percentile	SBP 1	SBP 2	SBP 3	SBP 4	SBP 5	SBP 6	SBP 7	DBP 1	DBP 2	DBP 3	DBP 4	DBP 5	DBP 6	DBP 7
6	50th	91	92	94	96	98	99	100	53	53	54	55	56	57	57
	90th	105	106	108	110	111	113	113	68	68	69	70	71	72	72
	95th	109	110	112	114	115	117	117	72	72	73	74	75	76	76
	99th	116	117	119	121	123	124	125	80	80	81	82	83	84	84
7	50th	92	94	95	97	99	100	101	55	55	56	57	58	59	59
	90th	106	107	109	111	113	114	115	70	70	71	72	73	74	74
	95th	110	111	113	115	117	118	119	74	74	75	76	77	78	78
	99th	117	118	120	122	124	125	126	82	82	83	84	85	86	86
8	50th	94	95	97	99	100	102	102	56	57	58	59	60	60	61
	90th	107	109	110	112	114	115	116	71	72	72	73	74	75	76
	95th	111	112	114	116	118	119	120	75	76	77	78	79	79	80
	99th	119	120	122	123	125	127	127	83	84	85	86	87	87	88
9	50th	95	96	98	100	102	103	104	57	58	59	60	61	61	62
	90th	109	110	112	114	115	117	118	72	73	74	75	76	76	77
	95th	113	114	116	118	119	121	121	76	77	78	79	80	81	81
	99th	120	121	123	125	127	128	129	84	85	86	87	88	88	89
10	50th	97	98	100	102	103	105	106	58	59	60	61	61	62	63
	90th	111	112	114	115	117	119	119	73	73	74	75	76	77	78
	95th	115	116	117	119	121	122	123	77	78	79	80	81	81	82
	99th	122	123	125	127	128	130	130	85	86	86	88	88	89	90
11	50th	99	100	102	104	105	107	107	59	59	60	61	62	63	63
	90th	113	114	115	117	119	120	121	74	74	75	76	77	78	78
	95th	117	118	119	121	123	124	125	78	78	79	80	81	82	82
	99th	124	125	127	129	130	132	132	86	86	87	88	89	90	90
12	50th	101	102	104	106	108	109	110	59	60	61	62	63	63	64
	90th	115	116	118	120	121	123	123	74	75	75	76	77	78	79
	95th	119	120	122	123	125	127	127	78	79	80	81	82	82	83
	99th	126	127	129	131	133	134	135	86	87	88	89	90	90	91

(cont.)

Table 1.2 (Cont.)

Age (year)	BP Percentile	Systolic BP (mm Hg) ←Percentile of Height→							Diastolic BP (mm Hg) ←Percentile of Height→						
		5th	10th	25th	50th	75th	90th	95th	5th	10th	25th	50th	75th	90th	95th
13	50th	104	105	106	108	110	111	112	60	60	61	62	63	64	64
	90th	117	118	120	122	124	125	126	75	75	76	77	78	79	79
	95th	121	122	124	126	128	129	130	79	79	80	81	82	83	83
	99th	128	130	131	133	135	136	137	87	87	88	89	90	91	91
14	50th	106	107	109	111	113	114	115	60	61	62	63	64	65	65
	90th	119	120	121	122	124	125	125	77	77	77	78	79	80	80
	95th	123	123	125	126	127	129	129	81	81	81	82	83	84	84
	99th	130	131	132	133	135	136	136	88	88	89	90	90	91	92
15	50th	107	108	109	110	111	113	113	64	64	64	65	66	67	67
	90th	120	121	122	123	125	126	127	78	78	78	79	80	81	81
	95th	124	125	126	127	129	130	131	82	82	82	83	84	85	85
	99th	131	132	133	134	136	137	138	89	89	90	91	91	92	93
16	50th	108	108	110	111	112	114	114	64	64	65	66	66	67	68
	90th	121	122	123	124	126	127	128	78	78	79	80	81	81	82
	95th	125	126	127	128	130	131	132	82	82	83	84	85	85	86
	99th	132	133	134	135	137	138	139	90	90	90	91	92	93	93
17	50th	108	109	110	111	113	114	115	64	65	65	66	67	67	68
	90th	122	122	123	125	126	127	128	78	79	79	80	81	81	82
	95th	125	126	127	129	130	131	132	82	83	83	84	85	85	86
	99th	133	133	134	136	137	138	139	90	90	91	91	92	93	93

The height percentiles are based on data available online at http://www.cdc.gov/growthcharts/. Adapted from National High Blood Pressure Education Program Working Group on High Blood Pressure in Children and Adolescents. The fourth report on the diagnosis, evaluation, and treatment of high blood pressure in children and adolescents. Pediatrics 2004; 114:555–576.

This is a work of the US government, published in the public domain by the American Academy of Pediatrics, available online at http://pediatrics.aappublications.org/cgi/content/full/114/2/S2/555 and http://www.nhlbi.nih.gov/health/prof/heart/hbp/hbp-ped.pdf.

Table 1.3 Blood Pressure Levels for Girls by Age (1–17 years) and Height Percentile.

Age (year)	BP Percentile	Systolic BP (mm Hg) ←Percentile of Height→							Diastolic BP (mm Hg) ←Percentile of Height→						
		5th	10th	25th	50th	75th	90th	95th	5th	10th	25th	50th	75th	90th	95th
1	50th	83	84	85	86	88	89	90	38	39	39	40	41	41	42
	90th	97	97	98	100	101	102	103	52	53	53	54	55	55	56
	95th	100	101	102	104	105	106	107	56	57	57	58	59	59	60
	99th	108	108	109	111	112	113	114	64	64	65	65	66	67	67
2	50th	85	85	87	88	89	91	91	43	44	44	45	46	46	47
	90th	98	99	100	101	103	104	105	57	58	58	59	60	61	61
	95th	102	103	104	105	107	108	109	61	62	62	63	64	65	65
	99th	109	110	111	112	114	115	116	69	69	70	70	71	72	72
3	50th	86	87	88	89	91	92	93	47	48	48	49	50	50	51
	90th	100	100	102	103	104	106	106	61	62	62	63	64	64	65
	95th	104	104	105	107	108	109	110	65	66	66	67	68	68	69
	99th	111	111	113	114	115	116	117	73	73	74	74	75	76	76
4	50th	88	88	90	91	92	94	94	50	50	51	52	52	53	54
	90th	101	102	103	104	106	107	108	64	64	65	66	67	67	68
	95th	105	106	107	108	110	111	112	68	68	69	70	71	71	72
	99th	112	113	114	115	117	118	119	76	76	76	77	78	79	79
5	50th	89	90	91	93	94	95	96	52	53	53	54	55	55	56
	90th	103	103	105	106	107	109	109	66	67	67	68	69	69	70
	95th	107	107	108	110	111	112	113	70	71	71	72	73	73	74
	99th	114	114	116	117	118	120	120	78	78	79	79	80	81	81
6	50th	91	92	93	94	96	97	98	54	54	55	56	56	57	58
	90th	104	105	106	108	109	110	111	68	68	69	70	70	71	72
	95th	108	109	110	111	113	114	115	72	72	73	74	74	75	76
	99th	115	116	117	119	120	121	122	80	80	80	81	82	83	83

(cont.)

Table 1.3 (Cont.)

Age (year)	BP Percentile	Systolic BP (mm Hg) ←Percentile of Height→							Diastolic BP (mm Hg) ←Percentile of Height→						
		5th	10th	25th	50th	75th	90th	95th	5th	10th	25th	50th	75th	90th	95th
7	50th	93	93	95	96	97	99	99	55	56	56	57	58	58	59
	90th	106	107	108	109	111	112	113	69	70	70	71	72	72	73
	95th	110	111	112	113	115	116	116	73	74	74	75	76	76	77
	99th	117	118	119	120	122	123	124	81	81	82	82	83	84	84
8	50th	95	95	96	98	99	100	101	57	57	57	58	59	60	60
	90th	108	109	110	111	113	114	114	71	71	71	72	73	74	74
	95th	112	112	114	115	116	118	118	75	75	75	76	77	78	78
	99th	119	120	121	122	123	125	125	82	82	83	83	84	85	86
9	50th	96	97	98	100	101	102	103	58	58	58	59	60	61	61
	90th	110	110	112	113	114	116	116	72	72	72	73	74	75	75
	95th	114	114	115	117	118	119	120	76	76	76	77	78	79	79
	99th	121	121	123	124	125	127	127	83	83	84	84	85	86	87
10	50th	98	99	100	102	103	104	105	59	59	59	60	61	62	62
	90th	112	112	114	115	116	118	118	73	73	73	74	75	76	76
	95th	116	116	117	119	120	121	122	77	77	77	78	79	80	80
	99th	123	123	125	126	127	129	129	84	84	85	86	86	87	88
11	50th	100	101	102	103	105	106	107	60	60	60	61	62	63	63
	90th	114	114	116	117	118	119	120	74	74	74	75	76	77	77
	95th	118	118	119	121	122	123	124	78	78	78	79	80	81	81
	99th	125	125	126	128	129	130	131	85	85	86	87	87	88	89

Age	Percentile	SBP by height percentile							DBP by height percentile						
12	50th	102	103	104	105	107	108	109	61	61	61	62	63	64	64
	90th	116	116	117	119	120	121	122	75	75	75	76	77	78	78
	95th	119	120	121	123	124	125	126	79	79	79	80	81	82	82
	99th	127	127	128	130	131	132	133	86	86	87	88	88	89	90
13	50th	104	105	106	107	109	110	110	62	62	62	63	64	65	65
	90th	117	118	119	121	122	123	124	76	76	76	77	78	79	79
	95th	121	122	123	124	126	127	128	80	80	80	81	82	83	83
	99th	128	129	130	132	133	134	135	87	87	87	89	90	90	91
14	50th	106	106	107	109	110	111	112	63	63	63	64	65	66	66
	90th	119	120	121	122	124	125	125	77	77	77	78	79	80	80
	95th	123	123	125	126	127	129	129	81	81	81	82	83	84	84
	99th	130	131	132	133	135	136	136	88	88	89	90	90	91	92
15	50th	107	108	109	110	111	113	113	64	64	64	65	66	67	67
	90th	120	121	122	123	125	126	127	78	78	78	79	80	81	81
	95th	124	125	126	127	129	130	131	82	82	82	83	84	85	85
	99th	131	132	133	134	136	137	138	89	89	89	90	91	92	93
16	50th	108	108	110	111	112	114	114	64	64	64	65	66	67	68
	90th	121	122	123	124	126	127	128	78	78	78	79	80	81	82
	95th	125	126	127	128	130	131	132	82	82	82	83	84	85	86
	99th	132	133	134	135	137	138	139	90	90	90	90	91	93	93
17	50th	108	109	110	111	113	114	115	64	64	64	65	66	67	68
	90th	122	122	123	125	126	127	128	78	78	78	79	80	81	82
	95th	125	126	127	129	130	131	132	82	82	82	83	84	85	86
	99th	133	133	134	136	137	138	139	90	90	90	91	92	93	93

The height percentiles are based on data available online at http://www.cdc.gov/growthcharts/. Adapted from National High Blood Pressure Education Program Working Group on High Blood Pressure in Children and Adolescents. The fourth report on the diagnosis, evaluation, and treatment of high blood pressure in children and adolescents. Pediatrics 2004; 114:555–576.

This is a work of the US government, published in the public domain by the American Academy of Pediatrics, available online at http://pediatrics.aappublications.org/cgi/content/full/114/2/S2/555 and http://www.nhlbi.nih.gov/health/prof/heart/hbp/hbp-ped.pdf.

appropriate-sized cuff, usually larger than the cuff used for measurement of the arm blood pressure in the same patient. Since the same-sized cuff is frequently used at both sites, the pressure values obtained may be higher in the legs than in the arms. Coarctation of the aorta is suspected when the systolic pressure is 20 mm Hg lower in the legs than in the arms.

Blood pressure must be recorded properly by listing on the patient's record the systolic and diastolic pressure values, the method of obtaining the pressure, the extremity used, and whether upper- and lower-extremity blood pressures were done simultaneously or sequentially. When using automated methods requiring nonsimultaneous measurement, recording the heart rate measured with each pressure reading may be helpful, since wide rate variations may give a clue to varying states of anxiety and may help in the interpretation of differing pressure values.

Pulse pressure. Pulse pressure (the difference of the systolic and diastolic pressures) normally should be approximately one third of the systolic pressure. A narrow pulse pressure is associated with a low cardiac output or severe aortic stenosis. Pulse pressure widens in conditions with an elevated cardiac output or with abnormal runoff of blood from the aorta during diastole. The former occurs in such conditions as anemia and anxiety, whereas the latter is found in patients with conditions such as patent ductus arteriosus or aortic insufficiency.

Pulse

In palpating the child's pulse, not only the rate and rhythm but also the quality of the pulse should be carefully noted, as the latter reflects pulse pressure. Brisk pulses reflect a widened pulse pressure, whereas weak pulses indicate reduced cardiac output and/or narrowed pulse pressure. Coarctation of the aorta, for example, can be considered from a comparison of the femoral with the upper-extremity pulses. Mistakes have been made, however, in interpreting the quality of femoral arterial pulses. Palpation alone is not sufficient either to diagnose or to rule out coarctation of the aorta. Blood pressures must be taken in both arms and one leg.

Respiratory rate and effort

The respiratory rate and respiratory effort should be noted. Normal values for the respiratory rate are given in Table 1.4. Although the upper limit of normal respiratory rate for an infant is frequently given as 40 breaths per minute, observed rates can be as high as 60 breaths per minute in normal infants; the respiratory effort in such infants is easy. Difficulty with breathing is indicated by intercostal or suprasternal retractions or by flaring of the alae nasae. Premature infants or neonates may show periodic breathing, so the rate should be counted for a full minute.

Table 1.4 Normal Respiratory Rates at Different Ages.*

Age	Rates
Birth	30–60 (35)
First year	30–60 (30)
Second year	25–50 (25)
Adolescence	15–30 (15)

*Respiratory rates (breaths/min) vary with changes in mental state and physical activity. Sleeping rates are slower and are indicated in parentheses. Depth of respirations and effort expended by the patient are equally or more important than the rate itself.

Cardiac examination
Inspection
Cardiac examination begins with inspection of the thorax. A precordial bulge may be found along the left sternal border in children with cardiomegaly. The upper sternum may bulge in children with a large left-to-right shunt and pulmonary hypertension or with elevated pulmonary venous pressure.

Palpation
Several findings may be discovered by palpation; the most important is the location of the cardiac apex, an indicator of cardiac size. Obviously, if the apex is in the right hemithorax, there is dextrocardia.

Point of maximal impulse. In infants and children under 4 years of age, the apex impulse, which is the most lateral place that the cardiac impulse can be palpated, should be located in the fourth intercostal space at the midclavicular line. In older children it is located in the fifth intercostal space at the midclavicular line. Displacement laterally or inferiorly indicates cardiac enlargement.

Thrills. These are best identified by palpation of the precordium with the palmar surfaces of the metacarpophalangeal and proximal interphalangeal joints. Thrills are coarse, low-frequency vibrations occurring with a loud murmur, and are located in the same area as the maximal intensity of the murmur. In any patient suspected of congenital heart disease, the suprasternal notch also should be palpated but with a fingertip. A thrill at this site indicates a murmur originating from the base of the heart, most commonly aortic stenosis, less commonly pulmonary stenosis. In patients with patent ductus arteriosus or aortic insufficiency, the suprasternal notch is very pulsatile.

Heaves. Forceful, outward movements of the precordium (heaves) indicate ventricular hypertrophy. Right ventricular heaves are located along the right sternal border, and left ventricular heaves are located at the cardiac apex.

Percussion
Percussion of the heart can substantiate estimation of cardiac size in addition to that obtained by inspection and palpation.

Auscultation of the heart
Auscultation of the heart provides perhaps the most useful diagnostic information and should be performed in a systematic way so as to obtain optimum information.

Instrumentation. A good stethoscope is a must. It should have short, thick tubing; snug-fitting earpieces; and both a bell and a diaphragm. Low-pitched sounds and murmurs are heard best with the bell, and high-pitched sounds with the diaphragm. For most children a 3/4-inch bell and a 1-inch diaphragm are suitable for auscultation, although an adult-sized bell and diaphragm are preferable if adequate contact can be made with the chest wall. A 1-inch in diameter, diaphragm can be used in all aged children, since only part of the diaphragm need be in contact with the chest wall to transmit sound. Smaller sized diaphragms provide poor sound transmission.

Position and technique. In infants, initially auscultate through the clothing despite the often-quoted admonition that auscultation should never be performed in such a manner. Sometimes removing the clothes disturbs the child and results in a fussy state that precludes adequate auscultation. After the initial measurement, the clothing can be removed for another listen. Make certain the chest pieces of the stethoscope are warm.

With children between the ages of 1 and 3 years, listening is easier if they are sitting in their parent's lap because children of this age are usually frightened by strangers. In older children, the physical examination can proceed as in adults.

When auscultating, sitting alongside the child is easiest. This position is neither fatiguing to the examiner nor threatening to the child.

Auscultation of the heart should proceed in an orderly, stepwise fashion. Both the anterior and posterior thorax are auscultated with the patient in the upright position. Then the precordium is reexamined with the patient reclining. Each of the five major areas (aorta, pulmonary, tricuspid, mitral, and back) is carefully explored. Both the bell and diaphragm should be used in auscultation of the heart. High-pitched murmurs and the first and second heart sounds are heard better with the diaphragm; low-pitched murmurs and the third heart sound are most evident with the bell. The diaphragm should be applied with moderate pressure; the bell must be applied with only enough pressure for uniform contact but not enough force to stretch the underlying skin into a "diaphragm," which alters the sensitivity to low frequencies. When auscultating the heart, attention is directed not only to cardiac murmurs but also to the quality and characteristics of the heart sounds.

Physiologic basis of auscultation. The events and phases of the cardiac cycle should be reviewed. Figure 1.2 represents a modification of a diagram by Wiggers and shows the relationship between cardiac pressures, heart sounds, and electrocardiogram. In studying this diagram, relate the events vertically as well as horizontally.

Systole. The onset of ventricular systole occurs following depolarization of ventricles and is indicated by the QRS complex of the electrocardiogram. As the ventricles begin to contract, the papillary muscles close the mitral and tricuspid valves. The pressure in the ventricles soon exceeds the atrial pressure and continues to rise until it reaches the diastolic pressure in the great vessel, at which point the semilunar valves open. The period of time between closure of the atrioventricular (AV) valves and the opening of the semilunar valves represents the *isovolumetric contraction period*. During this period, blood neither enters nor leaves the ventricles. During the next period, the ejection period, blood leaves the ventricles, and the ventricular pressure slightly exceeds the pressure in the corresponding great artery. As blood flow decreases, eventually the pressure in the ventricle falls below that in the great vessel, and the semilunar valve closes. This point represents the end of systole. The pressure in the ventricles continues to fall until it reaches the pressure of the corresponding atrium, at which time the AV valve opens. The period between closure of the semilunar valves and the opening of the AV valves is termed the *isovolumetric relaxation period* because blood neither enters nor leaves the ventricles.

Diastole. Diastole is divided into three consecutive phases:
Early. Early diastole is defined as the portion of ventricular diastole comprising the isovolumetric relaxation period, a time when ventricular pressures are falling but the volume is not changing because all cardiac valves are closed.

Mid. Mid-diastole begins with the opening of the AV valves; 80% of the cardiac output traverses the AV valves during mid-diastole. It has two distinct phases, a rapid and a slow filling phase. The rapid filling phase

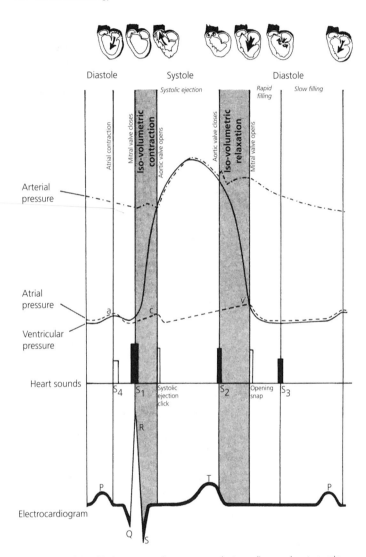

Figure 1.2 Relationship between cardiac pressures, electrocardiogram, heart sounds, and phases of the cardiac cycle. (Abbreviations: S₁, first heart sound; S₂, second heart sound, etc.)

comprises approximately the first 20% of diastole, during which about 60% of blood flow into the ventricle occurs. When a third heart sound (S_3) is present, it occurs at the boundary between the rapid and slow filling phases (see Fig. 1.2).

Late. Late-diastole begins with atrial contraction and the remaining 20% of ventricular filling occurs.

Interpretation of cardiac sounds and murmurs. The timing and meaning of cardiac sounds and murmurs are easily understood by considering their location within the cardiac cycle and the corresponding cardiac events. Although the origin of certain heart sounds remains controversial, in this chapter we discuss them as originating from valvar events.

Heart sounds. The first heart sound (S_1) represents closure of the mitral and tricuspid valves (Fig. 1.2) and occurs as the ventricular pressure exceeds the atrial pressure at the onset of systole. In children, the individual mitral and tricuspid components are usually indistinguishable, so the first heart sound appears single. Occasionally, two components of this sound are heard. Splitting of the first heart sound can be a normal finding, although patients with complete right bundle branch block show wide splitting, since tricuspid valve closure is delayed secondary to delayed right ventricular activation.

The first heart sound is soft if prolonged AV conduction occurs, which allows the valves to drift closed after atrial contraction, or if myocardial disease is present.

The first heart sound is accentuated in conditions with increased blood flow across an AV valve (as in left-to-right shunt) or in high cardiac output.

The second heart sound (S_2) is of great diagnostic significance, particularly in a child with a cardiac malformation. The normal second heart sound has two components which represent the asynchronous closure of the aortic and pulmonary valves. These sounds signal the completion of ventricular ejection. Aortic valve closure normally precedes closure of the pulmonary valve because right ventricular ejection is longer. The presence of the two components, aortic (A_2) and pulmonic (P_2), is called splitting of the second heart sound (Fig. 1.3).

The time interval between the components varies with respiration. Normally, on inspiration the degree of splitting increases, whereas on expiration it shortens. This variation is related to the greater volume of blood that returns to the right side of the heart during inspiration. Since ejection of this augmented volume of blood requires a longer time, the second heart sound becomes more widely split on inspiration.

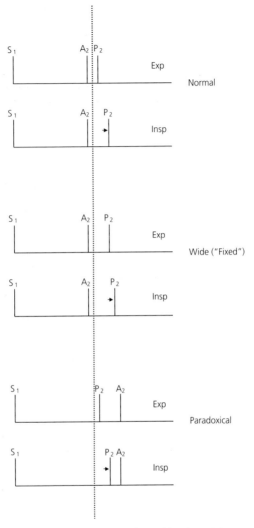

Figure 1.3 Respiratory variations in splitting of second heart sound. In a normal individual, P_2 (pulmonary component of second heart sound) is delayed on inspiration. Wide splitting occurs in conditions prolonging right ventricular ejection. Paradoxical splitting occurs in conditions delaying A_2 (aortic component of second heart sound). P_2 changes normally with inspiration. Thus, the interval between P_2 and A_2 narrows on inspiration and widens on expiration.

The second heart sound can be split abnormally:

Wide splitting. Conditions prolonging right ventricular ejection lead to wide splitting of the second heart sound because P_2 is delayed further than normal. This phenomenon is present in three hemodynamic states.

Conditions in which the right ventricle ejects an increased volume of blood (e.g., ASD–but not VSD).

Obstruction to right ventricular outflow (e.g., pulmonary stenosis).

Delayed depolarization of the right ventricle (e.g., complete right bundle branch block).

Paradoxical splitting. Paradoxical splitting of the second heart sound is probably of greater importance in understanding the physiology of heart sounds than in reaching a cardiac diagnosis in children. Conditions prolonging left ventricular ejection may delay the aortic component causing it to follow the pulmonary component (Fig. 1.3). Thus, as P_2 varies normally with respiration, the degree of splitting widens paradoxically on expiration and narrows on inspiration. Left ventricular ejection is prolonged in conditions in which the left ventricle ejects an increased volume of blood into the aorta (e.g., patent ductus arteriosus), in left ventricular outflow obstruction (e.g., aortic stenosis), and in delayed depolarization of the left ventricle (complete left bundle branch block).

Thus, wide splitting and paradoxical splitting of the second heart sound occur from similar cardiac abnormalities but on opposite sides of the heart. Paradoxical splitting is associated with severe left-sided disorders.

Intensity of P_2. In assessing a child with a cardiac anomaly, particular attention also should be directed toward the intensity of the pulmonary component (P_2) of the second heart sound. The pulmonic component of the second sound is accentuated whenever the pulmonary arterial pressure is elevated, whether this elevation is related to pulmonary vascular disease or to increased pulmonary arterial blood flow. In general, as the level of pulmonary arterial pressure increases, the pulmonic component of the second heart sound becomes louder and closer to the aortic component.

Single second heart sound. The finding of a single second heart sound usually indicates that one of the semilunar valves is atretic or severely stenotic because the involved valve does not contribute its component to the second sound. The second heart sound also is single in patients with persistent truncus arteriosus because there is only a single semilunar valve or whenever pulmonary arterial pressure is at systemic levels, and the aortic and pulmonary artery pressure curves are superimposed.

Third heart sound (S_3) may be present in a child without a cardiac anomaly but may be accentuated in pathologic states. This sound occurs early in diastole and represents the transition from rapid to slow filling phases. In conditions with increased blood flow across either the mitral valve (as in mitral insufficiency) or the tricuspid valve (as in ASD), the third heart sound may be accentuated. A gallop rhythm found in congestive cardiac failure often represents exaggeration of the third heart sound in the presence of tachycardia.

Fourth heart sounds (S_4) are abnormal. Located in the cardiac cycle late in diastole, they occur with the P wave of the electrocardiogram and exist synchronous to the atrial "a" wave. They are found in conditions in which either the atrium forcefully contracts against a ventricle with decreased compliance, as from fibrosis or marked hypertrophy, or when the flow from the atrium to the ventricle is greatly increased. The fourth heart sound may be audible as a presystolic gallop, particularly if tachycardia is present.

Systolic ejection clicks are abnormal and occur at the time the semilunar valves open. Therefore, they mark the transition from the isovolumetric contraction period to the onset of ventricular ejection. Ordinarily this event is not heard, but in specific cardiac conditions, a sound (systolic ejection click) may be present at this point in the cardiac cycle and because of its timing be confused with a split first heart sound.

Systolic ejection clicks indicate the presence of a dilated great vessel, most frequently from poststenotic dilation. These sharp, high-pitched sounds have a clicky quality. Ejection clicks of aortic origin are heard best at the cardiac apex or over the left lower thorax when the patient is in a supine position; they vary little with respiration. Aortic ejection clicks are common in patients with valvar aortic stenosis or a bicuspid aortic valve with concomitant poststenotic dilation. Ejection clicks may also originate from a dilated pulmonary artery, as present in pulmonary valvar stenosis or pulmonary arterial hypertension. Pulmonic ejection clicks are best heard in the pulmonary area when the patient is sitting; they vary in intensity with respiration. Ejection clicks in patients with a stenotic semilunar valve occur more commonly in mild or moderate cases; they may be absent in patients with severe stenosis.

Clicks are not associated with subvalvar stenosis since there is no poststenotic dilation.

Opening snaps are abnormal and occur when AV valves open. At this point, the ventricular pressure is falling below the atrial pressure, the isovolumetric relaxation period is ending, and ventricular filling is beginning. Ordinarily, no sound is heard at this time, but if the AV valve is thickened or fibrotic, a low-pitched noise may be heard when it opens. Opening snaps, rare in children, are almost always associated with rheumatic mitral valvar stenosis.

Murmurs. Cardiac murmurs are generated by turbulence in the normal laminar blood flow through the heart. Turbulence results from narrowing the pathway of blood flow, abnormal communications, or increased blood flow.

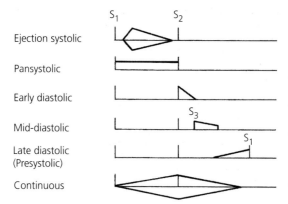

Figure 1.4 Classification of murmurs, showing location within cardiac cycle and usual contour. (Abbreviations: S_1, first heart sound; S_2, second heart sound; S_3, third heart sound.)

> Five aspects of a cardiac murmur provide knowledge of the underlying cause of turbulence: location in cardiac cycle (timing), location on thorax, radiation of murmur, loudness, and pitch and character.

Location in cardiac cycle (timing). Murmurs may be classified by their location within the cardiac cycle (Fig. 1.4). A murmur is heard only during that portion of the cardiac cycle in which turbulent blood flow occurs.

Systolic murmurs. Two types of systolic murmurs exist: holosystolic and systolic ejection.

Holosystolic murmurs (synonyms are pansystolic or systolic regurgitant) start with the first heart sound and continue into systole, often extending to the second heart sound. Therefore, these murmurs involve the isovolumetric contraction period.

> Only two conditions permit blood flow during isovolumetric contraction:
>   Ventricular septal defect.
>   Atrioventricular valve insufficiency (mitral, tricuspid, or the "common" valve in AV canal defect).

In VSD, flow occurs between the left and right ventricles from the onset of systole, whereas in AV valve insufficiency the high-pressure ventricle is in communication with the lower-pressure atrium from the time of the first heart sound.

Because holosystolic murmurs begin so close to the first heart sound, that sound may be masked at the location of maximal murmur intensity. This masking can be a clue to a holosystolic murmur, particularly in patients with rapid heart rate.

Systolic ejection murmur (SEM) results from turbulent forward blood flow across a semilunar valve (aortic, pulmonary, or truncal valve), a great vessel, or ventricular outflow tract. Since turbulent flow in these locations cannot begin until the semilunar valves open, an interval (the isovolumetric contraction period) exists between the first heart sound and the onset of the murmur. Although often diamond-shaped (crescendo/decrescendo), SEMs are distinguished by the delayed onset of the murmur after the isovolumetric contraction period.

Ejection murmurs are found in such conditions as ASD, aortic stenosis, and pulmonary stenosis. In contrast to holosystolic murmurs, the first heart sound is distinctly audible at the site where the SEM is best heard.

Diastolic murmurs can also be classified according to their timing in the cardiac cycle.

Early diastolic murmurs occur immediately following the second heart sound and include the isovolumetric relaxation period. During this time, blood can only flow from a higher-pressure great vessel into a lower-pressure ventricle.

> Early diastolic murmurs indicate regurgitation across a semilunar valve (aortic, pulmonary, or truncal valve insufficiency).

Usually decrescendo, their pitch depends on the level of diastolic pressure within the great vessel: high-pitched in aortic or truncal regurgitation and lower-pitched with pulmonary regurgitation (unless pulmonary hypertension is present).

Mid-diastolic murmurs (sometimes called inflow murmurs) occur at the time of maximal passive ventricular filling and usually result from increased forward blood flow across a normal AV valve. In children, they occur most commonly in conditions with increased pulmonary blood flow and therefore, with increased blood flow into the ventricles (as in ASD or VSD). These low-pitched rumbles are usually heard only with the bell of the stethoscope and are easily overlooked by an inexperienced examiner.

Late diastolic murmurs represent organic obstruction of an AV valve. These murmurs crescendo with a low pitch. Rheumatic mitral stenosis is the typical example.

Table 1.5 Characteristics of Murmurs.

Location in Cardiac Cycle	Type of murmur	
	Regurgitant	Forward Flow
Systolic	Holosystolic Begins with S_1 Includes isovolumetric contraction period	Ejection Follows S_1 Occurs after isovolumetric contraction period
Diastolic	Early diastolic Begins with S_2 Includes isovolumetric relaxation period	Mid- or late diastolic Follows S_2 Occurs after isovolumetric relaxation period
Continuous	Systole and diastole Continues during S_2	

S_1, first heart sound; S_2, second heart sound.

Continuous murmur. A continuous murmur indicates turbulence beginning in systole and extending into diastole. It may last throughout the cardiac cycle. Usually, it occurs when communication exists between the aorta and the pulmonary artery or other portions of the venous side of the heart or circulation.

Patent ductus arteriosus is the classic example, but continuous murmurs are heard with other types of systemic arteriovenous fistulae.

The similarities and differences between regurgitant murmurs and those due to forward blood flow, whether in systole or diastole, are summarized in Table 1.5.

Regurgitant murmurs begin with either the first or second heart sound and include the isovolumetric periods, whereas those related to abnormalities of forward flow begin after an isovolumetric period and may be associated with an abnormal cardiac sound (systolic ejection click or opening snap). A notable exception to these rules is the murmur associated with mitral valve prolapse, discussed in Chapter 10. Table 1.6 presents differential diagnosis of murmurs by timing.

Location on the thorax. The location of the maximal intensity of murmurs on the thorax (Fig. 1.5) provides information about the anatomic origin of the murmur:

(a) *Aortic area*: from the mid-left sternal border to beneath the right clavicle.
(b) *Pulmonary area*: the upper left sternal border and beneath the left clavicle.
(c) *Tricuspid area*: along the lower left and right sternal border.
(d) *Mitral area*: the cardiac apex.

Table 1.6 Differential Diagnosis of Murmurs by Location in Cardiac Cycle.

Location in Cardiac Cycle	Timing	Physiology	Possible Conditions
Systolic	Holosystolic	Flow, ventricle to ventricle Regurgitation, ventricle to atrium	VSD AV valve regurgitation (MR, TR, common AV valve regurgitation)
	Ejection	Flow, ventricle to artery	Semilunar valve, outflow tract, or branch pulmonary artery flow (normal) Increased pulmonary valve flow (e.g. ASD, AVM—abnormal)
		Stenosis, ventricle to artery	Semilunar valve stenosis (e.g., AS, PS, truncal valve stenosis), subvalvar stenosis, or supravalvar stenosis
	Mid- to late systolic	Regurgitation, ventricle to atrium, only with AV valve prolapse	Mitral valve prolapse with regurgitation
Diastolic	Early diastolic	Regurgitation, artery to ventricle	Semilunar valve regurgitation (AI, PI, truncal valve insufficiency)
	Mid- or late diastolic	Flow, atrium to ventricle	Increased flow via AV valve (e.g. Mitral mid-diastolic murmur in VSD, PDA, or severe MR; Tricuspid valve mid-diastolic murmur in ASD, AVM)
		Stenosis, atrium to ventricle	AV valve stenosis (e.g., MS, TS)
Continuous	Systolic accentuation	Flow, artery to artery	PDA Surgical systemic artery to pulmonary artery shunt
		Flow, artery to vein Flow, within artery	AVM Arterial bruit
	Respiratory accentuation	Flow, within vein	Venous hum

AI, aortic insufficiency (regurgitation); AS, aortic stenosis; ASD, atrial septal defect; AV, atrioventricular; AVM, arteriovenous malformation; MR, mitral regurgitation; MS, mitral stenosis; PDA, patent ductus arteriosus; PI, pulmonary insufficiency (or regurgitation); PS, pulmonary stenosis; TR, tricuspid regurgitation; TS, tricuspid stenosis; VSD, ventricular septal defect.

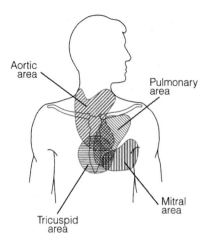

Figure 1.5 Primary areas of auscultation. (Reprinted from Pediatr Clin North Am, Vol 45, pelech AN, The cardiac murmur: When to refer? Pages 107–122, Copyright 1998, with permission from Elsevier.)

In these areas respectively, the murmurs of aortic stenosis, pulmonary stenosis, tricuspid insufficiency, and mitral insufficiency are found. In infants and children, listening over both sides of the back is essential. For example, the murmur of coarctation of the aorta is heard best in the left paraspinal area, directly over the anatomic site of the aortic narrowing. The murmur of peripheral pulmonary artery stenosis is heard over both sides of the back and axillae.

Radiation of murmurs. The direction of transmission of the murmur is also helpful, for it reflects the direction of turbulent flow, which often is along major blood vessels.

Murmurs originating from the aortic outflow area (e.g., aortic valvar stenosis) radiate toward the neck and into the carotid arteries.

Murmurs from the pulmonary outflow area are transmitted to the left upper back.

Mitral murmurs are transmitted toward the cardiac apex and left axilla; occasionally, mitral regurgitation is heard in the middle back.

Loudness. The loudness of a cardiac murmur is graded on a scale in which grade 6 represents the loudest murmur. Conventionally, loudness is indicated by a fraction in which the numerator indicates the loudness of the patient's murmur and the denominator indicates the maximum grade possible. Although somewhat arbitrary, the classification is based on sound intensity and chest wall vibration (thrills).

1/6 is very soft—heard only with careful attention
2/6 is not loud but is easily heard
3/6 is loud but no thrill can be palpated
4/6 is loud and associated with a thrill
5/6 is very loud
6/6 very loud—heard even with the stethoscope held just off the chest
  wall

The pitch of the murmur can be described as high, medium, or low. High-pitched murmurs (heard with a diaphragm) occur when a high-pressure difference in the turbulent flow exists, such as in aortic or mitral insufficiency. Low-pitched murmurs (heard with a bell) occur when there is a low-pressure difference, as in the mid-diastolic mitral inflow murmur accompanying a VSD.

The character of the murmur can be helpful in distinguishing certain causes. Harsh murmurs are typical of severe outflow stenosis when a large pressure difference is present, as in aortic valvar stenosis.

Normal murmurs. Distinction between a normal or functional (innocent) and a significant (organic) murmur can be difficult in some children. Although this text describes the characteristics of the commonly heard functional murmurs, only by experience and careful auscultation one can become proficient in distinguishing a functional murmur from a significant one.

Functional murmurs have four features which help to distinguish them from significant murmurs: (a) normal heart sounds, (b) normal heart size, (c) lack of significant cardiac signs and symptoms, and (d) loudness of grade 3/6 or less.

Some mild forms of cardiac abnormalities may have these features. Thus, the ability to categorize the murmur as a specific type of functional murmur is helpful.

Six types of normal or functional murmurs follow:
(1) *Still's murmur*. Often called "musical" or "twangy string," this soft (grade 1/6–3/6), low-pitched vibratory SEM is heard between the lower left sternal border and apex. Because of this location on the thorax, it may be misinterpreted as a VSD. It can be distinguished because it begins

after, not with, the first heart sound (as in VSD), and lacks the harsh quality of a VSD murmur.

(2) *Pulmonary flow murmur*. This soft (grade 1/6–3/6) low-pitched SEM is heard in the pulmonary area. The murmur itself may be indistinguishable from ASD. With this functional murmur however, the characteristics of the second heart sound remain normal, whereas in ASD the components of the second heart sound show wide, fixed splitting.

(3) *Normal neonatal pulmonary artery branch flow murmur*. This soft SEM is heard in many premature neonates, often at the time their physiologic anemia reaches its nadir, and in many term infants. It is characterized by a soft systolic flow murmur best heard in the axillae and back, and poorly heard, if at all, over the precordium. To avoid confusion with true pulmonary artery pathology, the synonym peripheral pulmonic stenosis, or PPS, should not be used.

(4) *Venous hum*. This murmur might be confused with a patent ductus arteriosus because it is continuous. It is heard best, however, in the right infraclavicular area. Venous hum originates from turbulent flow in the jugular venous system. Several characteristics distinguish it from patent ductus arteriosus: it can be louder in diastole and varies with respiration; it is best heard with the patient sitting; it diminishes and usually disappears when the patient reclines; and it changes in intensity with movements of the head or with pressure over the jugular vein.

(5) *Cervical bruit*. In children, a soft systolic arterial bruit may be heard over the carotid arteries. They are believed to originate at the bifurcation of the carotid arteries. The bruit should not be confused with the transmission of cardiac murmurs to the neck, as in aortic stenosis. Aortic stenosis is associated with a suprasternal notch thrill.

(6) *Cardiopulmonary murmur*. This sound (more along the mid left sternal border than right) originates from compression of the lung between the heart and the anterior chest wall. This murmur or sound occurs during systole, becomes louder in mid-inspiration and mid-expiration, and sounds close to the ear.

In most children with a functional cardiac murmur, a chest X-ray, electrocardiogram, or echocardiogram is unnecessary, as the diagnosis can be made with certainty from the physical examination alone. In a few patients these studies may be indicated to distinguish a significant and functional murmur. If it is a normal (innocent) murmur, the parents and the patient should be reassured of its benign nature. No special care is indicated for these children, and the child can be monitored at intervals dictated by routine pediatric care by their own medical provider. Many (not all) functional murmurs disappear in adolescence, and the murmurs may be accentuated during times of increased cardiac output, such as during fever and anemia.

Abdominal examination. The abdomen should also be carefully examined for the location and size of the liver and spleen. The examiner should be alert to the presence of situs inversus. The hepatic edge should be palpated and its distance below the costal margin measured. If the edge is lower than normal, the upper margin of the liver should be percussed to determine the span of the liver. In patients with a depressed diaphragm (e.g., from asthma), the liver edge is also depressed downward; in this instance, the upper extent of the liver is also depressed. The liver edge normally is palpable until 4 years of age. Pulsatile motion may be palpated over the liver in severe tricuspid regurgitation or transmitted through soft tissues from a hyperdynamic heart in the absence of AV valve regurgitation.

The spleen ordinarily should not be palpable. It may be enlarged in patients with chronic congestive cardiac failure or infective endocarditis.

LABORATORY EXAMINATION

Electrocardiography

Electrocardiography plays an integral part in evaluation of a child with cardiac disease. It is most useful in reaching a diagnosis when combined with other patient data. The electrocardiogram permits assessment of the severity of many cardiac conditions by reflecting the anatomic changes of cardiac chambers resulting from abnormal hemodynamics imposed by the cardiac anomaly.

For example, left ventricular hypertrophy develops in patients with aortic stenosis. The electrocardiogram reflects the anatomic change; and the extent of electrocardiographic change roughly parallels the degree of hypertrophy, yielding information about the severity of the obstruction. However, a pattern of left ventricular hypertrophy is not diagnostic of aortic stenosis because other conditions, such as systemic hypertension or coarctation of the aorta, also cause anatomic left ventricular hypertrophy and the associated electrocardiographic changes. Occasionally, electrocardiographic patterns are specific enough for diagnosis of a particular cardiac anomaly (e.g., anomalous left coronary artery, tricuspid atresia, or endocardial cushion defect).

The electrocardiogram is used to assess cardiac rhythm disturbances (see Chapter 10) and electrolyte abnormalities. Ambulatory electrocardiography (24-hour electrocardiogram or "Holter monitor") is used for surveillance of subclinical arrhythmias, to access the range and variability of heart rate, and to document the rhythm during symptoms. When symptoms suspected of originating from arrhythmia occur less frequently than daily, an event monitor allows recording of brief (1–2 minutes) electrocardiograms during symptoms for later transmission via telephone.

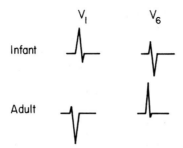

Figure 1.6 Comparison of the contour of QRS complex in leads V_1 and V_6 of infants and adults.

Developmental changes

The electrocardiogram of children normally changes with age; the greatest changes occur during the first year of life reflecting changes in the circulation. At birth the right ventricle weighs more than the left ventricle because during fetal life it supplied blood to the aorta by way of the ductus arteriosus and had a greater stroke volume than the left ventricle. As the child grows, the left ventricular wall thickens as systemic arterial pressure rises slowly; meanwhile, the right ventricular wall thins as pulmonary arterial pressure falls. These anatomic changes primarily affect those portions of the electrocardiogram reflecting ventricular depolarization (QRS complex) and repolarization (T waves).

Therefore, in infancy, the thicker than normal right ventricular wall directs the QRS axis more toward the right with tall R waves in lead V_1 and relatively deep S waves in lead V_6. With age, the QRS axis shifts toward the left, and leads V_1 and V_6 assume a pattern similar to that seen in adults (Fig. 1.6).

In interpreting the electrocardiogram of a child, these changes and others that occur with age must be considered. Table 1.7 shows the range of normal values for several electrocardiographic intervals and wave forms.

Technical factors

Analysis of an electrocardiogram should proceed in an orderly sequence to gain maximal information from the tracing. The speed and sensitivity of the recording should be noted, and variation from "standard" speed of 25 mm/s and amplitude of 10 mm/mV must be considered with comparison to normal values.

Rate and rhythm. The initial step should be to recognize any cardiac arrhythmias or major conduction abnormalities. These can usually be detected by answering the following three questions:

Table 1.7 Normal Values of Important Electrocardiographic Parameters.

Age	QRS Axis (degrees)	R Wave in V_1(mm)	S Wave in V_1(mm)	R Wave in V_6(mm)	S Wave in V_6(mm)
0–24 hours	137 (70–205)	16 (6–27)	10 (0–25)	4 (0–8)	4 (0–12)
1–7 days	125 (75–185)	17 (4–30)	10 (0–20)	6 (0–16)	3 (0–12)
8–30 days	108 (30–190)	13 (3–24)	7 (0–18)	8 (0–20)	2 (0–9)
1–3 months	75 (25–125)	10 (2–20)	7 (0–18)	9 (2–16)	2 (0–6)
3–6 months	65 (30–96)	10 (2–20)	7 (2–12)	10 (2–16)	1 (0–5)
6–12 months	65 (10–115)	10 (2–20)	8 (2–15)	12 (3–20)	1 (0–3)
1–3 years	55 (6–108)	9 (2–18)	10 (2–25)	12 (3–21)	1 (0–3)
3–5 years	62 (20–105)	7 (1–16)	13 (2–25)	13 (4–21)	1 (0–3)
5–8 years	65 (16–112)	7 (1–16)	14 (2–25)	14 (6–24)	1 (0–3)
8–12 years	62 (15–112)	6 (1–16)	14 (2–25)	14 (8–21)	1 (0–3)
12–16 years	65 (20–116)	5 (0–16)	15 (2–25)	13 (8–20)	1 (0–3)

Are there P waves?
Is each P wave followed by a QRS complex?
Is each QRS complex preceded by a P wave?

If the answer to any of these questions is no, the type of rhythm disturbance should be further investigated by following the instructions given in Chapter 10.

Components of the electrocardiogram. The next step is the analysis of each component of the electrocardiographic tracing. This is accomplished not by looking at each lead from left to right, as in reading a newspaper but by reading up and down, first assessing the P waves in each lead, then at the QRS in each lead, and finally at the T wave in each lead.

For each wave form, four features are analyzed: axis, amplitude, duration, and any characteristic pattern (such as the delta wave of Wolf–Parkinson–White syndrome). Using groups of leads, axis is analyzed: the limb leads are used to derive frontal–plane axes, and the chest or precordial leads are used for horizontal plane axes.

Confusion exists about the word axis. Commonly the term "the axis" is used to describe the QRS in the standard leads. But, just as the direction of the QRS can be described so can that of P and T waves; the principle is the same.

P wave. The P wave is formed by depolarization of the atria. Depolarization is initiated from the sinoatrial node located at the junction of the superior vena cava and right atrium. It generally proceeds inferiorly and leftward toward the

AV node located at the junction of the atrium and ventricle, low in the right atrium and adjacent to the coronary sinus. The direction of atrial depolarization also proceeds slightly anteriorly. Since atrial depolarization begins in the right atrium, the initial portion of the P wave is formed primarily from right atrial depolarization, while the terminal portion is formed principally from left atrial depolarization.

The following three characteristics of the P wave should be studied.

(1) *P wave axis*. The P wave axis indicates the net direction of atrial depolarization (Fig. 1.7). Normally, the P wave axis in the frontal plane is $+60°$ ($+15°$ to $+75°$), reflecting the direction of atrial depolarization from the sinoatrial to the AV nodes.

> Therefore, the largest P waves are usually in lead II; the P waves are normally positive in leads I, II, and aVF; always negative in lead aVR; and positive, negative, or diphasic in leads aVL and III.
>   In the horizontal plane, the P wave axis is directed toward the left (approximately lead V_5). Therefore, the P wave in lead V_1 may be positive, negative, or diphasic.

The P wave axis changes when the pacemaker initiating atrial depolarization is abnormally located. One example is mirror-image dextrocardia associated with situs inversus, in which the anatomic right atrium and the sinoatrial node are located on the left side, so atrial depolarization occurs from left to right. This leads to a P wave axis of $+120°$ with the largest P waves in lead III. Another example is junctional rhythm, in which atrial depolarization proceeds from the AV node in a superior-rightward direction.

(2) *P wave amplitude*. The P wave should not exceed 3 mm in height. Because most of the right atrium is depolarized before the left atrium, the early portion of the P wave is accentuated in right atrial enlargement.

> P waves taller than 3 mm indicate right atrial enlargement. This condition causes tall, peaked, and pointed P waves, usually found in the right precordial leads or in leads II, III, or aVF.

(3) *P wave duration*. The P wave should be less than 100 milliseconds in duration. When longer, left atrial enlargement or intraatrial block (much rarer) is present.

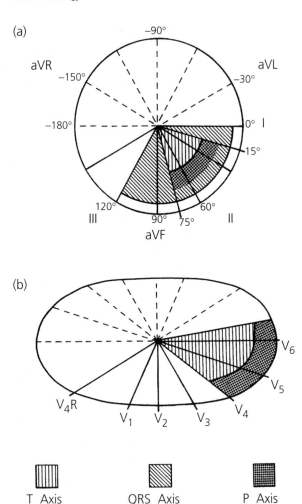

Figure 1.7 Electrocardiogram normal axes. Relationship of limb leads in frontal plane (a) and precordial leads in horizontal plane (b). The normal ranges for the P wave, QRS complex, and T wave axes in frontal plane and the P and T wave axes in horizontal plane are shown.

> In left atrial enlargement, the P wave is broad and notched, particularly in leads I, aVL, and/or leads V_5 and V_6; a broad negative component of the P wave may also exist in lead V_1 because the latter part of the P wave principally represents left atrial depolarization and because the left atrium faces the left precordial leads so the terminal P wave forces are accentuated and directed leftward.

PR interval. The PR interval is the time from the onset of the P wave to the onset of the QRS complex. It represents the transmission of the impulse from the sinoatrial node through the atria and then through the AV node and the Purkinje system.

> The normal values of PR interval measured in leads I, II, or III are
> 100–120 milliseconds in infancy,
> 120–150 milliseconds in childhood, and
> 140–220 milliseconds in adulthood.
> However, the PR interval varies with heart rate as well as age, becoming shorter with faster rates.

A PR interval longer than these values is caused by prolongation of AV nodal conduction, such as that caused by acute febrile illness or digoxin. The PR interval may also be shorter than normal if an ectopic focus for atrial depolarization exists, as in low atrial rhythm, or if an accessory conducting pathway into the ventricle with preexcitation is present, as in Wolf–Parkinson–White syndrome.

QRS complex. The QRS complex represents ventricular depolarization. Ventricular depolarization starts on the left side of the interventricular septum near the base and proceeds across the septum from left to right. Depolarization of the free walls of both ventricles follows. The posterior basilar part of the left ventricle and the infundibulum of the right ventricle are the last portions of ventricular myocardium to be depolarized.

The QRS complex should be analyzed for the following features:

(1) *QRS axis.* The QRS axis represents the net direction of ventricular depolarization. In children, the axis varies because of the hemodynamic and anatomic changes occurring with age. The value of the QRS axis in the frontal plane for various ages is shown in Table 1.7.

In neonates, the QRS axis range is $+70°$ to $+215°$, but with age the axis comes into the range of $0°$ to $+120°$. Most of the change occurs by 3 months of age (Fig. 1.7).

> Right axis deviation is diagnosed when the calculated value for the QRS axis is greater than the upper range of normal, which for older children is more than $+120°$. Right axis deviation is almost always associated with right ventricular hypertrophy or enlargement.
>
> Left axis deviation is indicated when the calculated QRS axis is less than the smaller value of the normal range. Left axis deviation is associated with myocardial disease or ventricular conduction abnormalities, such as those that occur in endocardial cushion defect, but rarely with left ventricular hypertrophy.

When the QRS axis lies between $-90°$ and $-150°$ ($+210°$ to $+270°$), deciding if this represents marked right axis deviation or marked left axis deviation is difficult. In such patients, the practitioner should interpret the location of the axis in light of the patient's cardiac anomaly.

Calculation of the direction of the mean QRS vector in the horizontal plane is more difficult, but the vector can be generally described as anterior, posterior, leftward, or rightward. Determination of the horizontal QRS axis can be combined with information about QRS amplitude to determine ventricular hypertrophy.

(2) *QRS amplitude*. In infants and children, little diagnostic information is obtained from the QRS amplitude of the six standard leads except when low voltage is present in these leads. Normally, the QRS complex in leads I, II, and III exceeds 5 mm in height, but if smaller, suggests conditions such as pericardial effusion.

In the precordial leads, QRS amplitude is used to determine ventricular hypertrophy. Leads V_1 and V_6 should each exceed 8 mm; if smaller, pericardial effusion or similar conditions may be present.

Ventricular hypertrophy is manifested by alterations in ventricular depolarization and amplitudes of the QRS complex. The term ventricular hypertrophy is partly a misnomer, as it applies to electrocardiographic patterns in which the primary anatomic change is ventricular chamber enlargement and to patterns associated with cardiac conditions in which the ventricular walls are thicker than normal.

> Generally, hypertrophy is the response to pressure loads upon the ventricle (e.g., aortic stenosis), whereas enlargement reflects augmented ventricular volume (e.g., aortic insufficiency).

Interpretation of an electrocardiogram for ventricular hypertrophy must be made relative to the normal evolution of the QRS complex, particularly to the amplitude of the R and S waves in leads V_1 and V_6 (Table 1.7).

Right ventricular hypertrophy. In right ventricular hypertrophy, the major QRS forces are directed anteriorly and rightward. This usually leads to right axis deviation, a taller than normal R wave in lead V_1 and a deeper than normal S wave in lead V_6.

Right ventricular hypertrophy can be diagnosed by either of the following criteria: (a) the R wave in lead V_1 is greater than normal for age or (b) the S wave in lead V_6 is greater than normal for age.

A positive T wave in lead V_1 in patients between the ages of 7 days and 10 years supports the diagnosis of right ventricular hypertrophy.

RVH/RVE criteria:
R in V_1 > normal for age
S in V_6 > normal for age
rSR' in V_1 with R' > R and R' > 5 mm
Upright T wave in V_1 between age 1 week and 12 years
RAD (right axis deviation of QRS frontal plane axis)

Differentiating RVH and RVE:
Patterns reflecting increases in right ventricular muscle mass ("hypertrophy") usually show a tall R wave in lead V_1 whereas patterns showing right ventricular enlargement usually show an rSR' pattern in lead V_1 and a qRs complex in lead V_6 with a large broad S wave. Usually, the R' exceeds 10 mm. This distinction is not absolute; variations occur.

Left ventricular hypertrophy. The major QRS forces are directed leftward and, at times, posteriorly. Left ventricular hypertrophy can be diagnosed by this "rule of thumb": (a) an R wave in lead V_6 > 25 mm (or >20 mm in children less than 6 months of age) and/or (b) an S wave in lead V_1 > 25 mm (or >20 mm in children less than 6 months of age) (Fig. 1.8).

Combined with ST segment changes and inversion of the T wave in lead V_6, this is referred to as a pattern of "strain" and may be seen in severe left ventricular outflow obstruction.

Distinction between left ventricular hypertrophy and left ventricular enlargement is difficult. Left ventricular hypertrophy may show a deep S wave in lead V_1 and a normal amplitude R wave in lead V_6, whereas left ventricular enlargement shows a tall R wave in lead V_6 associated with a deep Q wave and a tall T wave.

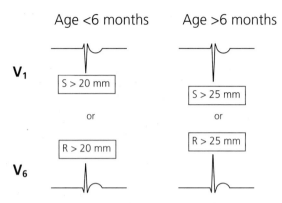

Figure 1.8 Electrocardiographic criteria for LVH/LVE by "rule of thumb."

Biventricular hypertrophy. This condition is diagnosed by criteria for both right and left ventricular hypertrophy or by the presence of large equiphasic R and S waves in the mid-precordial leads with a combined amplitude ≥70 mm (Katz–Wachtel phenomenon).

The electrocardiographic standards presented are merely guidelines for interpretation. The electrocardiograms of a few normal patients may be interpreted as ventricular hypertrophy; and indeed, with utilization of these standards only, the electrocardiograms of some patients with heart disease and anatomic hypertrophy may not be considered abnormal.

(3) *QRS duration*. The width of the QRS complex should be measured in lead V$_1$. The normal range is from 60 to 100 milliseconds; however, infants show shorter QRS intervals. If the QRS complex is greater than 100 milliseconds, a conduction abnormality of ventricular depolarization, such as right or left bundle branch block, is most likely present. In complete right bundle branch block, an rsR′ pattern appears in lead V$_1$, and the R′ is wide. In lead V$_6$, the S wave is frequently broad and deep. Right bundle branch block frequently results from operative repair of tetralogy of Fallot. Another example of prolonged QRS duration is Wolff–Parkinson–White syndrome.

Q wave. The Q waves should be carefully analyzed; abnormal Q waves may be present in patients with myocardial infarction. Normally, the Q wave represents primarily depolarization of the interventricular septum. It can be exaggerated if infarction of the left ventricular free wall exists. After the initial 20 milliseconds of the ventricular depolarization, the left ventricular free wall begins depolarizing. With left ventricular infarction, the right ventricular depolarization is unopposed and directed rightward. This creates a larger and longer Q wave in the left-side leads.

Q wave amplitude. Except in leads aVR, aVL, and V_1, the Q wave should not exceed 25% of the combined amplitude of the QRS complex. If it is larger, the initial QRS forces are accentuated, usually a result of either left ventricular myocardial damage or abnormal septal hypertrophy.

Q wave duration. The Q wave in leads I, II, and V_6 should be less than 30 milliseconds. If the Q wave duration is longer, myocardial infarction is suspected.

ST segment. The QRS complex returns to the baseline before forming the T wave. The segment (ST) between the QRS complex and the T wave should be isoelectric; but in normal children, particularly adolescents, it may be elevated 1 mm in the limb leads and 2 mm in the mid-precordial leads. It should not be depressed more than 1 mm.

Alterations in the ST segment beyond these limits occur because of myocardial ischemia (depression), pericarditis (elevation), or digoxin (coving depression). The ST segment and T wave are often considered as a unit but should be analyzed separately. ST–T abnormalities are not specific as they can occur in many conditions (e.g., electrolyte disturbances) or in normal children (so-called early depolarization).

T wave. The T wave represents repolarization of the ventricles. Whereas ventricular depolarization takes place from the endocardium to the epicardium, repolarization is considered to occur in the opposite direction. Thus, the direction of the T wave axis is generally that of the QRS axis.

T wave axis. The T wave axis in the frontal plane is normally between $+15°$ and $+75°$; in the horizontal plane, it is between $-15°$ and $+75°$ (Fig. 1.7). In neonates, it begins closer to $-15°$ and moves gradually toward $+75°$ during childhood. Thus in the horizontal plane, the T wave should always be positive in lead V_6. In V_1, the T wave is upright in the first 3 days of life and then becomes inverted until 10–12 years of age, when it again changes to positive.

When both the T wave and the QRS complex, showing either hypertrophy or conduction abnormalities, are abnormal, the T wave abnormalities are probably secondary to the QRS changes.

If, however, the T wave is abnormal while the QRS complex remains normal, the T wave changes represent primary repolarization abnormalities. These may be caused by a variety of factors, such as electrolyte abnormality, metabolic abnormality, pericardial changes, or medication effect.

T wave amplitude. There are no rigid criteria for the amplitude of T waves, although the general rule is the greater the amplitude of the QRS, the greater the T wave. The average T wave amplitude is approximately 20% of the average QRS amplitude. T waves normally range from 1 to 5 mm in standard leads and from 2 to 8 mm in precordial leads.

T wave amplitude is affected by serum potassium concentration. Hypokalemia is associated with low voltage T waves, and hyperkalemia is associated with tall, peaked, and symmetrical T waves. A variety of T wave patterns have been associated with other electrolyte abnormalities.

T wave duration. Best measured by the QT interval, defined as the time from onset of the Q wave to termination of the T wave, it varies naturally with heart rate. Therefore, it needs to be corrected for heart rate by measuring the interval between R waves (R–R). Thus, the equation representing this follows:

$$QT_c = \frac{QT}{\sqrt{R-R}},$$

where QT_c is corrected QT interval (seconds); QT is measured QT interval (seconds); and R–R is measured interval between R waves (seconds).

Males:

normal $QT_c \leq 440$ milliseconds

Females:

normal $QT_c \leq 450$ milliseconds

The QT_c normally does not exceed 440 milliseconds for males and 450 milliseconds for females. Hypercalcemia and digitalis shorten the QT_c; hypocalcemia lengthens it. Other medications may variably affect the QT_c.

Long QT syndrome (LQTS) is a familial condition associated with syncope, seizures, ventricular tachycardia, and sudden death.

U wave. In some patients, a small deflection of unknown origin, the U wave, follows the T wave. It can be prominent in patients with hypokalemia or hypothermia.

Chest radiography

Chest X-rays should be considered for every patient suspected of cardiac disease. Study of the X-ray films reveals information about cardiac size, the size of specific cardiac chambers, the status of the pulmonary vasculature, and the variations of cardiac contour, vessel position, and organ situs. Two views of the heart are usually obtained, posteroanterior and lateral.

Cardiac size

Size can be evaluated best on a posteroanterior projection.

> Cardiac enlargement indicates an augmented volume of blood in the heart. Any condition that places a volume load upon the heart (e.g., an insufficient valve or a left-to-right shunt) leads to cardiac enlargement proportional to the amount of volume overload.
>
> In contrast, ventricular hypertrophy, meaning increased thickness of the myocardium, does not show as cardiac enlargement on the roentgenogram, although it might change the contour of the heart.

Care must be taken in interpreting X-rays of neonates, particularly those obtained in intensive care units with portable equipment. Three factors in this situation can result in an image that falsely appears as cardiomegaly. The films are usually obtained in anteroposterior rather than posteroanterior projection; the X-ray source-to-film distance is short (40 inches rather than the standard 72 inches); and the infant is supine. (In all supine individuals, cardiac volume is greater.)

The anatomic position of the cardiac chambers in the roentgenographic views is shown in Fig. 1.9. Several important anatomic features are illustrated. The atria and ventricles, rather than being positioned in true right-to-left relationship, have a more anteroposterior orientation. The right atrium and right ventricle are anterior and to the right of the respective left-sided chambers. The interatrial and interventricular septae are not positioned perpendicular to the anterior chest wall but at a 45° angle to the left and 35% tilted away from the midline of the body.

In the posteroanterior projection, the right cardiac border is formed by the right atrium. Prominence of this cardiac border may suggest right atrial enlargement, but this diagnosis is difficult to make from the roentgenogram.

The left cardiac border is composed of three segments: the aortic knob, pulmonary trunk, and broad sweep of the left ventricle. The right ventricle does not contribute to the left cardiac border in this projection.

Prominence of the aorta or the pulmonary trunk may be found on this view. Enlargement of either of these vessels occurs in three hemodynamic situations: increased blood flow through the great vessel, poststenotic dilation, or increased pressure beyond the valve, as in pulmonary hypertension. A concave pulmonary arterial segment suggests pulmonary artery atresia or hypoplasia and diminished volume of pulmonary blood flow.

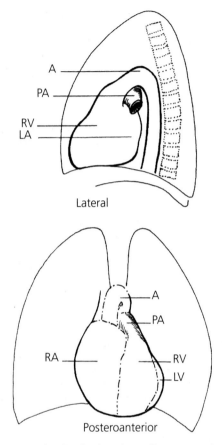

Figure 1.9 Relationship of cardiac chambers observed in posteroanterior and lateral chest X-rays. (Abbreviations: A, aorta; LA, left atrium; LV, left ventricle; PA, pulmonary artery; RA, right atrium; RV, right ventricle.)

On the lateral film the margins of the cardiac silhouette are formed anteriorly by the right ventricle and posteriorly by the left atrium. This view is preferred for showing left atrial enlargement because the left atrium is the only cardiac chamber that normally touches the esophagus. A barium swallow can be employed to delineate the esophagus. In a normal individual, the left atrium may indent the anterior esophageal wall, but the posterior wall is not displaced.

If both anterior and posterior walls are displaced, left atrial enlargement is present.

Normally, the lower part of the right ventricle abuts the sternum and air-filled lung extends down between the sternum and the right ventricle and pulmonary artery. When the latter retrosternal space is obliterated by cardiac density, right ventricular enlargement is present; however, in infants this space may also be obliterated by the thymus.

Both the electrocardiogram and the chest X-ray may be used to assess cardiac chamber size. Left atrial enlargement is best detected by chest X-ray, whereas ventricular or right atrial enlargement is better detected by electrocardiogram.

Cardiac contour

In addition to the search for information about cardiac size on the posteroanterior view of the heart, the practitioner should direct attention to distinctive cardiac contours, such as the boot-shaped heart of tetralogy of Fallot. In conditions with right ventricular hypertrophy, the cardiac apex may be turned upward, whereas conditions with left ventricular hypertrophy or dilation lead to displacement of the cardiac apex outward and downward toward the diaphragm.

Situs

Note situs of the heart, stomach, and especially the aortic arch. In infants with a prominent thymus, the aortic knob is usually obscured, and normal aortic arch position is inferred from the rightward displacement of the trachea in a properly positioned posteroanterior chest film. A right aortic arch is common in tetralogy of Fallot and truncus arteriosus and can be diagnosed by leftward displacement of the trachea.

Pulmonary vasculature

The status of the pulmonary vasculature is the most important diagnostic information derived from the chest X-ray; this function has not been replaced by the echocardiogram. The radiographic appearance of the lung blood vessels reflects the degree of pulmonary blood flow. Because many cardiac anomalies alter pulmonary blood flow, proper interpretation of pulmonary vascular markings is diagnostically helpful. It is one of the two major features discussed in this book for initiating the differential diagnosis.

The lung fields are assessed to determine if the vascularity is increased, normal, or diminished, reflecting augmented, normal, or decreased pulmonary blood flow respectively. As a check of the logic of interpretation, the vascular markings should be compared with cardiac size. If a large volume left-to-right shunt exists, the heart size has to be larger than normal.

Pulmonary vascular markings may be more difficult to analyze from portable films obtained in a neonatal care unit because X-ray exposure time is longer, resulting in blurred images from rapid respirations, and from the redistributed pulmonary blood volume in the supine patient.

With experience obtained from viewing a number of chest X-rays, the status of pulmonary vasculature can be judged. With increased vascularity, the lung fields show increased pulmonary arterial markings; the hilae are plump; and vascular shadows radiate toward the periphery. With decreased vascularity, the lungs appear dark or lucent; the hilum is small; and the pulmonary arterial vessels are stringy.

> Summary of chest X-ray parameters
> Situs (heart, stomach, and aortic arch)
> Cardiac size
> Cardiothymic silhouette, shape, and contour
> Pulmonary artery silhouette
> Pulmonary vascular markings (normal, increased, or decreased;
>   symmetric versus asymmetric)

Pulse oximetry

Because oxyhemoglobin and deoxyhemoglobin absorb light differently, spectrophotometry can be used to measure the percent of hemoglobin bound to oxygen.

Pulse oximeters utilize a light source and light sensor applied to the surface of a patient's skin to noninvasively compare the light absorption of moving blood (during arterial flow) with the light absorption of the nonmoving blood and tissue during arterial diastole (analogous to a reference sample).

Functional arterial oxygen saturation (SaO_2) in percent is calculated automatically and displayed along with pulse rate.

Pulse oximeters do not detect dysfunctional hemoglobin (e.g., methemoglobin and carboxyhemoglobin), so patients with important concentrations of these types of abnormal hemoglobin have a factitiously high SaO_2 compared with their true fractional saturation as measured from a blood sample using a standard laboratory co-oximeter.

Other factors affecting pulse oximeter results include skin pigmentation, poor skin perfusion, tachycardia, ambient light, and shifts in the oxyhemoglobin absorption spectrum that can accompany chronic cyanosis.

Neonates with cyanotic heart malformations (e.g., transposition of the great vessels) or obstructive lesions (e.g., coarctation of the aorta) may have differential cyanosis, a measurable inequality in the pulse oximetry readings from preductal (right hand) compared to postductal (foot) sites, even though the difference is not apparent by physical examination.

Blood counts

In infants and children with cyanotic forms of congenital cardiac disease, hypoxemia stimulates the bone marrow to produce more red blood cells (polycythemia), thus improving oxygen-carrying capacity. As a result, both the total number of erythrocytes and the hematocrit are elevated. The production of the increased red cell mass should be paralleled by an increase in hemoglobin. In a patient with cyanosis and normal iron stores, the hemoglobin should be elevated and the red cell indices normal.

Iron deficiency

In infancy, however, iron deficiency is common; it may be accentuated in cyanotic infants because of the increased iron requirements and by the fact that such infants may have poor appetites and a milk diet primarily. In such infants, the red cell indices reflect iron deficiency anemia because the hemoglobin value is low relative to the red blood count and the hematocrit. In fact, a cyanotic infant may have a hemoglobin value that is normal or even elevated for age and still suffer from iron deficiency.

An example is an infant with a hemoglobin of 16 g/dL and a hematocrit of 66%. The hematocrit value reflects the volume of red cells elevated in response to hypoxemia; the hemoglobin value primarily reflects the amount of iron available for its formation. In this infant the hemoglobin should be 22 g/dL. (Normally, the number for the hemoglobin value should be one third that of the number of the hematocrit value.)

The mean corpuscular volume is always low in iron deficiency, even if the hemoglobin is normal or above normal. An iron-deficient infant may improve symptomatically following administration of iron. Iron deficiency has been associated with an increased risk of stroke in severely polycythemic patients.

Patients with inoperable cyanotic heart disease should have hemoglobin and hematocrit values periodically measured; discrepancies between the two should be noted and managed. Similar information may be obtained by evaluating a blood smear. Serum iron testing is usually unnecessary.

Hyperviscosity

Although vascular resistance varies with viscosity, which itself varies with polycythemia, the effect is not clinically important until the hematocrit approaches 70%. In general, adolescents and young adults with inoperable cyanotic heart disease worsen with phlebotomy, probably because of its detrimental effects on oxygen-carrying capacity. Iron deficiency usually complicates repeated phlebotomy.

Anemia

Anemia may increase the cardiac workload in patients with congestive heart failure and may predispose tetralogy patients to have hypercyanotic spells. In cyanotic patients, severe anemia may lead to an important decrease in the oxygen-carrying capacity.

Echocardiography

Echocardiography, a powerful noninvasive diagnostic technique, requires a high degree of skill in performance and interpretation. This method adds considerable information regarding cardiac function and structure to that gained from history, examination, electrocardiogram, and chest radiography.

Echocardiography of pediatric patients is considerably different from that of adults, both in the technical performance required to obtain quality information in sometimes less than cooperative children and in the interpretation, which emphasizes anatomic relationships, connections, and physiologic principles more than the mere recording of chamber size and ventricular function. Because of poor acoustic penetration, the latter information is often the most that can be obtained from an adult patient without resorting to more invasive techniques, like transesophageal echo, in which the heart is imaged from a probe positioned in the esophagus instead of on the anterior chest wall. In most pediatric patients, excellent images are obtained using surface (transthoracic, or TTE) echo alone so that other techniques, such as transesophageal echo (TEE), are reserved for special circumstances (e.g., intraoperative echo) where surface images would be impossible to obtain. Infants and children are not routinely sedated for echocardiography since a complete and high-quality echocardiogram can usually be done without sedation.

Echocardiography is based on a familiar principle illustrated by bats, which emit ultrahigh frequency sound waves that are reflected from surfaces and are received back, allowing the bats to judge their surroundings and to avoid collision with objects. The principles of Doppler determination of the velocity of moving objects is applied to determine the speed and direction of blood flow.

Two-dimensional images

An echocardiogram is recorded by placing a transducer in an interspace adjacent to the left sternal border and at other locations on the chest and abdomen (Fig. 1.10). The small transducer contains a piezoelectric crystal that converts electrical energy to high-frequency sound waves. Thus, the transducer emits sound waves into the chest that strike cardiac structures; these sound waves (echoes) are then reflected back to the chest wall. The transducer

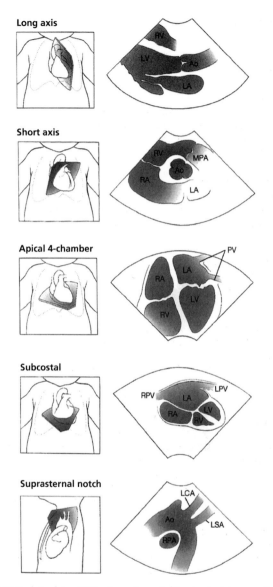

Figure 1.10 Two-dimensional (2D) echocardiography. Five standard views are shown. The left-sided illustrations show the sector-shaped plane of the ultrasound beam inscribed on the patient's chest; the right-sided illustrations show the corresponding 2D images of the heart and vessels. (Images courtesy of Agilent Technologies.)

receives sound (echoes) from the cardiac structures and reconverts them to electrical energy that is then recorded.

Because the frequency of the sound waves and the speed of sound in body tissues are constant, the interval between the emission of sound and the return of sound indicates the distance into the heart and back that the sound wave traveled. The ultrahigh frequency sounds are reflected only from interfaces between structures of different density, such as the interface between the ventricular cavity (blood) and the ventricular septum (muscle). The amount of sound returned depends on the nature of the substances on either side of the interface.

The reflecting surface must be perpendicular to the transducer; when a surface lies tangential, the sound waves are generally reflected in a different direction and are not received by the transducer. As the sound waves travel into the heart, at each interface some sound returns to the transducer, and some continues to the next structure where more is reflected, while some still continues. In this way, multiple sound waves are reflected at various distances from the surface of the chest; these echoes are used to generate two-dimensional images moving in real time.

M-mode

In M (movement) mode (Fig. 1.11), the vertical axis represents distance from the transducer on the surface of the chest and the horizontal axis represents time. The movements of cardiac structures can be recorded over several cardiac cycles. A simultaneous electrocardiogram assists in the timing of cardiac events.

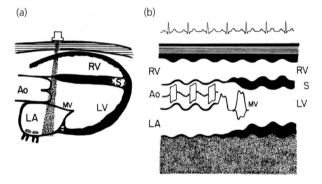

Figure 1.11 M-mode echocardiogram and two-dimensional (2D or cross-sectional) echocardiogram compared. The transducer beam passing through the cross-sectional view (a) corresponds to the same structures seen in the M-mode (b) during a "sweep" of the transducer from aorta to ventricles. (Abbreviations: Ao, aorta; LA, left atrium; LV, left ventricle; MV, mitral valve; RV, right ventricle; S, interventricular septum.)

Table 1.8 Echocardiographic Upper Limits of Left Ventricular (LV) Dimensions by Body Weight.

Body Weight (kg)	LV Diastolic Diameter (cm)	LV Diastolic Wall Thickness (mm)
4	2.5	5
8	3.0	6
15	3.5	7
30	4.5	9
60	5.0	10

Courtesy William S. McMahon, MD, based on published data, including Henry WL, Ware J, Gardin JM, et al. Echocardiographic measurements in normal subjects: Growth-related changes that occur between infancy and early adulthood. Circulation 1978;57:278–285.

Chamber size and wall thickness are usually measured by M-mode. Representative normal left heart values are shown in Table 1.8.

Cardiac function is estimated by M-mode. Although not true measures of contractility, left ventricular shortening fraction (percent change in diameter between diastole and systole; normal $\geq 28\%$) and ejection fraction (percent change in estimated volume; normal $\geq 55\%$) are often both used to describe systolic ventricular function. These values may vary with changes in afterload, preload, or contractility.

Calculation of Shortening Fraction (SF) and Ejection Fraction (EF)

$$SF\,(\%) = \frac{LVEDD - LVESD}{LVEDD} \times 100$$

$$EF\,(\%) \cong \frac{LVEDD^3 - LVESD^3}{LVEDD^3} \times 100$$

or

$$EF \cong SF \times 1.7$$

normal

$$SF \geq 28\%$$

$$EF \geq 55\%$$

LVEDD left ventricular end-diastolic diameter
LVESD left ventricular end-systolic diameter

Doppler

Doppler echocardiography provides information on the direction and speed (velocity) of moving blood. Three main types of Doppler echocardiography are commonly used.

Pulsed wave Doppler. Pulsed wave (PW) Doppler derives velocity information from discrete packets of ultrasound transmitted and then received by the transducer, allowing precise interrogation of small regions of a vessel or chamber. The main limitation of PW Doppler is the compromise between the depth of the structure to be Dopplered and the maximum velocity that can be measured—maximum velocity decreases as the distance to the target increases.

Continuous wave Doppler. Continuous wave (CW) Doppler uses simultaneous continuous transmission and receipt of ultrasound and provides highly accurate estimates of very-high velocity blood flow—for example, through a stenotic aortic valve—but cannot localize the source of the fastest velocities, as PW Doppler can.

Both PW and CW Doppler are commonly used to determine the following:

(1) *Pressure gradient*. Just as river water speeds up passing through a narrow rapids, Doppler velocities can be used to predict pressure gradients between two chambers according to a simplified form of the Bernoulli equation, given a constant flow rate.

$PG = V^2 \times 4,$

where PG is pressure gradient (millimeters of mercury; mm Hg); V is velocity (meters/second; m/s) of blood flow; and 4 is a constant.

This technique is commonly used to estimate the pressure gradient across a stenotic valve, such as aortic stenosis.

Also, the maximum velocity of blood regurgitating through an AV valve during systole (depending on atrial pressure) gives an approximation of the peak systolic pressure in the ventricle.
(2) *Flow (cardiac output)*. In areas where flow is laminar (most of the blood is moving at the same velocity at any given point in time), Doppler can be used to measure the change in this velocity throughout the systolic ejection period. The mean velocity (cm/s) during ejection through a normal semilunar valve of known area (cm^2) can be used to calculate the flow (cm^3/s of ejection) and combined with the heart rate to determine cardiac output (cm^3/s, or L/min).

Color (flow velocity mapping) Doppler. Color Doppler allows the generation of a color-coded display of real-time blood flow velocity and direction overlaid on the black-and-white two-dimensional image of the heart. Color Doppler allows visualization of jets of blood flow, such as in a small VSD or for grading the degree of insufficiency of a valve. Physiologic blood flow is easily demonstrated with color Doppler: by convention, flow away from the transducer is represented by blue and flow toward the transducer is red. The colors have no relationship to blood oxygen levels.

Specialized echocardiography

Transesophageal echocardiography. Both TTE and TEE are important diagnostic techniques in children. In general, in infants and children, the range of structures that can be evaluated is greater with TTE and the image quality comparable to TEE. For patients undergoing cardiac surgery or catheterization, TEE is often employed concurrently. TEE usually requires sedation and/or anesthesia whereas many centers do not routinely sedate children for TTE. The size of the available transesophageal transducer may limit the technique to larger infants.

Intracardiac echocardiography. Intracardiac echocardiography (ICE) utilizes a catheter-mounted transducer to acquire intravascular and intracardiac image and Doppler data during cardiac catheterization, usually electrophysiologic catheterization, and provides more precise localization of structures than fluoroscopy and angiography.

Tissue Doppler imaging. Tissue Doppler imaging, done at the time of TTE or TEE, uses Doppler principles to measure the velocity of the ventricular walls, rather than the movement of blood, as in standard Doppler, providing information about ventricular performance and regional wall motion abnormalities.

Three-dimensional echocardiography. Three-dimensional echocardiography (3D echo) generates a real-time pseudo-holographic representation of the heart using a "stack" of sequential 2D images, allowing enhanced images of complex structures such as AV valves and ventricular outflow tracts.

Magnetic resonance imaging (MRI and MRA)

This technique generates high-quality static images of the body that are similar to those of computed tomography except that ionizing radiation is not used. Rather, a powerful magnetic field surrounds the patient, and the chest is irradiated with radiofrequency pulses from nearby coils that produce alignment of the normally random arrangement of the atomic nuclei of paramagnetic elements. Since hydrogen in water and fat is the most common atom in the body, most images are created using the radiofrequency emitted from these hydrogen nuclei and received as induced current in surrounding coils.

A basic assumption of MRI is that the subject is stationary, a problem partly overcome during cardiac imaging by gating the acquisition of signals to respirations and the electrocardiogram.

Although multiple images can be acquired and "cinelooped" to create the illusion of movement, considerable time is required to create each image, so "real-time" images, such as those obtained with echocardiography, are not possible (see Table 1.9). Since the patient must lie still for the acquisition of all the multiple images, sedation is required for infants and small children, which, although MRI is noninvasive and involves no radiation, increases the relative risk of the procedure.

MRI can provide some data regarding pressure gradients, but the speed and ease of acquisition are not comparable to Doppler echocardiography. MRI does provide excellent images in large adolescents and adults where echocardiography is impossible, but patients with certain magnetic implants, such as artificial pacemakers and certain prosthetic devices, cannot be subjected to the intense magnetic field required. Intravenous nonionic contrast agents are often employed, especially with magnetic resonance arteriography.

Computed tomography

Computed tomography (CT) for cardiovascular imaging has many of the same advantages and disadvantages of MRI and MRA. Computed tomographic angiography (CTA) utilizes higher resolution, faster CT instruments, along with the intravenous administration of iodinated contrast, to obtain very high-quality images; however, the normally faster heart rates of children limit resolution and hemodynamic data is limited. CTA gated to the patient's electrocardiogram provides higher resolution images of moving cardiac structures, yet result in significantly higher radiation doses. See Table 1.9 comparing various imaging techniques.

Exercise testing

This technique is helpful in several situations but requires the cooperation of the child. Hence very young children are not candidates for testing. The authors usually limit exercise testing to children over the age of 6 years. Dobutamine challenge has been used as an alternative, with assessment of myocardial performance by echocardiography and myocardial perfusion using nuclear scans.

Indications

Pre- and postoperative assessment. Preoperative assessment of obstructive lesions (e.g., aortic stenosis) may benefit patients with borderline gradients because it helps decide the timing of intervention. Many patients have indications for intervention (surgery or catheterization) independent of exercise data.

Postoperative assessment. Postoperative assessment of cardiopulmonary function (using maximal oxygen consumption and/or exercise endurance time) helps in symptomatic patients and in those with mild systolic dysfunction. It can also aid in formulating sports or occupational recommendations for adolescents and adults with congenital heart disease.

Table 1.9 Comparison of Common Diagnostic Imaging Modalties in the Evaluation of Congenital Heart Disease Patients.

	CXR	Ba Eso	CT	CTA	MRI/MRA	Echo TTE	Echo TEE	Cath
Realtime	N	Y/N	N	N	N	Y	Y	Y
Hemodynamics	–	–	–	+	+	+++	++	++++
Availability	+++++	+++	+++	++	+	++	+	+
Interpretation	+	++	+++	+++++	+++++	+++++	+++++	+++++
Cost	+	++	+++	+++++	+++++	++	+++	+++++
Radiation	+	++	+++	+++++	–	–	–	+++++
Anesthesia and/or sedation	N	N	Y/N	Y/N	Y/N	N/Y	Y	Y
IV contrast	N	N	N/Y	Y	Y	N	N	Y
Heart rate effect	–	–	++	+++	++	–	–	–
Respiratory and movement effect	+	–	+	+	++	–	–	–
Most useful data/condition	Pulmonary blood flow, degree and symmetry	Vascular ring/sling	Rapid assessment aortic dissection; effusions	Detailed images. Short acquisition time	Detailed images; best for static structures	Realtime, chamber dimension, thickness, hemodynamics, anatomic relationships and situs	Enhanced images when TTE suboptimal, or intraop, intracath	Intervention. Diagnosis of PA htn and reactivity
Disadvantages	No direct hemodynamic data	No direct imaging of anomaly	Relatively low resolution	Heart rate, resp artifact	Heart rate, resp artifact	Acoustic windows become more limiting as pt size increases	Some structures imaged by TTE not seen by TEE	Radiation and contrast load. Vascular entry sites required

CXR, Chest radiograph; Ba Eso, Barium Esophagogram (table refers to fluoroscopically-performed examinations; simple studies can be accomplished with barium swallow at the time of an upright CXR in some patients); CT, computed tomography of the chest; CTA, computed tomographic, angiography; requires higher-resolution equipment than standard CT; MRI/MRA, magnetic resonance imaging/magnetic resonance arteriography; Echo TTE, echocardiogram, transthoracic; Echo TEE, echocardiogram, transesophageal; Cath, cardiac catheterization.

Myocardial ischemic syndromes. Suspected coronary artery insufficiency (e.g., Kawasaki disease with aneurysm or stenosis or postoperative anomalous coronary artery origin repair) is most sensitively assessed by a combination of electrocardiographic and nuclear perfusion studies done during a maximal exercise study. Exercise electrocardiography alone has a false-negative rate of 15% in adults.

Arrhythmias

Wolff–Parkinson–White syndrome. Patients with this condition may be at greater risk for life-threatening ventricular tachyarrhythmia if the delta wave persists at sinus rates of >180 bpm.

Premature ventricular contractions. If benign, these usually disappear at fast sinus rates during exercise.

Atrioventricular block. The rate reserve of the patient's natural subsidiary (backup) pacemaker can be assessed during exercise.

Suspected long QT syndrome. Patients with this condition do not show the usual shortening of the QT interval as the heart rate increases.

Tachyarrhythmia. Patients with documented tachyarrhythmia (SVT or VT) during exercise or those at risk during exercise (e.g., postoperative tetralogy of Fallot) may be candidates for drug treatment; exercise assesses the efficacy of the treatment.

Patients with a history of palpitations only usually have normal exercise tests and are better studied using outpatient electrocardiographic monitoring to document the rhythm during symptoms.

Syncope. Usually, only patients with a history of syncope during exercise need study.

Hypertension. Postoperative coarctation patients and some with other forms of systemic hypertension may register as normotensive (or borderline) at rest but may exhibit an exaggerated systolic hypertensive response to exercise.

Procedure
Specialized equipment is used for grading the workload and for continuously recording multilead electrocardiograms.

> Heart rate rises linearly to an age-related maximum (200–210 bpm for
> normal children and adolescents).
>   Systolic blood pressure rises to a normal maximum of 180–215 mm Hg,
> whereas diastolic pressure remains constant or falls slightly.

If indicated, pulse oximetry and oxygen consumption are measured.

Stress echocardiography allows determination of cardiac function or change
in gradients but can be technically challenging.

Spirometry before and after exercise is useful if exercise-induced bron-
chospasm is suspected.

A bicycle ergometer allows more precise setting of the workload but is often
limited to larger patients. A treadmill is more common. The Bruce protocol
involves increasing treadmill speed and inclination in stages every 3 minutes;
because smaller children are unable to run at the maximum speed (6 mph) of
the Bruce protocol, most pediatric laboratories use the modified Bruce protocol,
which limits the speed to a maximum of 3.4 mph.

Risks
Risks of syncope, arrhythmia requiring immediate treatment, or death are
higher in certain conditions, including hypertrophic cardiomyopathy, pulmonary vascular obstructive disease, severe aortic stenosis, uncontrolled hypertension, and severe dilated cardiomyopathy. The potential benefits of exercise
testing may not warrant the risk in many of these patients.

Cardiac catheterization
Cardiac catheterization requires a staff of trained specialists—pediatric cardiologists, radiologists, laboratory technicians, and nurses. As a diagnostic procedure it provides detailed information about the heart not found by other
techniques. Its use as a diagnostic technique has decreased as its application
for treatment (intervention) has expanded.

Diagnostic cardiac catheterization
Cardiac catheterization was used until recently to establish the diagnosis in
most children with cardiac malformation. Now, with the use of echocardiography and other noninvasive studies, the indications for diagnostic cardiac
catheterization have become targeted: to acquire specific anatomic (e.g., coronary artery anatomy in transposition), functional (e.g., pulmonary vascular resistance in an older child with a VSD), or histologic (cardiac biopsy in a transplant
patient) information.

Interventional therapeutic catheterization

Interventional catheterization began in the 1960s with the Rashkind atrial septostomy, which used a spherical latex balloon pulled forcefully through a patent foramen ovale to create a large ASD for palliation of d-transposition of the great vessels.

Currently, radial balloon dilation with sausage-shaped catheter-mounted balloons is commonly used to relieve obstruction in stenotic semilunar valves and nonvalved pathways (e.g., recurrent coarctation, stenotic pulmonary arteries).

Catheter-based methods for closure of patent ductus arteriosus and ASD are used widely, and devices for closure of certain VSDs are available.

Electrophysiologic catheterization

Electrophysiologic catheterization is performed to define the mechanism and characteristics of arrhythmias.

Radiofrequency ablation or cryoablation may be used to eliminate accessory electrical connections or automatic foci, thus curing certain arrhythmias.

Procedure

Cardiac catheterization is performed in children in a manner that ensures a quiet, controlled, and safe environment for the child; allows minimum discomfort, pain, and anxiety; and also achieves optimum data collection or treatment.

Anesthesia. Two basic approaches are used.

General anesthesia. Anesthesia, usually with endotracheal intubation in neonates, infants, and small children, allows precise control of airway and ventilation. This avoids pulmonary vascular resistance elevation that may accompany hypoventilation from oversedation.

Sedation. Sedation alone is successfully used in patients of all ages at many centers. This usually involves a combination of agents, including narcotics, benzodiazepines, phenothiazines, and ketamine.

Vascular access. Both the right and left sides of the heart may be catheterized either by percutaneous puncture (Seldinger technique) or by operative exposure ("cutdown") to major peripheral veins and arteries. The right side of the heart is accessed through veins in the inguinal area or upper body (e.g., internal jugular vein). The left side of the heart can be catheterized through two approaches: a venous catheter may be passed through the foramen ovale or ASD (or via a tiny defect created with a needle-tipped catheter) into the left atrium or an arterial catheter may be inserted into the brachial or femoral artery and passed retrograde across the aortic valve into the left ventricle. Arterial puncture and atrial septum puncture carry more risk than do venous studies.

Table 1.10 Normal Cardiac Catheterization Values.

Site	Oxygen Saturation (%)	Pressure (mm Hg)
RA	70 ± 5	mean 3–7
RV	70 ± 5	25/EDP 0–5
PA	70 ± 5	25/10, mean 15
LA, PCW	97 ± 3	mean 5–10
LV	97 ± 3	100/EDP 0–10
Aorta	97 ± 3	100/70, mean 85

EDP, end-diastolic pressure; LA, left atrium; LV, left ventricle; PA, pulmonary artery; PCW, pulmonary capillary wedge pressure; RA, right atrium; RV, right ventricle.

Technique. Once the catheter has been inserted into the vessel, it can be advanced into the heart and directed into various cardiac chambers and major blood vessels with the aid of fluoroscopy. At any of these sites, pressures can be measured, blood samples obtained, and contrast media injected.

Pressure data. The catheter is connected to a pressure transducer and the values obtained are compared with normal (Table 1.10) to evaluate stenotic lesions or pulmonary hypertension.

Oximetric data. Blood samples from each cardiac site are analyzed for oxygen content or hemoglobin saturation to determine if a shunt is present. Normally, the oxygen saturation in each right-sided cardiac chamber is similar, but an increase in the oxygen saturation in any chamber, compared with the preceding site, may mean a left-to-right shunt at that level. Normal variations in oxygen content occur, so a slight increase may not indicate a shunt. Multiple samples at each site are used to resolve this point.

Normally, the oxygen saturation of blood in the left atrium, the left ventricle, and the aorta should be at least 94%; if less, a right-to-left shunt is present.

Derived values. The pressure and oximetry data can be used to derive various measures of cardiac function.

Flow (cardiac output). This can be calculated using the Fick principle:

$$\text{Cardiac output (L/min)} = \frac{\text{Oxygen consumption (mL O}_2 / \text{min)}}{\text{Arteriovenous oxygen difference (mL/dL)} \times 10}$$

The patient's rate of oxygen consumption can be determined by analyzing a timed collection of the patient's expired air.

The arteriovenous oxygen difference is obtained by analyzing blood samples drawn from the arterial side of the circulation (aorta or peripheral artery) and from the venous side of the heart (usually the pulmonary artery). The oxygen content (mL of O_2/dL whole blood) is used, as the percent hemoglobin saturation alone cannot be used in this calculation.

Cardiac output determined by the Fick principle is widely used in analyzing catheterization data and has become the standard to which other methods of determining cardiac output, such as thermodilution, are compared.

Since many cardiac malformations have either a left-to-right or a right-to-left shunt, the blood flow through the lungs may differ from that through the body, even though the oxygen consumption in the body must equal the oxygen picked up in the lungs. The Fick principle may still be used for such patients:

$$Q_S = \frac{\dot{V}_{O_2}}{SA - MV},$$

where Q_S is systemic blood flow (L/min); $\dot{V}_{O_2}$ is oxygen consumption (mL O_2/min); and SA − MV is systemic arterial–mixed venous oxygen difference (mL O_2/L blood).

$$Q_P = \frac{\dot{V}_{O_2}}{PV - PA},$$

where Q_P is pulmonary blood flow (L/min); $\dot{V}_{O_2}$ is oxygen consumption (mL O_2/min); and PV − PA is pulmonary venous–pulmonary arterial oxygen difference (mL O_2/L blood).

Pulmonary/systemic blood flow ratio (Q_P/Q_S). Without assuming or measuring the oxygen consumption, the pulmonary blood flow (Q_P) can be expressed as a ratio of the systemic blood flow (Q_S):

$$\frac{Q_P}{Q_S} = \frac{SA - MV}{PV - PA},$$

where SA, MV, PV, and PA represent oxygen saturations (%).

Except for oxygen saturation (%), all other variables required for oxygen content calculation (e.g., hemoglobin concentration) cancel out of the equation.

Resistance. Systemic and pulmonary vascular resistances can be calculated from the hydraulic equivalent of Ohm's law:

$$R = \frac{P}{Q},$$

where R is resistance; P is mean pressure drop across a vascular bed; and Q is cardiac output.

Table 1.11 Normal Derived Cardiac Catheterization Values.

Cardiac Index (CI)*	3–5 L/min/m²
Pulmonary resistance (R_P)*	2units • m²
Systemic resistance (R_S)*	10–20 units • m²
Resistance ratio (R_P/R_S)	0.05–0.10

*Values indexed to body surface area.

Therefore

$$R_S = \frac{\overline{SA} - \overline{RA}}{Q_S},$$

where R_S is systemic vascular resistance (mm Hg/L/min); $\overline{SA}$ is mean systemic artery (aortic) pressure (mm Hg); $\overline{RA}$ is mean systemic vein (right atrial) pressure (mm Hg); and Q_S is systemic blood flow (L/min).

$$R_P = \frac{\overline{PA} - \overline{LA}}{Q_P},$$

where R_P is pulmonary vascular resistance (mm Hg/L/min); $\overline{PA}$ is mean pulmonary arterial pressure (mm Hg); $\overline{LA}$ is mean pulmonary vein (left atrium or pulmonary capillary wedge) pressure (mm Hg); and Q_P is pulmonary blood flow (L/min).

Resistance ratio (R_P/R_S) can similarly be calculated from the ratio of the mean pressure differences across the pulmonary and systemic beds, divided by the Q_P/Q_S:

$$\frac{R_P}{R_S} = \frac{(\overline{PA} - \overline{SA})\,(\overline{LA} - \overline{RA})}{Q_P/Q_S}.$$

Normalization of output and resistance. Resistance is normalized to body surface area, either by using cardiac index (CI) expressed as L/min/m² in place of cardiac output in the preceding formulas or by multiplying the raw resistance by the patient's body surface area, which yields resistance in mm Hg • min/L • m² or Wood units • m² (first described by Paul Wood in the 1950s). Resistance is also expressed as dyne • cm/s⁵, which can be converted from Wood units by multiplying by 80.

Normal indexed values are shown in Table 1.11.

Angiocardiography. Radio-opaque contrast material can be injected through the catheter into the cardiac chambers with serial X-ray images obtained digitally or on film (cine angiography), often in two projections simultaneously (biplane). The imaging system can be rotated around the patient so that angulated projections can be obtained to better visualize various structures (axial angiography). Excellent delineation of the cardiac anatomy can be obtained. Satisfactory details may be illustrated by injecting the material into the pulmonary artery and then imaging as the contrast passes through the left side of the heart (levophase).

Complications of cardiac catheterization. As with any procedure, cardiac catheterization may be associated with complications; the benefits from cardiac catheterization must clearly outweigh the risks.

Death. Death is extremely uncommon (<0.1%) in children beyond 1 year of age. The risk is higher in infants, particularly neonates, who are often critically ill and require catheterization so that a lifesaving catheter intervention or operation can be performed.

Vascular complications. Rarely, compromise of blood vessels used for catheter entry occurs. Temporary or permanent occlusion of the femoral vein or entire inferior vena cava may occur, which may cause transient venous stasis and edema in the lower extremities. Seldom dangerous, the major impact is the inability to reenter these vessels if the patient requires additional catheterization.

Femoral artery injury is more serious, as viability of the limb is at risk. Thrombolytic agents and heparin have been used in the acute management of patients with a pulseless extremity after catheterization.

Rarely, an arteriovenous fistula develops between adjacent vessels used for entry and requires surgery.

Arrhythmia. During most cardiac catheterizations, arrhythmias of some type occur, most often premature ventricular contractions; but these rarely compromise the patient because they tend to be transient. Occasionally, AV block that lasts for several hours occurs.

Radiation. The ionizing radiation dose received by most patients has fallen over the years with improved image-intensifier technology, even though procedure times have lengthened for patients having interventional procedures. Short- and long-term complications from radiation are rare.

ADDITIONAL READING

Driscoll DJ. Fundamentals of Pediatric Cardiology. Philadelphia: Lippincott Williams & Wilkins; 2006.

Lock JE, Keane JF, Perry SB. Diagnostic and Interventional Catheterization in Congenital Heart Disease. Boston: Kluwer Academic Publishers; 1999.

Moller JH, Hoffman JIE. (eds.) Pediatric Cardiovascular Medicine. New York: Churchill Livingstone; 2000.

Mullins C. Cardiac Catheterization in Congenital Heart Disease: Pediatric and Adult. Oxford: Blackwell; 2005.

Park MK, Guntheroth WG. How to Read Pediatric ECGs, 4th ed. St. Louis: Mosby; 2006.

Park MK. Pediatric Cardiology for Practitioners, 5th ed. St. Louis: Mosby; 2007.

Pelech AN. The cardiac murmur: When to refer? Pediatr Clin North Am 1998;45:107–122.

Chapter 2
Heart disease in special populations

This section presents the commonest conditions having demonstrated associations with congenital heart disease. This area of medicine is changing rapidly, particularly the understanding of genetic mutations in conditions which have traditionally only been described clinically.

Pediatric Cardiology, by W Johnson, J Moller © 2008 Blackwell Publishing,
ISBN: 978-1-4051-7818-1.

SYNDROMES ASSOCIATED WITH MATERNAL CONDITIONS

Maternal diabetes

Maternal diabetes may result in macrosomic, large-for-gestational-age infants who commonly have hypoglycemia and respiratory distress. Ventricular septal defect, especially a small muscular ventricular septal defect, may occur, but the classic cardiac problem of the infant of diabetic mother (IDM) is asymmetric hypertrophy of the interventricular septum. This condition can appear quite dramatic by echocardiography and can result in obstruction to the left ventricular outflow, but it almost always regresses completely by several weeks of age.

Fetal alcohol syndrome

Fetal alcohol syndrome may result from even a modest consumption of alcohol during gestation. The clinical spectrum is broad; classical features include unusual triangular facies, thin upper lip, absent philtrum, and small palpebral fissures, often with microphthalmia; hypoplastic nails; and a variety of neurodevelopmental abnormalities. Cardiac defects, usually atrial and ventricular septal defect or tetralogy of Fallot, occur in 15–40% of individuals.

Maternal HIV infection

Although no association between maternal or infant HIV infection and congenital cardiac malformations has been found, comparison with infants of non-HIV-infected mothers with similar risk factors, such as maternal illicit drug use, smoking, or alcohol use, showed that both groups have up to a 10-fold higher incidence of cardiac malformation (10% versus less than 1%).

Maternal inflammatory (collagen vascular) disease

In the absence of structural heart deformities, congenital complete atrioventricular block (CCAVB) is often associated with maternal connective tissue disease, classically systemic lupus erythematosus (SLE), although mothers with no history of lupus or related diseases may have autoantibodies of various types. In clinically well mothers who are antinuclear antibody (ANA) negative, the presence of a Sjogren's syndrome antibody, usually anti-Ro (anti-SS-A), may exist. Injury to the developing conduction system and, in rare cases, the myocardium, occurs when these maternal IgG autoantibodies cross the placenta and bind to fetal cardiac tissue. The risk of a mother with SLE giving birth to an infant with complete heart block has been estimated at 1 in 60; if maternal anti-SS-A antibodies are present, the risk is 1 in 20.

Maternal phenylketonuria

If not properly controlled by diet during gestation, maternal phenylketonuria may result in neurologic abnormality in the neonate. Cardiac malformations, usually tetralogy of Fallot or atrial or ventricular septal defects, occur in 20% of these neonates.

Maternal rubella infection

In the first trimester of pregnancy, maternal rubella infection often results in a newborn of low birth weight with multiple anomalies, including microcephaly, cataracts, and deafness. Hepatosplenomegaly and petechiae may be present in infancy. Cardiac lesions are often present, with patent ductus arteriosus occurring most commonly followed by peripheral pulmonary artery stenosis, ventricular septal defect, and pulmonary valve abnormalities. Maternal immunization prior to pregnancy prevents this problem.

Medications and other agents
Retinoic acid

Retinoic acid, other retinoids, and possibly very large exogenous doses of vitamin A have been associated with various fetal anomalies, including conotruncal defects and aortic arch anomalies.

Lithium

A common therapy for depression, lithium used during early gestation has been associated with Ebstein's malformation of the tricuspid valve, although recent studies show no consistent association.

Other drugs and environmental exposures

A variety of other therapeutic and nontherapeutic drugs, as well as various environmental exposures have been associated with some increased risk of cardiac malformation but the strength and consistency of the association is often weak and the amount and quality of the available data is often limited.

> Aside from this short list of cardiac teratogens, most cardiac disorders currently have not been consistently associated with specific agents.
> It is reasonable to reassure parents of affected children that their child's cardiac problem did not result from some perceived negligence on their part during pregnancy.

In the following sections, diagnostic features of a variety of syndromes will be described briefly and will include comments on the nature of the associated cardiac anomaly.

SYNDROMES WITH GROSS CHROMOSOMAL ABNORMALITIES

Down syndrome (trisomy 21)

This syndrome involves complete or partial duplication of chromosome 21 in all or some (mosaic) of the body cells of the affected individual.

Features

Features include slanted eyes; thick epicanthal folds; flattened bridge of the nose; thick, protuberant tongue; and a shortened anteroposterior diameter of the head. Common signs are short, broad hands; short, inward-curved fifth fingers; and a single transverse palmar crease (simian crease) together with a generalized hypotonia and joint hyperextensibility.

Cardiac anomalies

Anomalies are found in 40–50% of patients. Approximately, one-third are ventricular septal defects; one-third are endocardial cushion defects (usually the complete form of atrioventricular canal); and the remainder consist almost exclusively of patent ductus arteriosus, atrial septal defect, and tetralogy of Fallot. It is rare to find other cardiac lesions than these five diagnoses, especially aortic stenosis and coarctation of the aorta.

> Pulmonary vascular disease develops more rapidly in patients with Down syndrome than in other patients with a comparable cardiac malformation. Because some of these infants do not have the usual postnatal drop in pulmonary vascular resistance, their cardiac malformation may escape clinical detection until after irreversible pulmonary vascular disease occurs. An echocardiogram is advisable for all Down syndrome infants within a few weeks of birth, even in the absence of clinical findings of cardiac malformation.

Turner syndrome (45, X; monosomy X; Ullrich–Turner syndrome)

In this syndrome, a complete or partial absence of one of the X chromosomes in all or some (mosaicism) of the body cells is found.

Features

Though children have a female appearance, they also show abnormal gonadal development. Characteristically, they are short in stature (rarely over 60 inches or 152 cm) with a stocky build, webbing of the neck, a broad chest with widely spaced nipples, cubitus valgus, a low hairline, and edema of the hands and feet (a striking and diagnostic feature in neonates). Renal defects commonly occur and may be associated with hypertension. Gastrointestinal bleeding occurs rarely but can be catastrophic.

Turner syndrome occurs in 1 in 2500 female live births; the estimation is that 99% of all 45, X fetuses perish in utero.

Cardiac anomalies

Anomalies, almost exclusively left-sided cardiac lesions, occur in 35–55% of individuals. Coarctation of the aorta occurs in 20% of Turner syndrome patients and accounts for the greatest share (90%) of operations or interventions compared to other defects. Bicuspid aortic valve, with stenosis ranging from minimal to severe, occurs in up to 35% of Turner syndrome patients and may appear without coarctation. Anomalous pulmonary venous connection, hypoplastic left heart syndrome, mitral valve abnormalities, and aortic aneurysm occur rarely.

> Turner syndrome can be confused with the Noonan, LEOPARD, and related syndromes, but the cardiac findings do not overlap (see below).

Trisomy 18 syndrome
Features

Infants with an extra chromosome 18 have low birth weight, multiple malformations, and severe retardation. Although females live longer than males, these children usually die within weeks or months of birth. Overlapping of the flexed middle fingers by the second and fifth digits (camptodactyly) is very characteristic of this condition. Other features include micrognathia, low-set ears, rockerbottom feet, umbilical and inguinal hernias, and generalized hypertonia.

Cardiac anomalies

These are present in virtually all patients who are not mosaic. Usually, a ventricular septal defect is present, either as an isolated lesion or as a defect associated with the origin of both great vessels from the right ventricle. Patent ductus arteriosus and bicuspid semilunar valves are commonly associated malformations. Cardiac valves are usually not stenotic or insufficient yet often have a striking thickened appearance by echocardiography that is virtually pathognomonic. Pulmonary vascular disease may occur in infants who survive more than a few weeks.

Trisomy 13 syndrome
Features

Infants with an extra chromosome 13 have low birth weight and severe developmental retardation. Central facial anomalies, coloboma, and cleft lip and/or cleft palate are common. Microcephaly, prominent capillary hemangiomas, genitourinary defects, polydactyly, low-set ears, abnormally shaped skull, and rockerbottom feet are other characteristic anomalies.

Cardiac anomalies

These occur in 80% of those neonates with trisomy 13 syndrome. The most frequent lesion is ventricular septal defect, but atrial septal defect, patent ductus arteriosus, and cardiac malposition also commonly occur, often coexisting with the ventricular septal defect.

SYNDROMES WITH CHROMOSOMAL ABNORMALITIES DETECTABLE BY SPECIAL CYTOGENETIC TECHNIQUES

Digeorge syndrome and velocardiofacial syndrome
Features

First defined by the work of DiGeorge, Cooper, and others in the 1960s, DiGeorge syndrome classically involves variable degrees of thymic hypoplasia or aplasia, hypocalcemia from parathyroid hypofunction, and congenital heart malformations.

The syndrome appears to involve failure of proper migration of embryonic neural crest cells into the region of the third and fourth branchial arch clefts, which later form the heart, parathyroid, thymus, and other structures. Proper embryogenesis may depend on one or more genes encoding for embryonically active substances involved in cell migration or differentiation.

An association with the syndrome was noted in some families with gross chromosome 22 defects as early as 1980. A fluorescence in situ hybridization (FISH) probe to detect microdeletions of the q11 region became available only in the early 1990s. This technique is now commonly used and can identify more than 90% of affected individuals. Most occur as de novo sporadic deletions, but in approximately 10% of families with an affected child, one parent (usually the mother) is found to have the 22q11 deletion. Many of these parents have few or none of the phenotypic features. Of parents with the deletion, 50% of their offspring appear with deletion of chromosome 22q11, simulating autosomal dominant inheritance.

Physical findings include a bulbous nose, anteverted palpebral fissures, small- or low-set ears, cleft palate (many are subtle or submucous), and small stature.

> The prevalence of the deletion is estimated to be at least 1 in 4000 live births or 1 in 32 infants with a congenital cardiac malformation.

Immune and endocrine abnormalities that occasionally are problematic in infancy improve with age in most DiGeorge patients. When transfusion is indicated, irradiated blood products are recommended to prevent graft-versus-host disease.

Cardiac anomalies

The most common are the so-called conotruncal malformations: truncus arteriosus, interrupted aortic arch (especially type B), or tetralogy of Fallot with pulmonary atresia. Less common lesions include isolated right aortic arch, left arch with aberrant right subclavian artery, or ventricular septal defect.

Williams syndrome (Williams–Beuren syndrome)
Features

Almost all patients with Williams syndrome who display the characteristic appearance, neonatal hypercalcemia, and developmental delay have a "microdeletion" of the long arm of chromosome 7, which is detectable by FISH but not by standard chromosome analysis. One of the genes missing is responsible for a structural protein called elastin.

> Some patients with supravalvar aortic stenosis (SVAS) appear normal and test normally for both chromosomes and the FISH probe yet pass the cardiac anomaly in autosomal dominant fashion (first described by Eisenberg in 1964). Presumably, Williams syndrome patients have deletions of the elastin gene and other adjacent genes that may be responsible for their appearance and hypercalcemia, whereas normal-appearing supravalvar aortic stenosis patients suffer from deletion of a portion of the elastin gene or have a gene that is mutated. In these nonsyndromic patients, sometimes referred to as having Eisenberg type SVAS, clinical testing is not currently available.

The physical characteristics include a characteristic facial appearance, sometimes called elfin facies, with small, upturned nose with flattened bridge, long upper lip (philtrum), wide cupid-bow mouth, full cheeks, prominent forehead, and a brassy voice. A starburst or lacy pattern in the irises may be seen. The facies become more striking with age. Williams syndrome occurs in about 1 in 10,000 live births.

Cardiac anomalies

The characteristic cardiac lesion is supravalvar aortic stenosis, but patients may also have peripheral pulmonary artery stenosis or systemic arterial stenosis as isolated or combined lesions. Ostial involvement of the coronary arteries can occur. Renal artery stenosis and renal parenchymal dysgenesis can result in systemic hypertension.

OTHER SYNDROMES WITH FAMILIAL OCCURRENCE

Noonan syndrome and related conditions
Features

The chromosomes in most patients with Noonan syndrome are normal by standard karyotype testing. A variety of gene defects have been described including mutations in a family of genes that regulate basic functions such as cell differentiation, growth, and death (apoptosis; see Table 2.1).

Generally, inheritance is autosomal dominant, but affected individuals vary greatly in the degree of abnormality.

These patients typically present with short stature, hypertelorism, low-set ears, and ptosis, giving a rather characteristic facies.

Cardiac anomalies

The characteristic anomaly is valvar pulmonary stenosis with thickened "dysplastic" valve leaflets, but atrial septal defect and peripheral pulmonary stenosis also appear. The electrocardiogram usually shows a superiorly oriented QRS axis (around $-90°$). Ventricular tachycardia and a form of hypertrophic cardiomyopathy occur in some. In contrast to Turner syndrome, left-sided cardiac lesions (other than hypertrophic cardiomyopathy) are not seen.

Related syndromes

In some patients, there is apparent phenotypic overlap between Noonan and similar syndromes, including LEOPARD, cardiofaciocutaneous (CFC) syndrome, and Costello syndrome, and similar gene defects have been reported.

LEOPARD. Patients show many of the same features as Noonan syndrome, but skin lesions and deafness distinguish this syndrome. The term *LEOPARD* derives from the complex of clinical features: multiple Lentigines, Electrocardiographic conduction abnormalities, Ocular hypertelorism, Pulmonary stenosis, Abnormalities of genitalia, Retardation of growth, and sensorineural Deafness. Like Noonan syndrome, a consistent genetic pattern of dominant inheritance appears to occur.

Table 2.1 Summary of Genetic Disorders with Cardiac Malformations.

Syndrome	Clinical Features	Detectable by Std Chromo?	Detectable by FISH?	Mutation Analysis Clinically Available?	Inheritance	Frequency in Live Births	Patients with CHD	Most Common CHD
Down	Characteristic face, small stature, hypotonia (neonate)	Yes (+21)	—	—	—	1:650	40%	AVSD, VSD, ASD, PDA, TOF
DiGeorge	Bulbous nose, small ears, small stature ± hypocalcemia	No	Yes (22q11) in 80% of patients	—	Sporadic/AD*	1:2000–4000 (estimated)	75%	TA, IAA, TOF, R Arch
Noonan	Similar to Turner, but male or female	No†	No†	Yes†	Sporadic/AD*	1:2500	60%	PS, HCM
Turner	Female phenotype, "webbed" neck, short stature	Yes (XO)	—	—	—	1:5000 (1:2500 females)	35–55%	COA, Bic Ao, AS, PAPVR, HLHS
Trisomy 18	Rockerbottom feet; overlapping index finger	Yes (+18)	—	—	—	1:3000–5000	>99%	VSD, DORV

Trisomy 13	Rockerbottom feet; cleft lip (80%)	Yes (+13)	—	—	—	1:10,000	>80%	VSD, ASD
Williams	Elfin face ± hypercalcemia	No	Yes (7q11)	—	Sporadic/possibly AD*	1:10,000	75%	SVAS, Branch PA hypoplasia
Holt–Oram	Upper limb defects	No‡	No‡	Yes‡	Sporadic (40%), AD (60%)	1:100,000	95%	ASD, VSD, AVSD

*Most or many new cases are sporadic mutation but may be transmitted as autosomal dominant.

†Special testing for gene mutation (PTPN11; KRAS; SOS1; RAF1; etc.) may be clinically available; genetic heterogeneity; not all patients with Noonan syndrome or related phenotype have a described gene abnormality.

‡Special testing for gene mutation (TBX5) may be clinically available; genetic heterogeneity, not all patients with Holt–Oram syndrome phenotype have a described gene abnormality.

AD, autosomal dominant; AS, aortic stenosis; ASD, atrial septal defect; AVSD, atrioventricular septal defect (AV canal); Bic Ao, bicuspid aortic valve; CHD, congenital heart disease; COA, coarctation; DORV, double outlet right ventricle; FISH, fluorescence in situ hybridization analysis; HCM, hypertrophic cardiomyopathy; HLHS, hypoplastic left heart syndrome; IAA, interrupted aortic arch; PA, pulmonary artery; PDA, patent ductus arteriosus; PS, pulmonary stenosis; R Arch, right aortic arch; std chromo, standard chromosome analysis; SVAS, supravalvar aortic stenosis; TA, truncus arteriosus; TOF, tetralogy of Fallot; VSD, ventricular septal defect.

Cardiofaciocutaneous syndrome. This is distinguished by abnormally fragile hair and skin lesions, although the cardiac findings are similar to Noonan syndrome. Mental retardation is common.

Costello syndrome. At least a third of these children have atrial arrhythmias, usually a form of automatic atrial tachycardia, often coexisting with pulmonic stenosis and hypertrophic cardiomyopathy.

Limb/heart syndromes
Features
The association of congenital heart disease with deformities of the forearm was pointed out by Birch–Jensen in 1948. Subsequently, cases occurring with deformities of the hand or forearm bones were designated as having the Holt–Oram syndrome (Holt and Oram reported several cases in 1960) or ventriculoradial dysplasia.

Families transmitting Holt–Oram syndrome in autosomal dominant fashion have shown mutations of a gene, TBX5, located on the long arm of chromosome 12, but the manifestations are heterogenous, even among affected members of the same family.

Cardiac anomalies
These usually appear as an atrial septal defect in patients with carpal bone deformities and a ventricular septal defect in those with a deformed radius. Atrioventricular canal defects can occur in some families.

Syndromes frequently associated with congenital heart malformations are summarized in Table 2.1.

Other diseases related to a gene-determined metabolic defect lead to generalized signs and symptoms in which involvement of the heart may occur. Marfan syndrome, glycogen storage disease type II (Pompe), and Hurler syndrome are discussed in Chapter 9.

ADDITIONAL READING

GeneTests: Medical Genetics Information Resource (database online). Copyright, University of Washington, Seattle. 1993–2007. Available from http://www.genetests.org. Accessed 2007.

Jenkins KJ, Correa A, Feinstein JA, et al., for the American Heart Association Council on Cardiovascular Disease in the Young. Noninherited risk factors and congenital cardiovascular defects: Current knowledge: A scientific statement from the American Heart Association Council on Cardiovascular Disease in the Young: Endorsed by the American Academy of Pediatrics. Circulation June 12, 2007;115(23):2995–3014.

Jones KL. Smith's Recognizable Patterns of Human Malformation, 6th ed. Philadelphia: Elsevier Saunders; 2006.

Online Mendelian Inheritance in Man, OMIM (TM). McKusick–Nathans Institute of Genetic Medicine, Johns Hopkins University (Baltimore, MD) and National Center for

Biotechnology Information, National Library of Medicine (Bethesda, MD); 2007. Available from www.ncbi.nlm.nih.gov/omim/.

Pierpont ME, Basson CT, Benson DW Jr, et al., for the American Heart Association Congenital Cardiac Defects Committee, Council on Cardiovascular Disease in the Young. Genetic basis for congenital heart defects: Current knowledge: A scientific statement from the American Heart Association Congenital Cardiac Defects Committee, Council on Cardiovascular Disease in the Young: Endorsed by the American Academy of Pediatrics. Circulation June 12, 2007;115(23):3015–3038.

Chapter 3
Classification and pathophysiology

CLASSIFICATION

Although congenital cardiac malformations may be classified in various ways, a clinically useful classification is based on two clinical features: the presence or absence of cyanosis and the type of pulmonary vascularity as determined by chest X-ray (increased, normal, or diminished).

Six subgroups of malformations are therefore possible and within each subgroup the malformations result in similar hemodynamic alterations.

The 13 most common cardiac malformations are classified in Table 3.1 and represent the major diagnoses present in 80% of children with congenital cardiac disease. Certain exceptions to this classification occur in infancy and are discussed later.

PATHOPHYSIOLOGY

Hemodynamic principles

Four hemodynamic principles describe the pathophysiology of these common conditions: (1) communication at ventricular or great vessel level, (2) communication at atrial level, (3) obstructions, and (4) valvar insufficiency (regurgitation).

In addition, pulmonary hypertension leads to characteristic clinical and laboratory findings.

Pediatric Cardiology, by W Johnson, J Moller © 2008 Blackwell Publishing, ISBN: 978-1-4051-7818-1.

Table 3.1 Classification of Major Cardiac Malformations.

Pulmonary Vascularity	Acyanotic	Cyanotic (Right-to-Left)
Increased	*Left-to-right shunts* VSD, PDA, ASD, AVSD	*Admixture lesions* d-TGV, TAPVR, truncus
Normal	*Obstructive lesions* AS, PS, COA *Cardiomyopathy*	None
Decreased	None	*Obstruction to pulmonary blood flow + septal defect* TOF, tricuspid atresia, Ebstein's malformation

AS, aortic stenosis; ASD, atrial septal defect; AVSD, atrioventricular septal defect (AV canal); COA, coarctation; d-TGV, d-transposition of the great vessels; PDA, patent ductus arteriosus; PS, pulmonary stenosis; TAPVR, total anomalous pulmonary venous return; TOF, tetralogy of Fallot; VSD, ventricular septal defect.

Communication at ventricular or great vessel level

The first principle concerns conditions with a communication between the great vessels (e.g., patent ductus arteriosus) or between the ventricles (e.g., ventricular septal defect).

> The direction and magnitude of flow through such a communication depend on the size of the communication and the relative resistances to systemic and pulmonary blood flow.

When the size of the defect or communication approaches or exceeds the diameter of the aortic root (nonpressure-restrictive defects), the systolic pressures in the ventricles and great vessels are equal. Pressures on the right side of the heart are elevated to systemic levels.

> In patients with a large communication at the ventricular or great vessel level, the direction and magnitude of the shunt depend upon the relative pulmonary and systemic vascular resistances.
>
> These resistances in turn are directly related to the caliber and number of pulmonary and systemic arterioles.

Normally, systemic vascular resistance rises slowly with age, whereas the pulmonary vascular resistance shows a sharp fall in the neonatal and infancy period. This fall in pulmonary vascular resistance is partially related to regression of the thick-walled pulmonary arterioles of the fetal period to the adult pattern of pulmonary arterioles, which have a wide lumen.

Pulmonary vascular resistance falls in all infants following birth, but in infants with a large communication, the fall in pulmonary vascular resistance profoundly affects the patient.

In a patient with a large communication, the systolic pressure of the pulmonary artery (P) remains constant, determined largely by the systemic arterial pressure. Therefore, according to the formula $P = R_P \times Q_P$, as the pulmonary vascular resistance (R_P) falls in infancy, pulmonary blood flow (Q_P) increases. If some factor, such as the development of pulmonary vascular disease, increases pulmonary vascular resistance, the pulmonary blood flow decreases, but the pulmonary arterial pressure remains constant.

In defects or communications smaller than the diameter of the aortic root (pressure-restrictive defects), the relative systemic and pulmonary vascular resistances determine the direction of blood flow through the communication, as in large defects; but the size of the defects does not allow pressure equilibration. Therefore, a systolic pressure difference exists across the communication.

The impedance to blood flow through a small defect is a major determining factor governing the magnitude of the blood flow through it. Therefore, if pulmonary and systemic resistances are normal and the aortic and left ventricular systolic pressures are higher than the pulmonary arterial and right ventricular systolic pressures, respectively, then the shunt in these small-sized communications is from the aorta to the pulmonary artery, or from the left ventricle to the right ventricle.

Communication at the atrial level

The second hemodynamic principle governs shunts that occur at the atrial level. Most atrial communications leading to signs and symptoms are large; thus atrial pressures are equal. Therefore, pressure differences cannot be the primary determinant of blood flow through the atrial communication.

The direction and magnitude of blood flow through the defect are determined by the relative compliances of the atria and the ventricles.

In contrast to the shunts at the ventricular or great vessel level, which are influenced by the relative resistances of the pulmonary and systemic beds and therefore by systolic events, shunts at the atrial level are governed by factors influencing ventricular filling (diastolic events).

Compliance describes volume change per unit pressure change. At any given pressure, the more compliant the ventricle is the greater the volume that it can receive.

Ventricular compliance depends upon the thickness of the ventricular wall and on factors, such as fibrosis, that alter the stiffness of the ventricle. Usually a thinner ventricular wall means the ventricle is more compliant.

Normally, the left ventricle is thicker-walled and less compliant than the thin-walled right ventricle. This difference in compliance favors blood flow from the left atrium to the right atrium in patients with atrial communication. In addition, this direction of blood flow is favored because the valveless vena cavae add to the capacitance and compliance of the right atrium.

The direction and volume of an atrial-level shunt can be altered by changes in the degree of thickness of the ventricular walls or by other factors, such as myocardial fibrosis.

Right ventricular compliance increases during infancy as a result of the changes in pulmonary vascular resistance. During fetal life, the right ventricle develops systemic levels of pressure and ejects a large portion of its output across the ductus arteriosus into the aorta. The right ventricle is thick-walled and, at birth, weighs twice as much as the left ventricle. Since ventricular compliance is affected by the thickness of the ventricular wall, the right ventricle is relatively less compliant at birth.

Following birth, the pulmonary vascular resistance decreases and right ventricular systolic pressure falls to a normal level (25 mm Hg). Consequently, the right ventricular wall thins; and, by 1 month, the left ventricular weight exceeds that of the right ventricle. The thinning of the wall is associated with an increase in right ventricular compliance. Although this sequence occurs in every neonate, in those with an atrial septal defect, as right ventricular compliance increases, so does the volume of left-to-right shunt.

Obstructions

The third hemodynamic principle concerns cardiac conditions with obstruction to blood flow.

In infants and children, the primary response to obstruction is hypertrophy, not dilation. Pressure increases in the chamber proximal to the obstruction, leading to hypertrophy of that chamber.

In children, a normal level of pressure is usually maintained distal to the obstruction since the cardiac output is also usually maintained. Many of the signs and symptoms of patients with obstruction are related to the pressure elevation proximal to the obstruction, not to low pressure distal to the obstruction.

Valvar insufficiency (regurgitation)

The fourth principle governs conditions with valvar insufficiency.

> In valvar insufficiency, the chamber on either side of the insufficient valve is enlarged and the volume of blood in each chamber is larger than normal because the chambers are handling not only the normal cardiac output but also the regurgitant volume.

In contrast to conditions with obstruction, where the response is hypertrophy, the response to the increased volume is usually chamber enlargement. The major signs and symptoms of these patients are related to enlargement of the chambers.

Pulmonary hypertension

Pulmonary hypertension indicates an elevation of pulmonary arterial pressure. As indicated by the equation $P = R \times Q$, pressure (in this case pulmonary arterial pressure) equals the resistance (R_P) to blood flow through the lungs and the volume of pulmonary blood flow (Q_P). Therefore, for any given level of pressure, various combinations of pressure and blood flow may be present.

Large communication

Pulmonary arterial pressure may be elevated primarily from increased pulmonary blood flow secondary to a left-to-right shunt, as in a large ventricular septal defect or patent ductus arteriosus.

Elevated resistance to blood flow through the lungs

The elevated resistance may occur at either of two sites in the pulmonary circulation: at a precapillary site (usually the pulmonary arterioles) or at a postcapillary site (such as the pulmonary veins, the left atrium, or the mitral valve).

Precapillary site. Pulmonary hypertension results from narrowing of the pulmonary arterioles.

Developmental (physiologic) pulmonary hypertension. At birth the pulmonary arterioles show a thick medial coat and a narrow lumen, so the pulmonary resistance is elevated. With time the media of the arteriole thins, the lumen widens, and the pulmonary resistance falls. The arterioles of neonates and young infants are responsive to various influences, such as oxygen and acidosis, so that with hypoxia they contract further and with administration of oxygen they dilate. Such responsiveness remains longer in infants with cardiac malformations associated with increased pulmonary blood flow and elevated pressures.

Pathologic pulmonary hypertension. Pulmonary resistance may also be elevated because of acquired lesions in the pulmonary arterioles.

In patients with large pulmonary blood flow and elevated pulmonary arterial pressure, pulmonary vascular obstructive disease develops over time, leading to medial thickening and intimal proliferation.

These changes develop at a variable rate and influence the clinical findings, the operative results, and mortality of patients. If pulmonary vascular resistance is fixed or poorly reactive to maneuvers usually producing relaxation of pulmonary arterioles, such as hyperventilation or high concentrations of inspired oxygen, the operative risk is high, and the pulmonary resistance remains elevated following operation.

Postcapillary site. Pulmonary arterial pressure can be elevated by malformations that cause obstruction to blood flow beyond the pulmonary capillary (e.g., in the pulmonary veins or left atrium or across the mitral valve). The classic example is mitral stenosis, in which the pulmonary arterial pressure is passively elevated because of elevation of left atrial pressure and the subsequent elevation of pulmonary venous and capillary pressures.

Some patients with obstruction at this level show reflex pulmonary arteriolar vasoconstriction, further elevating pulmonary arterial pressure. In such patients without an intracardiac communication, pulmonary artery systolic pressure may exceed systemic levels. If the obstruction has not been longstanding, pulmonary pressures usually return rapidly to normal postoperatively.

Differentiation of these two sites leading to elevated pulmonary arterial pressure can usually be done clinically, although both show right ventricular hypertrophy and a loud P_2.

In the postcapillary form, usually signs of pulmonary venous hypertension, such as pulmonary edema and Kerley B lines, are present.

Right heart catheterization also allows differentiation by measurement of the pulmonary capillary wedge pressure. Wedge pressure is obtained by advancing an end-hole catheter as far into the pulmonary artery as possible; the pulmonary artery is occluded, so the pressure recorded reflects the pressure in the vascular bed beyond the catheter (i.e., pulmonary venous pressure).

In pulmonary hypertension secondary to a postcapillary obstruction, the wedge pressure is elevated, whereas in that of precapillary origin, the wedge pressure is normal.

CLINICAL CORRELATION

During the evaluation of patients with cardiac anomalies, a variety of information is obtained clinically. The signs, symptoms, and laboratory data divide conveniently into three categories to permit a better understanding of the physiologic significance of the findings and of the patient's condition. In the first category are findings indicating the cardiac diagnosis; in the second, the severity of the condition; and in the third, features that suggest an etiology.

Diagnosis

The findings, usually auscultatory, that relate directly to the abnormality indicate the diagnosis. These usually stem from the turbulent flow through the defect or abnormality (e.g., the continuous murmur of a patent ductus arteriosus or the aortic systolic ejection murmur of aortic stenosis).

Severity

Findings that reflect the effect of the malformation upon the circulation help assess the severity of the malformation. Often symptoms, electrocardiographic and roentgenographic findings, and certain auscultatory findings belong to this category.

Since several malformations have similar effects upon the circulation (e.g., ventricular septal defect and patent ductus arteriosus both place increased volume load on the left atrium and left ventricle), similar secondary clinical features are found in each.

In the above example, clinical and laboratory evidence will indicate enlargement of these chambers, and the degree of enlargement will roughly parallel the magnitude of symptoms and laboratory changes. For either of these conditions, if the communication is sufficiently large and pulmonary blood flow is excessive, then congestive cardiac failure, apical mid-diastolic murmur, left ventricular hypertrophy, and cardiomegaly are found.

Etiology

The type of cardiac malformation is a useful clue to a possible etiology (e.g., the unequal upper-extremity blood pressures of supravalvar aortic stenosis are common in patients with Williams syndrome).

Chapter 4
Acyanosis and increased pulmonary blood flow (left-to-right shunt)

Pediatric Cardiology, by W Johnson, J Moller © 2008 Blackwell Publishing,
ISBN: 978-1-4051-7818-1.

The combination of increased pulmonary vascular markings and absence of cyanosis indicates the presence of a cardiac defect that permits the passage of blood from a left-sided cardiac chamber to a right-sided cardiac chamber.

Four cardiac defects account for most instances of left-to-right shunt and half of all instances of congenital heart disease: (1) ventricular septal defect, (2) patent ductus arteriosus, (3) atrial septal defect of the ostium secundum type, and (4) atrioventricular (AV) canal (endocardial cushion) defect.

In the first two conditions (ventricular septal defect and patent ductus arteriosus), the direction and magnitude of the shunt are governed by factors influencing shunts at either the ventricular level or the great vessel level: relative resistances if the defect is large and relative pressures if the communication is small. In most cases, the resistances and pressures on the right side of the heart and pulmonary arterial system are less than those on the left side of the heart, causing a left-to-right shunt.

In the second two conditions (atrial septal defect and endocardial cushion defect) since the shunt occurs at the atrial level in atrial septal defect and endocardial cushion defect, ventricular compliances influence the shunt. The left-to-right shunt in these patients is caused by the fact that the right ventricle normally is more compliant than the left.

In certain circumstances, the shunt in these four malformations may become right-to-left; this state, sometimes called Eisenmenger syndrome, will be discussed more fully below.

The clinical and laboratory findings of any given condition vary considerably with the volume of pulmonary blood flow, the status of pulmonary vasculature, and the presence of coexistent cardiac anomalies.

Although most patients with these malformations are asymptomatic, poor growth and symptoms of congestive cardiac failure occur in the 5% of patients with greatly increased blood flow, as in ventricular septal defect and patent ductus arteriosus. A tendency to frequent respiratory infections and episodes of pneumonia also is present in those with a large shunt.

In this section, the factors governing flow through ventricular septal defects and through atrial septal defects will be discussed in greater detail. This information should be carefully studied and mastered, for it can be applied in subsequent sections for understanding more complex anomalies that also have a communication between the two sides of circulation.

VENTRICULAR SEPTAL DEFECT

Ventricular septal defect (Fig. 4.1), the most frequently occurring congenital cardiac anomaly, accounts for nearly one fourth of all cases. It is a component of the cardiac anomaly in about one-half of all patients with a cardiac malformation.

Isolated ventricular septal defects causing clinical concern are most frequently located in the area of the membranous portion of the ventricular septum;

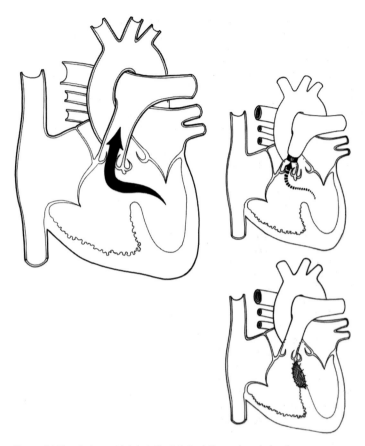

Figure 4.1 Ventricular septal defect. Central circulation and surgical options.

however, occasionally they are found above the crista supraventricularis or in the muscular portion of the septum.

Asymptomatic small defects in the muscular interventricular septum create characteristic murmurs in the neonate and young infant as pulmonary resistance falls and represent the most common cardiac "defect" (reported in as many as 5% of neonates, as detected by highly sensitive echocardiography). Most of these small muscular defects close spontaneously within the first few months of life.

As a result of the defect, shunting of blood occurs between the ventricles. When the size of the defect approaches the size of the aortic annulus, flow is governed by the relative pulmonary and systemic vascular resistances. When the defect is smaller, blood flows from the left to the right ventricle because of the higher systolic pressure in the left ventricle.

As two physiologic mechanisms influence the shunt in ventricular septal defect, the clinical findings, natural history, and operative considerations for the two different sizes of defects will be considered separately.

Large ventricular septal defect

In patients whose ventricular septal defect approaches the size of the aorta, the resistance to outflow from the heart is determined primarily by the caliber of the arterioles of the respective vascular beds.

Since the systemic arterioles have a thick muscular coat and narrow lumen and the pulmonary arterioles have a thin coat and wide lumen, the systemic resistance is greater than the pulmonary resistance.

> In a normal individual (someone without a left-to-right shunt), this difference in systemic and pulmonary resistances is reflected by systemic arterial pressure in the range of 110/70 mm Hg and by pulmonary arterial pressure of 25/10 mm Hg.
>
> Because the pulmonary and systemic blood flows are the same in a normal person, therefore, the resistance in the pulmonary arteriolar bed is a fraction of that in the systemic vasculature.

Since the flow through a larger defect is governed by resistances, any condition that increases resistance to left ventricular outflow, such as coarctation of the aorta or aortic stenosis, increases the magnitude of the left-to-right shunt; whereas any abnormality that obstructs right ventricular outflow, such as co-existent pulmonary stenosis, as in tetralogy of Fallot, or pulmonary arteriolar disease, decreases the magnitude of the left-to-right shunt. If the resistance to right ventricular outflow exceeds the resistance to left ventricular outflow, the shunt is in a right-to-left direction.

> Before and at birth the pulmonary vascular resistance is elevated and is greater than the systemic vascular resistance. In a neonate, the pulmonary arterioles are thick-walled and histologically resemble systemic arterioles. The elevation of pulmonary vascular resistance before birth is supported by observations of the fetal circulation: the right ventricular output enters the pulmonary artery, the major portion flows into the aorta through the ductus arteriosus, and only a small portion enters the gasless high-resistance lungs. The systemic vascular bed has relatively low

resistance because of the highly vascular placenta. The proportions of flow in utero to each vascular bed depend on the relative resistances.

Immediately after birth, the lungs expand with air, dropping the pulmonary vascular resistance; and as the placenta is disconnected from the systemic circuit, the systemic resistance nearly doubles. The pulmonary arterioles continue to change gradually. The media becomes thinner and the lumen becomes wider (Fig. 4.2). Thus, the pulmonary vascular resistance falls, almost reaching adult levels by the time the child is close to 8 weeks of age.

Although this sequence occurs in every individual, this decrease in pulmonary vascular resistance has profound effects on patients with ventricular septal defect. In patients with a large ventricular septal defect, the medial layer does not undergo regression either as quickly as or as much as that of normal individuals so that at any age the pulmonary vascular resistance is higher than normal yet is lower than the systemic resistance.

In patients with a large isolated ventricular septal defect, the systolic pressure in both ventricles and both great vessels is the same, with the right-sided pressures elevated to the same levels as those normally present on the left side of the heart. Because systolic pressure in the aorta is regulated at a constant level by baroreceptors, the pulmonary artery pressure (P) is also relatively fixed in a large ventricular septal defect. According to $P = R_P \times Q_P$, as the pulmonary vascular resistance (R_P) falls, the volume of pulmonary blood flow (Q_P) increases. This occurrence contrasts with the events occurring in an infant without a shunt, who has constant pulmonary blood flow (Q_P); therefore, according to $P = R_P \times Q_P$, as pulmonary resistance (R_P) falls following birth, so does the pulmonary arterial pressure (P).

Among patients with a large ventricular septal defect, as the pulmonary resistance falls as a consequence of the maturation of the pulmonary vessels, the volume of pulmonary blood flow increases no matter what the level of the pulmonary arterial pressure. At birth, little flow across the defect may exist, but as the neonate and young infant grows, the pulmonary blood flow increases.

Large ventricular septal defects place two major hemodynamic loads upon the ventricles: increased pressure load on the right ventricle and increased volume load on the left ventricle.

In a large defect the right ventricle develops a level of systolic pressure equal to that of the left ventricle. The right ventricular workload is proportional to the level of pulmonary arterial pressure ($P = R \times Q$); pulmonary arterial hypertension results either from increased pulmonary arterial resistance or from increased pulmonary blood flow. Regardless of the origin of pulmonary hypertension, the right ventricle is thick-walled; but its state does not really change

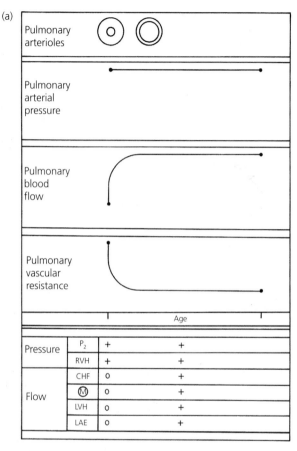

Figure 4.2 Changes in pulmonary arterial pressure, pulmonary blood flow, and pulmonary vascular resistance in (a) an infant with a large ventricular septal defect and (b) a normal infant. Correlation with major clinical findings reflecting pulmonary arterial pressure and pulmonary blood flow. (Abbreviations: CHF, congestive heart failure; LAE, left atrial enlargement; LVH, left ventricular hypertrophy; M, murmur; P_2, pulmonary component of second heart sound; RVH, right ventricular hypertrophy.)

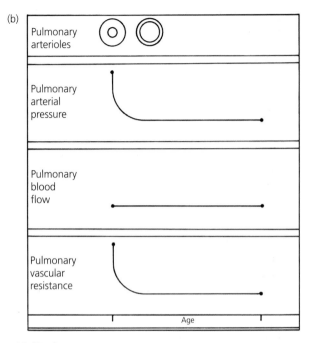

Figure 4.2 (*Cont.*)

from fetal life when it also developed high levels of pressure. Since the pressure remains elevated postnatally, the normal evolution of the right ventricle to a thin-walled, crescent-shaped chamber does not occur. The right ventricle is able to tolerate and to maintain these levels of pressure without the development of cardiac failure.

In ventricular septal defect and left-to-right shunt, a volume overload of the left ventricle exists because this chamber not only must maintain the systemic blood flow but must also eject blood through the ventricular septal defect into the lungs. When the ventricles contract, the flow from the left ventricle through the ventricular septal defect is directed almost entirely into the pulmonary artery, and the right ventricle has little excess volume load. The augmented pulmonary blood flow returns through the left atrium to the left ventricle.

To accommodate the increased pulmonary venous return, the left ventricle dilates (Fig. 4.3). As dilation occurs, the radius and circumference of the left ventricle increase and the myocardial fibers lengthen. Both the Laplace and Starling laws describe this relationship.

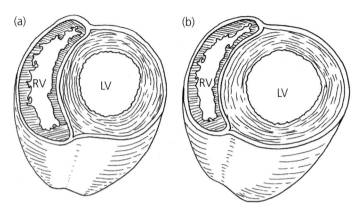

Figure 4.3 Cross-section through ventricles. (a) Normal contour; (b) dilated left ventricle in ventricular septal defect. (Abbreviations: LV, left ventricle; RV, right ventricle.)

The Laplace relationship (Fig. 4.4) states that in a cylindrical object, as the radius increases, the tension (T) in the wall must also increase to maintain pressure ($T = P \times R$). Therefore as the left ventricle dilates and increases its radius, it must develop increased wall tension to maintain ventricular pressure. If the left ventricle becomes greatly dilated, the myocardium cannot develop sufficient tension to maintain the pressure volume relationship, causing congestive cardiac failure.

Starling's law states that as myocardial fiber stretches, cardiac function increases up to a certain point only, beyond which function falls.

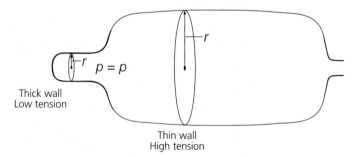

Figure 4.4 Balloon illustrating the Laplace relationship. The pressure (p) in both the wide and narrow portions of the balloon is the same, but the wall tension (T) is greater where the radius (r) is greater.

The signs and symptoms of a large ventricular septal defect vary with the relative vascular resistances and the volume of pulmonary blood flow. In evaluating a patient with a large ventricular septal defect, the physician should seek diagnostic information that permits definition of pulmonary blood flow (Q_P) and pulmonary artery pressure (P) so that he or she can estimate pulmonary vascular resistance (R_P).

History
In many patients with a large ventricular septal defect, the murmur may not be heard until the first postnatal visit. By that age the pulmonary vascular resistance has fallen sufficiently that enough blood flows through the defect to generate the murmur.

Patients with a larger-sized defect develop congestive cardiac failure by 2–3 months of age. By this time the pulmonary arterioles have matured sufficiently to permit a large volume of pulmonary blood flow. As a consequence, left ventricular dilation develops and results in cardiac failure and its symptoms of tachypnea, slow weight gain, and poor feeding.

Physical examination
Holosystolic murmur. The classic auscultatory finding is a loud holosystolic murmur heard best in the third and fourth left intercostal spaces. Usually associated with a thrill, the murmur is widely transmitted. The murmur begins with the first heart sound and includes the isovolumetric contraction period of the cardiac cycle. Since the ventricles are in communication, blood shunts from the left to the right ventricle from the onset of systole. The murmur usually lasts until the second heart sound. The loudness of the murmur does not directly relate to the size of the defect; loudness depends on other factors, such as volume of blood flow through the defect. However, large defects tend not to produce loud holosystolic murmurs.

Mid-diastolic murmur. In patients with a large ventricular septal defect and a large volume of pulmonary blood flow, the volume of pulmonary venous blood crossing the mitral valve into the left ventricle during diastole greatly increases. When the volume of blood flow across the mitral valve exceeds twice normal, a mid-diastolic inflow murmur may be heard, often following the third heart sound. Low pitched, it is best heard at the cardiac apex. The loudness roughly parallels the volume of pulmonary blood flow.

Loud P_2. Patients with a large ventricular septal defect have pulmonary hypertension related to various combinations of pulmonary blood flow and increased pulmonary vascular resistance. Regardless of the cause, pulmonary hypertension is indicated by an increased loudness of the pulmonary component of the second heart sound. The louder the pulmonary component, the higher the pulmonary arterial pressure.

In the presence of a diastolic murmur, the loud pulmonic valve closure primarily relates to increased pulmonary flow. The absence of a mitral murmur indicates that the pulmonary hypertension is secondary to increased pulmonary vascular resistance.

Clinical evidence of cardiomegaly. This may be present in those patients with increased pulmonary blood flow; it is indicated by a laterally and inferiorly displaced cardiac apex or by a precordial bulge.

Congestive cardiac failure. Tachypnea, tachycardia, and dyspnea (especially with poor feeding and diaphoresis increasing during feeding in infants) suggest congestive cardiac failure. Cardiomegaly and hepatomegaly support the diagnosis. Peripheral edema and abnormal lung sounds are not typical signs of congestive cardiac failure in infants.

Electrocardiogram

The electrocardiogram reflects the types of hemodynamic load placed upon the ventricles: left ventricular volume overload related to increased pulmonary blood flow and right ventricular pressure overload related to pulmonary hypertension.

The electrocardiogram varies depending upon the hemodynamics: left ventricular and left atrial enlargement (Fig. 4.5) reflect the increased pulmonary blood flow.

Right ventricular hypertrophy indicates right ventricular systolic hypertension paralleling the pulmonary arterial pressure increase.

Biventricular enlargement/hypertrophy exists in patients with a large volume of pulmonary blood flow and pulmonary hypertension due to a large defect.

Isolated right ventricular hypertrophy and right axis deviation occur in patients with pulmonary hypertension related to increased pulmonary vascular resistance of any cause. The increased pulmonary vascular resistance limits pulmonary blood flow, and therefore a pattern of left ventricular hypertrophy is absent.

Chest X-ray

Chest X-ray (Fig. 4.6) shows normal appearing pulmonary vasculature at birth, but soon thereafter, the vascularity increases. The radiographic appearance of the heart varies according to the magnitude of the shunt and the level of

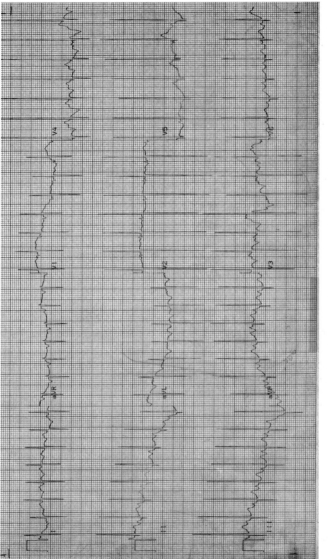

Figure 4.5 Electrocardiogram in ventricular septal defect. Normal QRS axis. Biphasic P waves in V_1 indicate left atrial enlargement. Pattern of left ventricular hypertrophy/enlargement in a 6-week-old infant. Deep Q wave and tall R wave in lead V_6 indicate volume overload of left ventricle.

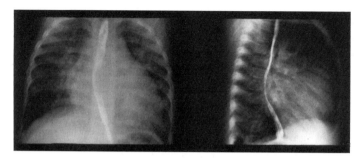

Figure 4.6 Chest X-ray in ventricular septal defect. Cardiomegaly and increased pulmonary vascular markings. The lateral view shows left atrial enlargement, outlined by barium within the esophagus.

pulmonary arterial pressure. Ranging from normal to markedly enlarged, the size varies directly with the shunt's magnitude.

The cardiac enlargement results from the increased flow that causes enlargement of both the left atrium and the left ventricle. The left atrium is a particularly valuable indicator of pulmonary blood flow because this chamber is easily assessed using the lateral projection. By itself the right ventricular hypertrophy does not contribute to cardiac enlargement. The pulmonary artery can be enlarged because of the volume of pulmonary blood flow or because of pulmonary hypertension. There is no characteristic contour of the heart in ventricular septal defect.

> Summary of clinical findings. The primary finding of ventricular septal defect is a holosystolic murmur along the left sternal border. The secondary features of ventricular septal defect reflect the components of the equation $P = R \times Q$. The pulmonary arterial pressure (P) is indicated by the loudness of the pulmonary component of the second heart sound and by the degree of right ventricular hypertrophy on the electrocardiogram. Pulmonary blood flow (Q) is indicated by a history of congestive cardiac failure, an apical diastolic murmur, left ventricular hypertrophy on the electrocardiogram, cardiomegaly, and left atrial enlargement on chest X-ray. The changes with age of the secondary features are shown in Fig. 4.2a.

Natural history
An uncorrected large ventricular septal defect may follow one of three courses in a patient.

Pulmonary vascular disease. Pulmonary vascular disease may develop. The initiating factors causing the development of medial hypertrophy and later intimal proliferation are unknown, but they are probably related to the fact that the arterioles are being submitted to high levels of pressure and, to a lesser degree, to elevated blood flow. The anatomic changes can develop in pulmonary arterioles of children as young as 1 year. The early changes of medial hypertrophy are generally reversible if the ventricular septal defect is corrected, but the intimal changes are permanent. The pathologic changes of the pulmonary arterioles are usually progressive unless the course is interrupted by operation. From experience, children with Down syndrome appear to develop irreversible (or if reversible, a more reactive and problematic) elevation of pulmonary vascular resistance within the first 6 months of life.

The result of these anatomic changes is progressive elevation of pulmonary vascular resistance (Fig. 4.7). The pulmonary arterial pressure does not increase, but instead stays constant because the ventricles are in free communication. Therefore the volume of pulmonary blood flow decreases.

Eventually the pulmonary vascular resistance may become greater than systemic vascular resistance, at which time the shunt becomes right-to-left through the defect and cyanosis develops (Eisenmenger syndrome).

The progressive rise in pulmonary vascular resistance can be followed clinically by observing the changes in the secondary features of ventricular septal defect. Those features reflecting elevated pulmonary arterial pressure, right ventricular hypertrophy, and loudness of the pulmonary component remain constant, whereas those reflecting pulmonary blood flow change (Fig. 4.7).

The clinical findings reflecting the excessive flow through the left side of the heart gradually disappear. Congestive cardiac failure lessens; the diastolic murmur fades; the electrocardiogram no longer shows the left ventricular hypertrophy; and the cardiac size is reduced on chest X-ray. The heart size becomes normal because the total volume of blood flow is normal. The right ventricle is hypertrophied, but this does not cause enlargement. For many patients with cardiac disease, the disappearance of congestive cardiac failure and the presence of a normal heart size is favorable; but in this instance, the changes are ominous.

Infundibular pulmonary stenosis. Infundibular pulmonary stenosis may develop. In certain patients with a large ventricular septal defect, infundibular stenosis may develop and progressively narrow the right ventricular outflow tract. In such patients, this stenotic area represents a major resistance to outflow into the lungs; the pulmonary vascular resistance is often normal (Fig. 4.8). The shunt in these patients is influenced by the relationship between the systemic vascular resistance and the resistance that is imposed by the infundibular stenosis. Eventually the latter may exceed the former so that the shunt becomes

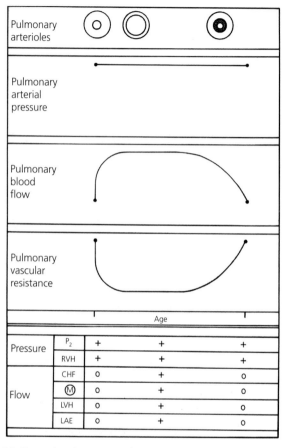

Figure 4.7 Changes in pulmonary arterial pressure, pulmonary blood flow, and pulmonary vascular resistance in a patient with a large ventricular septal defect who develops pulmonary vascular disease. Correlation with major clinical findings reflecting pulmonary arterial pressure and pulmonary blood flow. (Abbreviations: CHF, congestive heart failure; LAE, left atrial enlargement; LVH, left ventricular hypertrophy; M, murmur; P₂, pulmonary component of second heart sound; RVH, right ventricular hypertrophy.)

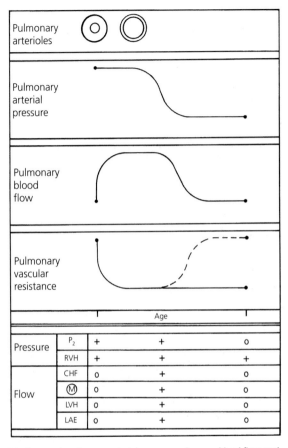

Figure 4.8 Changes in pulmonary arterial pressure, pulmonary blood flow, and pulmonary vascular resistance in a patient with a large ventricular septal defect who develops infundibular pulmonary stenosis. Correlation with major clinical findings reflecting pulmonary arterial pressure and pulmonary blood flow. Dashed line indicates resistance imposed by infundibular stenosis. (Abbreviations: CHF, congestive heart failure; LAE, left atrial enlargement; LVH, left ventricular hypertrophy; M, murmur; P_2, pulmonary component of second heart sound; RVH, right ventricular hypertrophy.)

right-to-left and cyanosis develops. The clinical picture of these patients then resembles tetralogy of Fallot.

In these patients, the loudness of the pulmonary component becomes normal or is reduced and delayed, but right ventricular hypertrophy persists because the right ventricle is still developing systemic levels of pressure. The features related to pulmonary blood flow—congestive cardiac failure, apical diastolic murmur, left ventricular hypertrophy on the electrocardiogram, cardiomegaly, and left atrial enlargement on chest X-ray—disappear as the pulmonary blood flow is reduced.

Regardless of whether the resistance to pulmonary blood flow resides in the infundibulum or the pulmonary arterioles, the hemodynamic effects are similar; but the prognosis is dissimilar.

Spontaneous closure. Spontaneous closure of the ventricular septal defect may occur. The exact incidence of spontaneous closure is unknown, but up to 5% of large ventricular septal defects and at least 50% of small defects undergo spontaneous closure; others become smaller. The spontaneous closure occurs by two basic mechanisms: by adherence of the septal leaflet of the tricuspid valve to the ventricular septum, thereby occluding the perimembranous ventricular septal defect or creating a mobile and partially restrictive so-called aneurysm of the membranous septum or by closure of a muscular defect by ingrowth of myocardium and then fibrous proliferation.

Most instances of spontaneous closure occur by 3 years of age when the pulmonary vascular resistance is still near-normal levels.

As the closure of the ventricular septal defect occurs, the systolic murmur softens; and the secondary features reflecting pulmonary arterial pressure become normal (Fig. 4.9). The pulmonary component becomes normal and the right ventricular hypertrophy disappears. Those features reflecting pulmonary blood flow also gradually disappear. Thus, eventually the systolic murmur disappears; and no residual cardiac abnormalities exist, although the heart may remain large for some months. Some liken the gradual resolution of cardiomegaly to the process of a patient "growing into" their own heart size, rather than calling it an active reduction in heart size.

Echocardiogram

A large ventricular septal defect appears as an area of "dropout" within the septum by cross-sectional two-dimensional (2D) echocardiography.

Perimembranous infracristal defects appear near the tricuspid valve septal leaflet and the aortic valve right coronary cusp.

Small defects, especially those within the trabecular (muscular) septum, may not be apparent by 2D, but color Doppler demonstrates a multicolored jet traversing the septum, representing the turbulent shunt from left to right ventricle.

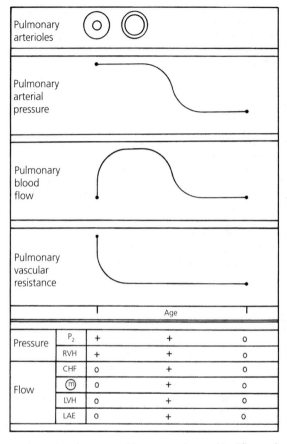

Figure 4.9 Changes in pulmonary arterial pressure, pulmonary blood flow, and pulmonary vascular resistance in a patient with a large ventricular septal defect that undergoes spontaneous closure. Correlation with major clinical findings reflecting pulmonary arterial pressure and pulmonary blood flow. (Abbreviations: CHF, congestive heart failure; LAE, left atrial enlargement; LVH, left ventricular hypertrophy; M, murmur; P₂, pulmonary component of second heart sound; RVH, right ventricular hypertrophy.)

Inlet ventricular septal defect, located near the AV valves, is seen in endocardial cushion defect.

The maximum velocity of the blood traversing the defect, as determined using spectral Doppler, is used to estimate the interventricular pressure difference. Large defects lead to high right ventricular pressure that is reflected as low-velocity flow across the defect. In the presence of normal right ventricular systolic pressure, small defects have high-velocity shunts, reflecting the large interventricular pressure difference. Small ventricular septal defects in neonates may have low-velocity flow, indicating that pulmonary resistance and right ventricular pressure have not yet fallen. Low-velocity shunt, or right-to-left shunt, is seen in older patients with pulmonary vascular obstructive disease or right ventricular outflow obstruction.

In patients with a large ventricular septal defect, 2D echocardiography reveals left atrial and left ventricular enlargement. Left ventricular systolic function may appear hyperdynamic because of the increased stroke volume associated with a large ventricular septal defect.

Cardiac catheterization

Cardiac catheterization may be indicated in patients with multiple ventricular septal defects and congestive cardiac failure, suspected elevation of pulmonary vascular resistance, or suspected associated anomalies. The purposes of the procedure are to define the hemodynamics, to identify coexistent cardiac anomalies, and to localize the site(s) of the ventricular septal defect(s).

A large increase in oxygen saturation is found at the right ventricular level. The pulmonary arterial and right ventricular systolic pressures are identical to those in the aorta and the left ventricle. If the pulmonary vascular resistance is increased, the increase in oxygen saturation at the right ventricular level is less, and the pulmonary arterial pressure remains the same.

Left ventriculography is indicated to locate the position of the ventricular septal defect(s) because location influences operative repair. Aortography may also be performed to exclude a coexistent patent ductus arteriosus, which can be a silent partner.

Operative considerations

Patients with a large ventricular septal defect and congestive cardiac failure should be treated with diuretics, inotropes, and/or afterload reduction and with aggressive nutritional support (discussed in Chapter 11). Fluid restriction (which also means caloric restriction) is usually counterproductive. Although these measures improve the clinical status, many patients frequently show persistent findings of cardiac failure, indicating need for operative treatment. Two operative procedures are available.

Corrective operation. Corrective operation for closure of the ventricular septal defect is indicated in infancy for those patients with persistent cardiac failure and pulmonary hypertension. Cardiopulmonary bypass is instituted; the right atrium is opened; and by working through the tricuspid valve, the ventricular septal defect is closed using a patch of Dacron or pericardium. This technique avoids a transmural scar in the ventricular myocardium. The operative mortality risk in infants is less than 0.25%. The long-term results of the procedure are excellent; virtually no patients who had normal or reactive pulmonary vascular resistance preoperatively develop late pulmonary vascular obstructive disease. Almost no patients develop endocarditis or arrhythmia late postoperatively.

Banding of the pulmonary artery. Banding of the pulmonary artery is a palliative procedure that causes an increase in the resistance to blood flow into the lungs. Therefore, the pulmonary artery pressure and volume of blood flow returning to the left side of the heart are reduced, improving congestive cardiac failure. Pulmonary artery deformity and stenosis may persist after removal of the band.

Because the risk for operative ventricular septal defect closure is low (usually less than that for banding and subsequent reoperation for debanding with defect closure), corrective surgery is preferable. For some cardiac malformations with a large ventricular communication (e.g., single ventricle), pulmonary artery banding is indicated as temporary or permanent palliation.

Small or medium ventricular septal defects

The size of ventricular septal defects varies considerably. The previous section discussed those defects whose diameter approached the size of the aortic annulus. This section discusses smaller ventricular septal defects.

The direction and magnitude of blood flow in a small- or medium-sized ventricular septal defect depend upon the size of the defect and the relative resistances of the systemic and pulmonary vascular beds. The pulmonary arterial pressures are lower than the systemic pressures because the defect limits the transmission of left ventricular systolic pressure to the right side of the heart. Such defects are pressure-restrictive.

Whereas in a large ventricular septal defect the level of pulmonary arterial pressure is determined by systemic arterial pressure, in a small- or medium-sized defect the pulmonary arterial pressure is determined by a combination of pulmonary vascular resistance and pulmonary blood flow. In most of these patients the pulmonary vascular resistance falls normally with age. Pulmonary vascular disease may occur; but if it does, it appears at a slower rate than with a large defect and only in those few patients who have a large volume of left-to-right shunt despite a pressure-restrictive defect.

In general, the volume of pulmonary blood flow varies with the size of the defect and the level of pulmonary vascular resistance. Since beyond infancy most children have normal pulmonary vascular resistance, the shunt is directly related to the size of the defect. In some patients the defect is so small that the shunt is undetectable by oximetry data, whereas in other patients the pulmonary blood flow is three times the systemic blood flow.

History

Most of the patients in this category have a small defect which has little effect on pulmonary blood flow and none on pulmonary artery pressure. Most patients with a small- or medium-sized ventricular septal defect are asymptomatic. Heart disease is usually detected by the discovery of a murmur either before discharge from the newborn nursery or, more commonly, at the first postnatal visit. However, the occasional patient with a large pulmonary blood flow may have frequent respiratory infections and pneumonia. Relatively few of them develop congestive cardiac failure. The growth and development of most patients are normal.

Physical examination

Usually no evidence of cardiomegaly is found on physical examination.

There are two categories of murmurs associated with small VSDs.

Some murmurs are holosystolic, loud (grades 3/6–4/6), may be accompanied by a thrill, and are heard along the left sternal border. These are more likely from membranous VSDs.

Other murmurs are less loud (grade 2/6), squirty in quality, heard best more toward the apex, and are usually caused by muscular VSDs.

Muscular defects may functionally "close" during each systole as the surrounding myocardium constricts the VSD lumen until the shunt is obliterated in middle to late systole. This results in the murmur being shorter in duration than those associated with membranous VSDs. The "squirty" quality of the murmur is probably due to constantly changing pitch as the blood accelerates through the narrowing defect.

As in those patients with a large defect, defining pulmonary arterial pressure by the loudness of the pulmonary component of the second sound (P_2) and defining pulmonary blood flow by the presence of an apical diastolic murmur is important. In patients with a small defect, P_2 is normal and diastole is clear;

those with a medium-sized defect may have an accentuated P_2 and a soft apical mid-diastolic murmur.

Electrocardiogram
In many patients in this category, the electrocardiogram is normal, reflecting that the volume of pulmonary blood flow and level of pulmonary arterial pressure are normal or near normal. A pattern of left ventricular hypertrophy indicates an increased volume of pulmonary blood flow with little change in pulmonary arterial pressure. A few patients with elevation of pulmonary arterial pressure and pulmonary blood flow have a pattern of biventricular hypertrophy.

Chest X-ray
The cardiac size, left atrial size, and pulmonary vascularity directly parallel the volume of pulmonary blood flow. The heart and lung fields usually are normal or show some increase in vascularity and size, but not to the degree found in patients with large ventricular septal defect and severe pulmonary overcirculation.

> Summary of clinical findings. In ventricular septal defect, the magnitude of the shunt depends upon the size of the defect and the relative levels of pulmonary and systemic vascular resistances. A loud, harsh, holosystolic murmur along the left sternal border is the hallmark of ventricular septal defect. The other clinical and laboratory findings reflect alterations of hemodynamics. Alterations in the second sound, the presence of an apical diastolic murmur, and changes in the electrocardiogram and chest X-ray reflect the magnitude of shunt and the level of pulmonary arterial pressure.

Natural history
Patients with a small- or medium-sized ventricular septal defect, pulmonary blood flow less than twice systemic blood flow, and normal pulmonary arterial pressure are considered to have a normal life expectancy.

They are at relatively low risk for infective endocarditis. A few with perimembranous defects (less than 1% of patients) develop aortic valve prolapse and insufficiency.

Most patients are not at risk for development of pulmonary vascular disease. Some patients with a larger volume of pulmonary blood flow or with elevated pulmonary arterial pressure may develop pulmonary vascular changes.

The defects do not enlarge, and at least 50% undergo spontaneous closure, usually in early childhood, but in rare instances it occurs in adulthood.

Echocardiogram

Small ventricular septal defects, especially those within the trabecular (muscular) septum, may not be apparent by 2D but are easily viewed using color Doppler where they appear as a multicolored jet traversing the septum, representing the turbulent shunt from left to right ventricle.

The maximum velocity of the blood traversing the defect, determined using spectral Doppler, is used to estimate the interventricular pressure difference—a large defect allows elevated right ventricular systolic pressure, reflected as low-velocity flow across the defect. In the presence of normal right ventricular systolic pressure, a small defect has a high-velocity Doppler signal, reflecting the large interventricular pressure difference. Small ventricular septal defects in neonates may have low-velocity flow, indicating that neither pulmonary resistance nor right ventricular pressure has yet fallen. Low-velocity shunt, or right-to-left shunt, is seen in older patients with pulmonary vascular obstructive disease or right ventricular outflow obstruction.

In patients with a small ventricular septal defect, 2D echocardiography shows normal left atrial and left ventricular size. Left ventricular and left atrial size may be moderately increased because of the volume overload associated with a moderate-sized ventricular septal defect.

Cardiac catheterization

In patients with clinical evidence of an obvious, small ventricular septal defect, cardiac catheterization is not indicated. Cardiac catheterization to verify the diagnosis and to determine the volume of pulmonary blood flow and level of pulmonary arterial pressure may be indicated in patients with moderate-sized defects and clinical evidence of pulmonary overcirculation and hypertension. Therefore, careful oximetry and pressure data are obtained. Many of these patients may have minimal or no symptoms.

Catheterization is performed before 4 or 5 years of age, since spontaneous closure or narrowing of the defect is less likely after that age, yet surgical closure of the defect can be prophylactic against pulmonary vascular disease. Catheterization is performed at an earlier age (within the first year of life) if cardiac failure or other symptoms develop or if risk factors for accelerated pulmonary vascular disease, such as Down syndrome, are present.

Operative considerations

The rate of operative mortality and morbidity for patients with a small defect usually exceeds the rate of problem development in the unoperated patient. Therefore, operation is not recommended for these patients. Patients with either elevated pulmonary arterial pressure or pulmonary blood flow twice normal should have operative closure. Closure, which can be performed at a low risk, eliminates the risk of development of pulmonary vascular disease and bacterial endocarditis. Patients who develop aortic valve prolapse or insufficiency should undergo ventricular septal defect closure to prevent progressive insufficiency.

> Summary. In ventricular septal defect, the magnitude of the shunt depends upon the size of the defect and the relative levels of pulmonary and systemic vascular resistances. A holosystolic murmur along the left sternal border is the hallmark of ventricular septal defect. The other clinical and laboratory findings reflect alterations of hemodynamics. Alterations in the second sound, the presence of an apical diastolic murmur, and changes in the electrocardiogram and chest X-ray reflect the magnitude of shunt and the level of pulmonary arterial pressure.

PATENT DUCTUS ARTERIOSUS

Patent ductus arteriosus (Fig. 4.10) represents the persistence of the fetal communication between the aorta and the pulmonary trunk. The ductus arteriosus

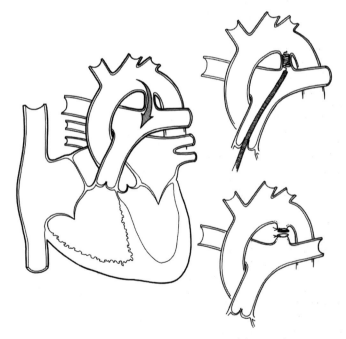

Figure 4.10 Patent ductus arteriosus. Central circulation and closure options.

is formed from the embryonic left sixth aortic arch and connects the proximal descending aorta beyond the left subclavian artery and the proximal left pulmonary artery.

Normally, the ductus arteriosus functionally closes by the fourth day of life. Although the mechanisms for closure of the ductus are largely unknown, rising oxygen tension and withdrawal of endogenous prostaglandins are factors influencing closure.

Pharmacologic ductal closure can be accomplished in premature infants by administration of indomethacin, a prostaglandin synthase inhibitor. Ductal patency can be maintained for palliation of certain cardiac malformations by administration of prostaglandin.

The direction and magnitude of flow through the ductus depend upon the size of the ductus and the relative systemic and pulmonary vascular resistances.

In fetal life the ductus is large, and since the pulmonary vascular resistance exceeds systemic vascular resistance, blood flow is from right to left.

Following birth, if the ductus arteriosus remains patent, the shunt occurs from the aorta into the pulmonary artery. In patients with a large patent ductus arteriosus, pressures are equal in the aorta and the pulmonary artery, and blood flows into the pulmonary artery because the pulmonary resistance is normally less than systemic resistance. In patients with a smaller ductus arteriosus, the shunt also occurs left to right because of pressure differences between the great vessels.

The hemodynamics resemble ventricular septal defect. As pulmonary vascular resistance falls following birth, the volume of pulmonary blood flow increases. If the volume of pulmonary blood flow is large, congestive cardiac failure occurs because of the excessive volume load placed upon the left ventricle.

History

Patent ductus arteriosus occurs more frequently in females and in prematurely born children. The defect is also common in children with Down syndrome. In children whose mothers had rubella during the first trimester of pregnancy, patent ductus arteriosus is the most commonly observed cardiac anomaly. Patent ductus arteriosus occurs more commonly in children born at high altitudes (above 10,000 feet), emphasizing the role of oxygen in closure of the ductus.

The course of patients with patent ductus arteriosus is variable, depending upon the size of the ductus and the volume of pulmonary blood flow. Many patients are asymptomatic; the ductus is identified only by the presence of a murmur. On the other hand, congestive cardiac failure can develop early in infancy because of volume overload of the left ventricle, although this typically does not occur for at least 2–3 months. In prematurely born infants, cardiac failure may develop at an earlier age because pulmonary vascular resistance reaches normal levels at an earlier age.

Symptomatic children may also present a history of frequent respiratory infections and easy fatigability.

Physical examination
Continuous murmur
The classical physical finding is a machinery type murmur best heard over the upper left chest inferior to the clavicle. The murmur may be associated with a thrill or prominent pulsations in the suprasternal notch. Blood flows through the ductus arteriosus throughout the cardiac cycle because of the pressure or resistance difference between the systemic or pulmonary vascular circuits. The murmur may not continue through the entire cardiac cycle, but generally it does extend well into diastole except in the first few months of life. At this age the murmur may be confined to systole, perhaps because the diastolic pressure in the pulmonary artery is closer to that in the aorta than at older ages.

Wide pulse pressure
This physical finding resembles that of aortic insufficiency. The aortic systolic pressure is elevated because of an increased stroke volume and the diastolic pressure is lowered because of the flow into the pulmonary circuit. Peripheral arterial pulses are prominent. In patients with a small patent ductus arteriosus, the blood pressure readings are normal; however, those patients with a larger flow show wide pulse pressure. Prominent radial arterial pulses in a neonate or small infant suggest either patent ductus arteriosus or coarctation of the aorta. If the femoral pulses are bounding, coarctation is not usually present, but a large ductus can palliate coarctation (e.g., infants with coarctation palliated with prostaglandin are expected to have bounding femoral pulses).

Mid-diastolic murmur and second heart sound
As in ventricular septal defect, the severity of patent ductus arteriosus may be assessed from two findings: the intensity of the pulmonic component of the second heart sound and the presence of an apical diastolic murmur. The pulmonary component of the second heart sound is accentuated in pulmonary hypertension, either from increased pulmonary blood flow or from increased pulmonary vascular resistance. An apical mid-diastolic murmur suggests a large left-to-right shunt through the patent ductus arteriosus, resulting in a large volume of blood crossing a normal mitral valve.

Systolic ejection click
Frequently, an aortic systolic ejection click is heard because the aorta is dilated.

Findings in elevated pulmonary resistance
In an occasional patient (usually older) the pulmonary resistance exceeds the systemic resistance so that blood flow occurs from the pulmonary artery into the

aorta. Such patients have a soft systolic murmur, a loud pulmonic second sound, and differential cyanosis involving the lower extremities, a finding almost never appreciated by visual inspection but usually easily demonstrated by comparing upper- and lower-extremity pulse oximetry or arterial blood gases.

Electrocardiogram

The electrocardiographic patterns in patent ductus arteriosus are similar to those in ventricular septal defect since in both the potential hemodynamic burdens are volume overload of the left ventricle and pressure overload of the right ventricle.

As in patients with ventricular septal defect, one of four patterns may be present:

Normal. In patients with a small patent ductus arteriosus, a normal electrocardiogram indicates near-normal pulmonary blood flow, pulmonary arterial pressure, and pulmonary vascular resistance.

Left ventricular and left atrial enlargement. In many patients with patent ductus arteriosus, the major hemodynamic burden is volume overload of the left atrium and left ventricle (Fig. 4.11). In such patients, pulmonary arterial pressure is near normal. In general, the left ventricular hypertrophy is manifested by a QRS complex in lead V_6 with a sizable Q wave and a very tall R wave followed by a tall T wave.

Biventricular enlargement/hypertrophy. In infants and children with increased pulmonary arterial pressure, right ventricular hypertrophy coexists with the pattern of left ventricular enlargement/hypertrophy. This is manifested by patterns of left and right ventricular hypertrophy or tall (70 mm) equiphasic QRS complexes in the mid-precordial leads.

Isolated right ventricular hypertrophy. Isolated right ventricular hypertrophy may be present in those patients with a major elevation of pulmonary vascular resistance secondary to pulmonary vascular disease. The elevated resistance reduces pulmonary blood flow so that left ventricular enlargement/hypertrophy is not present.

Chest X-ray

In patent ductus arteriosus, chest X-ray (Fig. 4.12) reveals increased pulmonary vascularity and left atrial and left ventricular enlargement; however, cardiac and left atrial size vary from normal to greatly enlarged, depending upon the volume of shunt. A normal-sized heart is found in patients either with a small ductus or with markedly increased pulmonary vascular resistance. Usually, both the aorta and the pulmonary trunk are enlarged, although in infants the thymus may obscure the aortic knob.

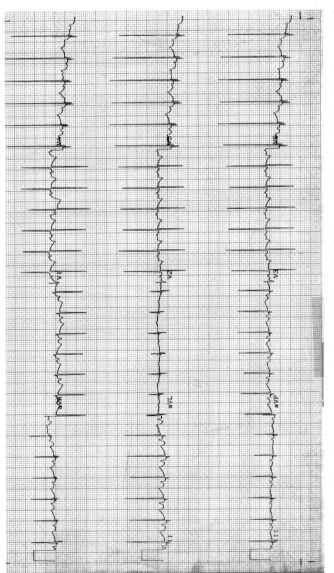

Figure 4.11 Electrocardiogram in patent ductus arteriosus. Normal QRS axis. Biphasic P waves in V_1 consistent with left atrial enlargement. Left ventricular hypertrophy/enlargement manifested by deep Q wave and tall R wave in lead V_6.

(a)

(b)

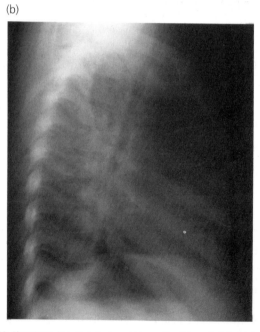

Figure 4.12 Chest X-ray in patent ductus arteriosus. Cardiomegaly, left atrial enlargement, and increased pulmonary vasculature.

Patent ductus arteriosus is the only major cardiac malformation with a left-to-right shunt causing aortic enlargement. The aorta is enlarged because it carries not only the systemic output but also the blood to be shunted through the lungs.

In each of the other cardiac malformations discussed in this section on left-to-right shunts, the aorta is normal or appears small.

Therefore, if a distinctly enlarged aorta is present and a left-to-right shunt is suspected, patent ductus arteriosus must receive serious consideration.

Summary of clinical findings. The primary features of patent ductus arteriosus include the continuous murmur and the findings associated with a wide pulse pressure. The secondary features are explained by the relationship $P = R \times Q$. Pulmonary arterial pressure is indicated by the intensity of the pulmonic component of the second heart sound and by the degree of right ventricular hypertrophy on the electrocardiogram. Flow is reflected by electrocardiographic evidence of left ventricular hypertrophy, the chest X-ray findings of cardiomegaly and left atrial enlargement, or the development of congestive cardiac failure. The presence of an apical diastolic murmur also reflects increased flow but may be obscured by the continuous murmur.

Natural history

The course of patients with patent ductus arteriosus resembles that previously described for patients with ventricular septal defect.

Patients with a small- or medium-sized patent ductus arteriosus do well and have few complications.

Pulmonary vascular disease can develop in patients with a large patent ductus arteriosus and in those with elevated pulmonary arterial pressure and blood flow. As pulmonary vascular resistance rises, the volume of pulmonary blood flow falls. Eventually, the pulmonary vascular resistance can exceed the systemic vascular resistance, so the shunt becomes right to left. Such patients have differential cyanosis manifested by cyanosis of the lower extremities and normal color of the upper extremities.

Similar to patients with ventricular septal defect who develop pulmonary vascular disease, the congestive cardiac failure improves; the diastolic murmur fades; and the left ventricular hypertrophy and cardiomegaly disappear as the pulmonary vascular resistance increases.

Echocardiogram

The patent ductus may appear quite large by 2D echocardiography with a diameter exceeding that of the individual branch pulmonary arteries or aortic arch, especially in newborn infants who are ill or who are receiving prostaglandin.

In such a large ductus, the velocity of the shunt is low, less than 1 m/s, because little pressure difference exists between the great vessels. However, the direction of shunting provides important clues to the physiology.

In infants with a normal postnatal fall in pulmonary vascular resistance, the shunt is continuous from aorta to pulmonary artery, with no demonstrable shunt from pulmonary artery to aorta.

In infants with abnormally high pulmonary resistance, such as those with "primary pulmonary hypertension of the newborn," or obstruction to pulmonary venous return, as in some types of total anomalous pulmonary venous connection, the ductal shunt is predominately from pulmonary artery to aorta. A to-and-fro, or "bi-directional," shunt is commonly seen in situations where pulmonary vascular resistance and systemic vascular resistance are similar, as in complete transposition (elevated pulmonary resistance) or large systemic arteriovenous malformation (decreased systemic vascular resistance).

A small ductus in an older patient may appear as a narrow jet of multicolored echoes, representing high-velocity turbulent flow, from aorta to pulmonary artery. In these patients with normal pulmonary artery pressure, Doppler shows a continuous signal from aorta to pulmonary artery at high velocity; the maximum velocity helps estimate the pulmonary artery systolic pressure when one calculates the pressure difference between this and the measured systolic blood pressure (equivalent to aortic pressure).

Treatment
Prostaglandin synthase inhibitors (indomethacin or ibuprofen)

For most patent ductus arteriosus occurring in premature infants, closure is accomplished by oral or intravenous administration of a prostaglandin synthase inhibitor. Three doses of indomethacin (q 12 hours) or ibuprofen (q 24 hours) achieve ductal closure in greater than 80% of premature infants, although subsequent dose courses can be given to improve success. Renal insufficiency and thrombocytopenia are relative contraindications.

In adults, children, and infants older than 2 weeks, drug therapy is unsuccessful; but a variety of other techniques are available for closure. In asymptomatic infants, some have suggested delay in closure until the child is 1 year old; although the risk of waiting is extremely low, the potential occurrence of spontaneous closure is extremely unlikely. The ductus should be closed regardless of age and patient size if it causes congestive cardiac failure. In older children it should be closed when recognized.

Operative division and ligation of the ductus arteriosus

This is the time-honored treatment, first performed in 1938 by two groups of surgeons in the United States and Europe who were working independently.

Classically, the procedure involves a left lateral thoracotomy but does not involve cardiopulmonary bypass. The risk of ligation and division of patent ductus arteriosus is extremely small; the results are generally excellent. The operation can be performed in the smallest of prematures who fail to respond to indomethacin treatment.

Thorascopic (endoscopic) closure of the ductus can be performed in any patient's past late infancy to avoid thoracotomy. Operative risks may be higher than with thoracotomy, possibly because of limited exposure.

Transcatheter closure

Using a variety of implantable devices, transcatheter closure has become a standard therapy. Currently, occlusion of the ductus with catheter-delivered spring wire coils covered with thrombogenic Dacron strands (Gianturco coils) has been the most widely and successfully used nonsurgical technique.

Incomplete closure, embolism of dislodged coils to distant sites (requiring extended procedure for retrieval), and prolonged radiation exposure remain the most frequent complications. Long-term efficacy data suggest that the results and the risks are at least as good as surgical closure.

The technique is usually limited to larger children and adults because of the size of the delivery devices; the length and shape of the ductus arteriosus are factors in successful coil occlusion.

Otherwise, for patients having operative closure of patent ductus arteriosus, cardiac catheterization and angiocardiography are not indicated because the physical and laboratory findings are so characteristic of the disease. In infants, however, aortography may be required to rule out suspected associated defects, such as aortic arch obstruction, vascular rings or sling, or aorticopulmonary window, which may be difficult to exclude by clinical means and echocardiography.

Summary. Patent ductus arteriosus is an abnormal communication between the aorta and the pulmonary artery. It occurs more frequently in prematurely born infants and term infants with respiratory disease, Down syndrome, or congenital rubella syndrome. The hemodynamics and many clinical findings resemble those of ventricular septal defect because both lesions place an excessive volume load on the left ventricle and may elevate pulmonary arterial pressure. The characteristic finding is a continuous murmur, combined with findings reflecting the flow and pressure characteristics. Closure of the ductus is indicated in almost all patients and is associated with low risk.

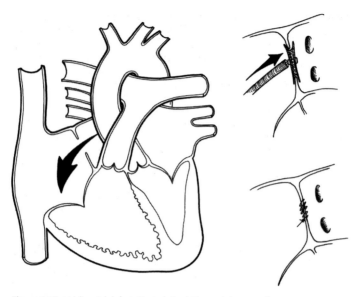

Figure 4.13 Atrial septal defect. Central circulation and closure options.

ATRIAL SEPTAL DEFECT

Atrial septal defect (Fig. 4.13) is most frequently located in the area of the fossa ovalis; defects in this location have been termed ostium secundum type defect.

Less frequently, atrial septal defect is of the sinus venosus type when it is located immediately below the entrance of the superior vena cava into the right atrium. This type may be associated with partial anomalous pulmonary venous connection of the right upper pulmonary veins to the right atrium.

Atrial septal defect is distinguished from patent foramen ovale, a small opening or potential opening between the atria in the area of the fossa ovalis. In many infants and one-fourth of older patients, the foramen ovale does not anatomically seal and remains a potential communication. In conditions that raise left atrial pressure or increase left atrial volume, the foramen ovale may stretch open to the point of incompetence, resulting in a communication that permits flow of blood from the left atrium to the right atrium because of the higher pressure in the former. A right-to-left shunt may occur, particularly if right atrial pressure is elevated.

> Atrial septal defect is usually large and allows equalization of the atrial pressures. During diastole, pressure is equal in the atria and the ventricles so that the direction and the magnitude of the shunt depend only upon the relative compliances of the ventricles.

Ventricular compliance is determined by the thickness of the ventricular wall and the stiffness of the myocardium, which might be altered by fibrosis. Normally, the right ventricle is more compliant (i.e., more distensible than the left ventricle), since it is much thinner than the left ventricle. At any filling pressure, the right ventricle accepts a greater volume of blood than the left ventricle (Fig. 4.14).

In most patients with atrial septal defect, the relative ventricular compliances allow a left-to-right shunt through the defect so that the pulmonary blood flow is at least three times the systemic blood flow. Factors altering ventricular compliance affect the magnitude and the direction of the shunt. For example, myocardial fibrosis of the left ventricle, developing from coronary arterial disease, increases the left-to-right shunt. In contrast, right ventricular hypertrophy, as from pulmonary stenosis, reduces the volume of left-to-right shunt and, if significant, leads to a right-to-left shunt.

In atrial septal defect, the right-sided cardiac chambers and the pulmonary trunk are enlarged. The clinical features of atrial septal defect reflect the enlargement of these chambers and the augmented blood flow through the right-sided cardiac chambers and lungs. In patients with atrial septal defect, the pulmonary arterial pressure is usually normal during childhood.

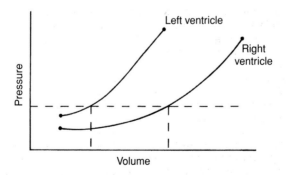

Figure 4.14 Schematic illustration of right and left ventricular compliance.

History

Several factors obtained in the history may be useful in diagnosing atrial septal defect.

Atrial septal defect of the ostium secundum type occurs two to three times more frequently in females.

Most children are asymptomatic and rarely develop congestive cardiac failure during infancy and childhood because the major hemodynamic abnormality, volume overload of the right ventricle, is well tolerated.

The right ventricle is crescent shaped and therefore has a large surface area for its resting volume. By altering its shape, the right ventricle can increase its volume without changing myocardial fiber length.

According to the Laplace law, $T = P \times r$, ventricular wall tension (T) varies directly with increasing pressure (P) and radius (r).

In the right ventricle, the pressure is relatively low and the radius is relatively large. Therefore, although the volume increases the radius, in comparison to the already large radius this increase adds relatively little to the level of tension required to maintain the pressure–volume relationship.

The right ventricle is better able to maintain its pressure–volume relationships as the volume increases than is the left ventricle.

On occasion, relatively asymptomatic neonates with atrial septal defect manifest cyanosis in the first week of life and then become acyanotic. The other condition that typically gives such a history is Ebstein's malformation of the tricuspid valve. The transient neonatal cyanosis indicates a right-to-left shunt at the atrial level. Right ventricular compliance in the neonate is decreased because the right ventricle is thick-walled, since before birth the right ventricle has developed systemic pressure. The right ventricular hypertrophy alters compliance (Fig. 4.14) and leads to a right-to-left shunt. As pulmonary resistance falls, right ventricular compliance and architecture change; so the shunt becomes left to right.

Typically, atrial septal defect is first recognized as late as the preschool physical examination because the murmur is soft and is mistaken for a functional murmur or is obscured during the examination of an active or fearful toddler.

Physical examination

The major cardiac findings are related to increased blood flow through the right side of the heart. Enlargement of the right ventricle may cause a precordial bulge.

The auscultatory features of atrial septal defect are usually diagnostic.

Accentuated first heart sound

Accentuated first heart sound is found in the tricuspid area.

A systolic ejection murmur

A systolic ejection murmur that results from turbulence due to the increased output of the right ventricle is located in the pulmonary area. The murmur varies from grade 1/6 to 3/6 and is rarely associated with a thrill. The systolic murmur of atrial septal defect resembles a functional pulmonary flow murmur but is distinguished by the characteristics of the second heart sound and the presence of a diastolic murmur.

Abnormalities of the second heart sound

Abnormalities of the second heart sound are important for diagnosis of atrial septal defect. Classically, wide, fixed splitting of the second heart sound is present.

Wide splitting. Wide splitting results from a marked delay of the pulmonic component because right ventricular ejection is prolonged, relative to the increased volume of blood that it must eject. Any condition in which the right ventricle ejects a larger quantity of blood has wide splitting.

Fixed splitting. Fixed splitting means that no variation occurs in the degree of splitting between inspiration and expiration. Fixed splitting indicates the presence of atrial communication. Because the degree of shunt is determined by the relative ventricular compliances, the relative volume of blood entering each ventricle is constant regardless of the total volume of blood entering the atria from the systemic and pulmonary veins. During inspiration an increased systemic venous return enters the total volume of blood in the atria, so during this phase of respiration, less blood flows left to right. During expiration, systemic venous return diminishes, yet the left-to-right shunt increases because pulmonary venous return is enhanced. But in each state the relative amount of blood entering each ventricle is constant, so duration of ejection for each ventricle is also constant.

> Fixed splitting of the second heart sound indicates an interatrial communication; it is present in any cardiac abnormality with an atrial communication. On occasion the murmur may be scarcely audible; but with fixed splitting of the second heart sound, one can make this clinical diagnosis.

A mid-diastolic murmur. A mid-diastolic murmur along the lower left and right sternal border is caused by increased blood flow across the tricuspid valve.

Electrocardiogram

Although the electrocardiogram may be normal in cases of atrial septal defect of the ostium secundum type, it usually reveals abnormalities.

The right atrium and right ventricle are anatomically enlarged in atrial septal defect and the electrocardiogram reflects these changes.
1. Right atrial enlargement
2. Right axis deviation, usually +120° to +150°
3. Right ventricular enlargement/hypertrophy
4. An rsR' pattern in lead V_1

The pattern of the QRS complex in lead V_1 is important in the diagnosis of atrial septal defect (Fig. 4.15). In 95% of patients with atrial septal defect, an rsR' pattern is present in lead V_1, with the R' being tall and broad. Lead V_6 shows a qRs pattern and a prominent and broad S wave. Diagnosing atrial septal defect is difficult in the absence of this electrocardiographic finding.

This particular QRS pattern has also been called incomplete right bundle branch block, but in this circumstance it reflects the increased right ventricular volume. No anatomic abnormality of the conduction system is present. An rSr' pattern may be found in lead V_1 of some normal children and in some children with other forms of congenital cardiac anomalies not associated with right ventricular enlargement, but the r' is neither tall nor broad.

A rule of thumb for electrocardiographic diagnosis of right ventricular enlargement is that the r' must be taller than the r and taller than 5 mm. This sign is less reliable in infants less than 2 months of age.

Chest X-ray

Chest X-ray reveals increased pulmonary vascularity and enlargement of the right side of the heart (Fig. 4.16). On the posteroanterior view, the pulmonary trunk is prominent, as is the right cardiac border (right atrium). On the lateral view, the right ventricle is enlarged. The left atrium is not enlarged since it is readily decompressed by the atrial communication. Therefore, the absence of displacement of the esophagus or other signs of left atrial enlargement in the presence of increased pulmonary blood flow indicates an atrial communication.

Summary of clinical findings. In atrial septal defect, the fixed splitting of the second heart sound indicates the presence of an atrial communication. The other findings—pulmonary ejection murmur, tricuspid diastolic murmur, rsR' on electrocardiogram, cardiomegaly, and increased pulmonary blood flow—each reflect the augmented volume of

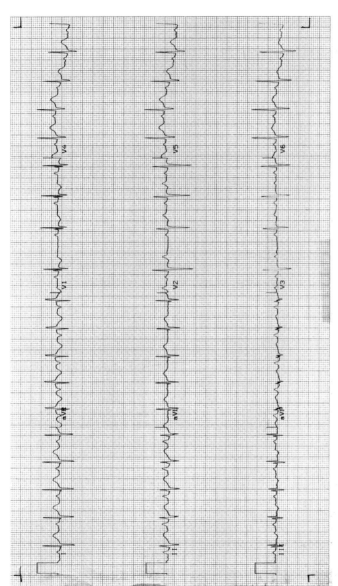

Figure 4.15 Electrocardiogram in atrial septal defect. Right atrial enlargement shown by tall P waves. rSR' pattern in lead V_1 indicates incomplete right bundle branch block. Right ventricular hypertrophy/enlargement manifested by large R' wave in lead V_1 and deep S wave in lead V_6.

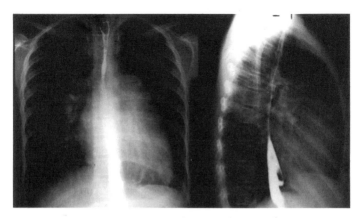

Figure 4.16 Chest X-ray in atrial septal defect. Left: Posteroanterior view. Cardiomegaly and increased pulmonary blood flow; enlarged pulmonary artery segment. Right: Lateral view. Enlargement of right ventricle indicated by obliteration of retrosternal space. As outlined by barium in the esophagus, left atrial enlargement is not present.

flow through the right side of the heart. In virtually all patients with an atrial septal defect, the flow through the right side of the heart is at least three times normal, and the pulmonary arterial pressure is normal. Thus, assessment of the severity of the condition is of less concern than in the case of most other forms of left-to-right shunts.

Natural history

Children with atrial septal defect rarely develop pulmonary arterial hypertension and usually remain asymptomatic. The lack of symptoms stems from the fact that excess pulmonary blood flow returning to the left atrium passes left to right across the atrial defect, the left ventricle does not receive excess blood flow, and therefore congestive heart failure does not develop as in ventricular septal defect. The excess volume load is carried entirely by the right ventricle, which because of its adaptable shape tolerates volume overload much better than the left ventricle. As long as pulmonary resistance remains normal, the right ventricular pressure is also normal. In adulthood the incidence of pulmonary vascular disease increases with each decade, although it rarely reaches the degree found in patients with ventricular septal defect or patent ductus arteriosus. Ultimately, pulmonary hypertension leads to right ventricular dysfunction, right heart failure, atrial arrhythmias, and development of right-to-left shunt. The average life span of those with untreated atrial septal defect is in the mid-50s.

One interesting observation in atrial septal defect is the rarity of infective endocarditis, probably because of the absence of jet lesions in this condition and the fact that no significant pressure gradient between the atria is found. Therefore, patients with atrial septal defect of the secundum type do not require prophylaxis for endocarditis.

Echocardiogram

An area of "dropout" can be seen within the atrial septum by 2D echocardiography. This is best seen when the transducer is placed over the epigastrium, a subcostal view that profiles the atrial septum and shows the fossa ovalis. Low-velocity left-atrium-to-right-atrium shunt is demonstrated by Doppler, reflecting the presence of similar atrial pressures.

Partial anomalous pulmonary venous connections of various types can occur in association with atrial septal defect in the region of the fossa ovalis and must be excluded using color Doppler. Sinus venosus atrial septal defects are separated from the true fossa ovalis by atrial septum; the defect appears close to the entrance of the superior vena cava into the right atrium. Partial anomalous pulmonary venous connection, frequently associated with sinus venosus atrial septal defect, consists of the right upper pulmonary vein joining the base of the superior vena cava at the right atrial junction and may be viewed by color Doppler.

The right atrium, right ventricle, and pulmonary arteries are all dilated in the presence of a large atrial septal defect, yet the left heart remains normal in size.

When "physiologic" tricuspid regurgitation and pulmonary valve insufficiency are present, the right ventricular and pulmonary artery pressures are measured as normal.

Echocardiography is useful in excluding possible associated anomalies like persistent left superior vena cava.

Cardiac catheterization

In most patients, cardiac catheterization is not performed as the diagnosis is easily made by other means. Catheterization is reserved to answer specific anatomic or hemodynamic questions, or to perform interventional closure of this defect. In most children with isolated fossa ovalis ("secundum") defects, cardiac catheterization is not indicated unless device closure is planned. Patients with suspected partial anomalous pulmonary venous connection, particularly those with a sinus venosus defect, may benefit from catheterization.

Cardiac catheterization reveals a large increase in oxygen saturation at the atrial level from the left-to-right shunt; this is maintained throughout the right side of the heart. In children, the pulmonary arterial pressure is usually normal. A pressure gradient of 10–20 mm Hg, caused by increased blood flow and not by an anatomic obstructive condition, may appear between the right ventricle and the pulmonary artery. The atrial pressures are equal, with left atrial pressure lower than normal. If contrast material is injected into the pulmonary artery, the pulmonary veins fill after 2 or 3 seconds. This means can be used to identify a coexistent anomalous pulmonary venous connection, although determination of the precise site of connection may be difficult since pulmonary overcirculation dilutes the pulmonary venous contrast.

Operative considerations

In most children with clinically recognizable atrial septal defect, the defect should be closed, either surgically, or by transcatheter (device) techniques.

Patients with an atrial septal defect and pulmonary blood flow less than twice normal may not require closure. The optimum age for closure is by approximately 5 years, since many fossa ovalis defects have either closed or narrowed sufficiently by then to preclude intervention, and spontaneous closure is unlikely after that age.

Surgical closure

Although the operation requires cardiopulmonary bypass, the operative risk is very low, and usually the hospital stay is brief. The most common short-term complication is postpericardiotomy syndrome. Few patients experience long-term complications.

Catheter-delivered devices

Formed from fabric with a support skeleton of metal and usually resembling umbrellas or double umbrellas linked in a dumbbell configuration, catheter-delivered devices have become a standard option for many children with fossa ovalis type atrial septal defects.

Current devices can be deployed via relatively small catheters yet the risk of vascular injury can be minimized by planning for closure after infancy; yet few infants have indications for closure, and many defects may narrow or close spontaneously after the first year.

Multiple defects or those defects which are not surrounded by a complete rim of atrial septum may not be suitable for closure with standard devices. Children with partial anomalous pulmonary venous return are not candidates for device closure and should have surgery. Transesophageal echocardiography at the time of catheterization is helpful in identifying children with these anatomic barriers to device closure.

Long-term safety and efficacy data suggest comparable results to surgical closure.

Summary. Atrial septal defect occurs more frequently in females, usually remains undiscovered until later in life than most forms of congenital heart disease, and rarely results in cardiac failure in the pediatric age range. Physical examination, electrocardiogram, chest X-ray, and echocardiography are usually sufficient to diagnose the condition in preparation for closure. Large atrial septal defects should be closed by operation or interventional catheterization during childhood to prevent complications in adulthood.

ENDOCARDIAL CUSHION DEFECT

Endocardial cushion defect (AV canal defect or AV septal defect) (Fig. 4.17) is a term encompassing a spectrum of cardiac malformations with a range of defects in the formation of the endocardial cushions. Developmentally, the endocardial cushions contribute to the lower portion of the atrial septum, the upper portion of the ventricular septum, and the mitral and tricuspid valves. Therefore, defective development of various portions of the endocardial cushions results in several types of malformations.

The defects classified in this group actually represent a spectrum of malformations. The simplest malformation, ostium primum defect or incomplete AV canal, consists of an atrial septal defect located low in the atrial septum, adjacent to the mitral valve annulus, which is often associated with a cleft in the anterior leaflet of the mitral valve leading to mitral insufficiency.

In other cases the ostium primum type of defect is continuous with a larger defect in the adjacent ventricular septum. In these instances the defect crosses both the mitral and tricuspid valvar annulae, causing deficiencies of the septal leaflets of both the tricuspid and mitral valves. This form of endocardial cushion defect is called complete AV canal.

Three major hemodynamic abnormalities are found.

The first is the volume overload on the right atrium and right ventricle and pulmonary overcirculation, as in patients with a left-to-right shunt at the atrial level. Even if the endocardial cushion defect involves portions of the ventricular septum, more of the shunt occurs above the level of the AV valves at the atrial level.

The second abnormality is mitral insufficiency, which leads to increased left ventricular volume because the left ventricle handles not only the normal cardiac output but also the regurgitated volume. In contrast to the usual patient with a mitral insufficiency, left atrial enlargement is not usually present because the left atrium is decompressed by the atrial septal communication.

The third abnormality relates to the varying degrees of pulmonary hypertension. Generally, the more deficient the ventricular septum is, the higher the level of pulmonary arterial pressure, even though little ventricular shunt may

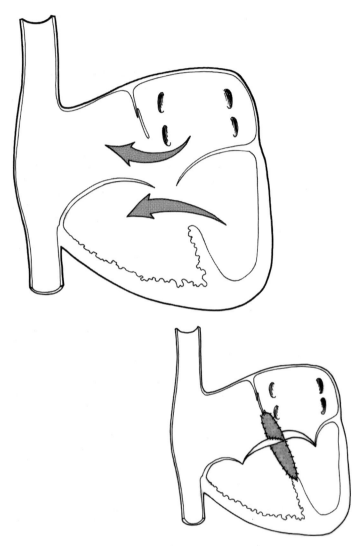

Figure 4.17 Endocardial cushion defect (atrioventricular canal defect or AV septal defect). Central circulation and surgical repair.

be found. The pulmonary hypertension is related to varying contributions of pulmonary vascular resistance and blood flow.

History
The histories of patients with endocardial cushion defect vary considerably. In general, symptoms appear earlier in patients with more extensive endocardial cushion defects and abnormalities of the mitral valve. Infants with the complete form of AV canal frequently develop congestive cardiac failure in the first few weeks or months of life, whereas patients with the ostium primum type of defect may be asymptomatic, as in the ostium secundum atrial septal defect.

When present, the symptoms are usually those related to congestive cardiac failure, poor growth, and frequent respiratory infections. Mild cyanosis may be related to right-to-left shunt from either the considerable pulmonary over-circulation with some intrapulmonary right-to-left shunting, the streaming of inferior vena caval blood through the defect, or the development of pulmonary vascular disease. Frequently, the murmur is heard early in life, even if the patient is asymptomatic.

Endocardial cushion defect is frequently found in association with Down syndrome (trisomy 21). Therefore, when evaluating a child with this particular trisomy and cardiac disease, the first diagnostic consideration is endocardial cushion defect.

Physical examination
The general appearance of the child may be normal, but infants with congestive cardiac failure may be scrawny, dyspneic, and tachypneic. In patients with cardiac enlargement, the precordium bulges and the cardiac apex are displaced toward the left and inferiorly.

The auscultatory findings vary, but characteristically they reflect mitral insufficiency and left-to-right shunt at the atrial level. In patients with ostium primum defect and cleft mitral valve, five findings may be present.

Apical holosystolic murmur of mitral insufficiency
This murmur radiates to the axilla and may be associated with a thrill. The absence of a murmur of mitral insufficiency does not preclude a cleft mitral valve.

Apical mid-diastolic murmur
This murmur is present in patients with larger amounts of mitral insufficiency.

Pulmonary systolic ejection murmur
This murmur is similar in characteristics and origin to the pulmonary flow murmur of atrial septal defect of the ostium secundum type.

Wide, fixed splitting of S$_2$

The second heart sound reveals these characteristic findings of an atrial communication. The pulmonic component of the second sound may be accentuated if associated pulmonary hypertension coexists.

Tricuspid diastolic murmur

Because of the left-to-right shunt at the atrial level, a large blood flow crosses the tricuspid valve.

Although these are the expected findings, a murmur of ventricular septal defect is found in some patients.

Surprisingly, a few patients with pulmonary vascular disease have minor murmurs, but the pulmonic component of the second heart sound is accentuated.

Electrocardiogram

The electrocardiogram in endocardial cushion defect is diagnostic (Fig. 4.18).

Five features are commonly observed:
(1) Left axis deviation. Left axis deviation is related to the abnormal position of the conduction system in the ventricle. The bundle of His displaced inferiorly by the septal defect enters along the posterior aspect of the ventricular septum. Ventricular depolarization proceeds inferiorly to superiorly and generally leftward. This leads to left axis deviation. The QRS axis may range from 0° to −150°; greater degrees of left axis deviation occur in patients with increasing degrees of right ventricular hypertrophy secondary to elevated pulmonary arterial pressure.
(2) Prolonged PR interval. Prolonged PR interval is probably related to the longer course of the bundle of His and the developmentally abnormal AV node.
(3) Atrial enlargement.
(4) Ventricular enlargement/hypertrophy. Often biventricular enlargement/hypertrophy is present; the left ventricular hypertrophy indicates excess volume in the left ventricle, and right ventricular enlargement/hypertrophy arises from combinations of excess right ventricular volume and increased pulmonary arterial pressure. Despite the abnormal ventricular conduction sequence, the precordial leads accurately predict ventricular hypertrophy.
(5) rSR′ pattern. rSR′ pattern is found in lead V$_1$ because of increased right ventricular volume.

The last three features reflect the cardiac hemodynamics and vary according to the relative volume and the pressure loads on the respective ventricles. They are

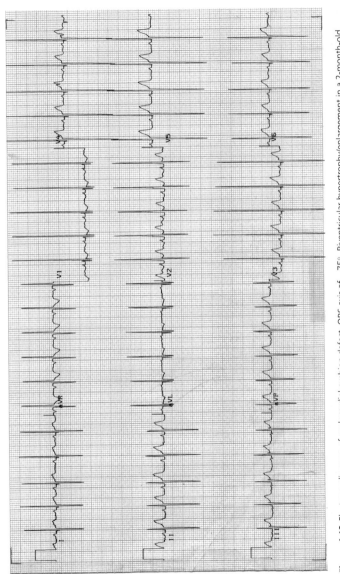

Figure 4.18 Electrocardiogram of endocardial cushion defect. QRS axis of −75°. Biventricular hypertrophy/enlargement in a 2-month-old infant. rSR' pattern in lead V_1.

therefore helpful in assessing the hemodynamic characteristics of the particular defect.

Chest X-ray

In addition to the increase in pulmonary vascularity, varying degrees of cardiomegaly are observed. Cardiac size increases because of the left-to-right shunt and also because of the mitral insufficiency with its resultant left ventricular enlargement. As a result of the mitral insufficiency, the heart is often enlarged out of proportion to the increased pulmonary vascular markings (Fig. 4.19). Left atrial enlargement may be present, although it is not as prominent as that observed in ventricular septal defect with a shunt of comparable magnitude. The right-sided cardiac chambers are also enlarged.

> Summary of clinical findings. Although the clinical and laboratory findings vary considerably, the electrocardiographic features are most diagnostic for endocardial cushion defect. The auscultatory, electrocardiographic, and chest X-ray findings reflect the three potential hemodynamic

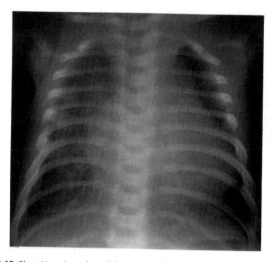

Figure 4.19 Chest X-ray in endocardial cushion defect. Cardiomegaly and increased pulmonary vasculature.

abnormalities: mitral insufficiency, pulmonary hypertension, and left-to-right shunt at the atrial level.

Natural history

Patients with complete endocardial cushion defect develop intractable cardiac failure in infancy and present a difficult management problem. They also develop pulmonary vascular disease during childhood. Patients with an ostium primum defect and mild mitral insufficiency are asymptomatic into adulthood, although pulmonary vascular disease may develop or mitral valve insufficiency may progressively worsen.

Echocardiogram

The 2D echocardiogram is easily interpreted in complete endocardial cushion defect: a four-chamber or apical view demonstrates AV valves with a large common central leaflet that spans the large "dropout" in both atrial and ventricular septa. The degree of AV valve regurgitation can be judged using color Doppler, and associated lesions, such as persistent left superior vena cava or patent ductus arteriosus, can be ruled out.

Partial forms of AV canal defect may show two apparently discrete AV valve rings without the normal "offset" in the septal leaflets of the AV valves created by the slightly more apical position of the tricuspid annulus that is seen in normal patients. Partial canal defects vary in severity from patients with a very large "primum" atrial septal defects to mildly affected children, whose only apparent abnormality is a cleft within the leaflet of the mitral valve, which may produce mitral regurgitation.

In endocardial cushion defect with pulmonary overcirculation, the left atrium and left ventricle do not appear dilated unless the patient also has considerable mitral regurgitation.

Cardiac catheterization

This is not always performed if the anatomy and physiology can be clearly illustrated by echocardiogram. A large increase in oxygen saturation is found at the atrial level. Occasionally, an additional increase is found at the ventricular level, but the atrial increase is so large that it obscures the ventricular component of the shunt. Slight right-to-left shunt may be detectable, either at the atrial level or at the intrapulmonary level (because of pulmonary overcirculation and edema). A large right-to-left shunt suggests pulmonary resistance greater than systemic resistance or an associated defect (e.g., a communication between the coronary sinus and left atrium). The pulmonary arterial pressure ranges from normal to systemic levels, the latter suggesting a complete AV canal.

Left ventriculography reveals a characteristic abnormality of the left ventricle termed gooseneck deformity. The medial border of the left ventricle, when viewed on an anteroposterior film, appears scooped out because of the lower margin of the endocardial cushion defect and the presence of abnormal chordal attachment to the septum. Mitral insufficiency is also demonstrated by the study. In a left anterior oblique projection or four-chamber view of a left ventriculogram, the common atrioventricular valve can be outlined.

Operative considerations

In patients with an ostium primum type of defect and a cleft mitral valve who are asymptomatic or who have few symptoms, operation can be delayed and can be performed at a low risk. The defect is closed; and the cleft of the mitral valve is sutured, which may greatly reduce the degree of mitral insufficiency.

In patients with complete AV canal, corrective operation can be indicated in very young symptomatic infants who often respond poorly to medical management. The authors routinely send infants such as these for operation at 2–3 months of age. The risk of pulmonary vascular disease developing within the first 6–9 months of life is high, especially in Down syndrome.

The operative results are good in almost all, although some infants have such deficient anatomy of the mitral valve that prosthetic replacement of the mitral valve is required. Surgically induced AV block is uncommon but is more likely with this lesion than in closure of perimembranous ventricular septal defect. Banding of the pulmonary artery is beneficial in a few instances, especially for patients with greatly unbalanced ventricular or AV valve size.

Summary. Endocardial cushion defect encompasses a group of anomalies involving specific portions of the atrial and ventricular septa and adjacent AV valves. The clinical and laboratory findings reflect the atrial left-to-right shunt and the mitral regurgitation. The electrocardiogram showing left axis deviation, atrial and ventricular hypertrophy, and incomplete right bundle branch block is quite diagnostic. X-ray studies reveal enlargement of each cardiac chamber. The anatomic details of the anomaly are clearly identified by echocardiography. The anatomic features of the defect complicate operative correction.

Table 4.1 Summary of Defects with Acyanosis and Increased Pulmonary Blood Flow (Left-to-Right Shunt).

Malformation	Gender Prevalence	Major Associated Syndrome	Congestive Cardiac Failure	Age Murmur First Heard	Pulse Pressure	Thrill	Murmur	Degree Splitting of S_2
			History				Physical Examination	
Atrial septal defect	F > M	Holt-Oram	Rare	5 years	Normal	Rare	Grade I–III systolic ejection murmur, pulmonary area; Tricuspid mid-diastolic rumble	Fixed, wide splitting
Ventricular septal defect	M > F	Trisomy 21, 13, 18	± Onset 1–2 mo	6 wks	Normal	Precordial	Grade IV harsh holosystolic, left sternal border; Mitral mid-diastolic rumble	Normal
Patent ductus arteriosus	F > M	Low birth weight Rubella	± Onset 1–2 mo	Infancy	Wide	Upper precordial (±); SSN (±)	Continuous (older) or systolic ejection (neonate); Apical mid-diastolic rumble	Normal
Endocardial cushion defect	F = M	Trisomy 21	± Onset 1–2 mo	Infancy	Normal	Apical (±)	Grade I–IV apical holosystolic murmur; Systolic ejection murmur, pulmonary area; Mid-diastolic rumble	Fixed, wide splitting

continued

Table 4.1 (*Cont.*)

		Electrocardiogram			Chest X-ray	
Malformation	Axis (QRS)	Atrial Enlargement	Ventricular Hypertrophy/ Enlargement	Other	Left Atrial Enlargement	Aortic Enlargement
Atrial septal defect	Normal or right	None or right	Right	Incomplete RBBB (RSR' in V₁)	Absent	Absent
Ventricular septal defect	Normal or right	None or left	None (small defect); Left (medium defect); Biventricular (large defect); Right (high R_P)		Present	Absent
Patent ductus arteriosus	Normal	None or left	None (small defect); Left (medium defect); Biventricular (large defect); Right (high R_P)		Present	Present
Endocardial cushion defect	Left	Right, left or both	Biventricular	Incomplete RBBB (RSR' in V₁) First-degree heart block	Present	Absent

F, female; M, male; mo, months; RBBB, right bundle branch block; R_P, pulmonary vascular resistance; S_2, second heart sound; SSN, suprasternal notch; wks, weeks; ± may be present or absent.

SUMMARY OF LEFT-TO-RIGHT SHUNTS

Certain generalizations can be made concerning the cardiac conditions with left-to-right shunts that aid in understanding their hemodynamics and that can be applied to other lesions, such as those with admixture.

Shunts occurring distal to the mitral valve have certain general characteristics. The flow through the defect depends upon either the size of the defect or the relative resistances of the pulmonary and systemic vascular systems. Therefore, systolic events influence the shunt primarily. Volume load is placed upon the left side of the heart and can lead to congestive cardiac failure. Left atrial enlargement, apical diastolic murmur, and left ventricular hypertrophy are other manifestations of the excess volume in the left side of the heart.

Shunts occurring proximal to the mitral valve have other characteristics. The shunt depends upon the relative compliance of the ventricles and therefore is influenced predominantly by diastolic events. Congestive heart failure is uncommon in uncomplicated cardiac anomalies because the volume load is placed on the right ventricle. Left atrial enlargement is absent. The electrocardiogram shows a pattern of right ventricular volume overload, and a tricuspid diastolic murmur may be present.

The features and classic findings of the four major acyanotic conditions associated with increased pulmonary blood flow are presented in Table 4.1.

Chapter 5
Obstructive lesions

Although conditions leading to obstruction of blood flow from the heart are common in children, those causing inflow obstruction, such as mitral stenosis, are rare in comparison. In this chapter therefore, the emphasis will be upon aortic stenosis, pulmonary stenosis, and coarctation of the aorta.

> Each of these obstructive conditions has two major effects upon the circulation:
> (1) Blood flow through the obstruction is turbulent, leading to a systolic ejection murmur and dilation of the great vessel beyond the obstruction and
> (2) Systolic pressure is elevated proximal to the obstruction, leading to myocardial hypertrophy proportional to the degree of obstruction.

Pediatric Cardiology, by W Johnson, J Moller © 2008 Blackwell Publishing,
ISBN: 978-1-4051-7818-1.

The severity of obstruction varies considerably among patients. The smaller the orifice size of the obstruction, the greater the level of pressure required to send the cardiac output past the obstruction. This principle is represented by the following equation:

$$\text{Orifice size} = \text{Constant} \times \frac{\text{Cardiac output}}{\sqrt{\text{Pressure difference across obstruction}}}$$

> The primary response to the obstruction is myocardial hypertrophy, not ventricular dilation.

During childhood the heart usually maintains the elevated ventricular systolic pressure without dilation; however, eventually ventricular enlargement may develop because of the development of myocardial fibrosis. Such fibrotic changes in the ventricle occur because of an imbalance between the myocardial oxygen demands and the available supply. In most children, coronary arterial blood flow is normal, but with ventricular hypertrophy, myocardial oxygen requirements are increased.

Myocardial oxygen requirements are largely devoted to the development of myocardial tension and therefore are related directly to the level of ventricular systolic pressure and the number of times per minute the heart must develop that level of pressure. Thus, elevated ventricular systolic pressure and tachycardia can increase myocardial oxygen consumption considerably.

When a patient with an obstructive lesion exercises, severe increases in myocardial oxygen requirements occur for two reasons: (1) During exercise, cardiac output increases; so according to the relationship shown earlier, ventricular systolic pressure also increases. (2) With exercise, the heart rate increases.

If these increased myocardial oxygen requirements cannot be met, myocardial ischemia occurs and ultimately can lead to myocardial fibrosis. These myocardial changes occur over a period of time and can lead to signs and symptoms. With the development of sufficient fibrosis, the contractile properties of the ventricle are affected so that ventricular dilation and cardiac enlargement develop.

As a group, the obstructive conditions are associated with normal pulmonary vascularity because the cardiac output from both sides of the heart is normal and there is no intracardiac shunt.

Children with obstructive lesions usually show few symptoms, but severe degrees of obstruction lead to congestive cardiac failure in infancy.

COARCTATION OF THE AORTA

Coarctation of the aorta (Fig. 5.1) is a narrowing of the descending aorta that occurs opposite the site of the ductus arteriosus.

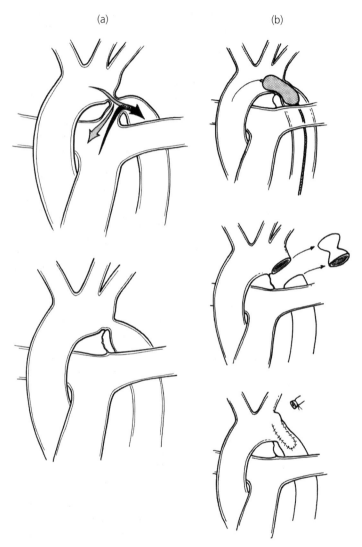

Figure 5.1 Coarctation of aorta. (a) Central circulation before and after ductal closure and (b) repair options.

Aortic coarctation has traditionally been defined by its relationship to the ductus arteriosus, whether patent or ligamentous. This relationship has been described as either preductal or postductal. However, virtually all coarctations of the aorta are located juxtaductal (i.e., occurring in the wall of the aorta opposite the ductus arteriosus).

Coarctation may occur either as a localized constriction of the aorta or as tubular hypoplasia of the aortic arch and proximal descending aorta. In general, patients with tubular hypoplasia of the aortic arch develop cardiac failure in infancy. The coarctation in older children is usually discrete and is located distal to the origin of the left subclavian artery. Preoperative treatment and correction depend more on the associated lesions, such as arch hypoplasia, than on the precise relationship of ductus to aortic narrowing.

The descending aorta beyond the coarctation usually shows poststenotic dilation. At least 50% of patients have a coexistent bicuspid aortic valve.

Coarctation of the aorta offers mechanical obstruction to blood flow from the left ventricle. The pressure proximal to the coarctation is elevated, whereas that beyond the obstruction is either normal or lower than normal; this blood pressure difference is the major diagnostic feature of this condition. In response to the pressure difference between the proximal and distal compartments of the aorta, collateral arterial vessels develop between the high-pressure ascending and the low-pressure descending aorta.

Collateral vessels develop in any vascular system when a pressure difference exists. These vessels represent enlargement of naturally occurring small arteries bridging the high- and low-pressure components. Blood flows through these bridging vessels, and the volume of flow slowly increases, leading to the eventual dilation of the vessels. The internal mammary and intercostal arteries are the most frequently occurring collateral vessels in coarctation of the aorta.

Left ventricular hypertrophy develops in response to the elevated systolic pressure proximal to the coarctation.

History

Although most children with coarctation of the aorta are asymptomatic throughout childhood, 10% develop congestive cardiac failure during the neonatal period or early infancy. In the latter group, recognition of the lesion is important because proper management can be lifesaving.

Older children rarely develop congestive cardiac failure; instead they have complaints, such as headaches, related to the systemic hypertension in the upper portion of the body. The very common childhood and adolescent symptom of chest pain, benign in most youngsters, occurs occasionally in coarctation patients and may be an ominous sign of myocardial ischemia secondary to severe left ventricular hypertrophy.

Coarctation of the aorta predominates in males at a ratio of 1.5–1. When coarctation of the aorta occurs in a female, consider Turner syndrome and perform chromosome analysis when appropriate. Some Turner syndrome patients exhibit very subtle findings and often escape clinical detection.

If coarctation of the aorta does not lead to congestive cardiac failure, the condition is often unrecognized until preschool age, when the murmur is heard, or at a later age, when hypertension is detected.

Physical examination

Most patients show normal growth and development; many have an athletic physique. In neonates or infants, the signs of congestive cardiac failure may be present and profound. Mild degrees of acrocyanosis and mottling of the skin may be present because of pulmonary edema and poor perfusion, but these signs are common in healthy children.

Clinical diagnosis of coarctation of the aorta rests on the recognition of a blood pressure differential between the upper and lower extremities. This information may be gathered by palpation of both the radial and the femoral arteries. If a substantial difference between the two is found, one should suspect coarctation of the aorta.

In addition, finding very sharp and brisk radial pulses in infants should lead one to consider the diagnosis of coarctation of the aorta; radial pulses are ordinarily difficult to palpate in this age group.

Regardless of whether the femoral pulses feel diminished or not, the blood pressure should be taken in both arms and a leg in any child with a cardiac murmur. Many cases of coarctation of the aorta have been missed because the "femoral arteries were palpable."

The blood pressure may be obtained by the flush method, by direct auscultatory means, or with the aid of automated devices (see Chapter 1). Blood pressure cuffs of appropriate width must be used. The largest cuff that fits the extremity should be used. In a patient without cardiac disease, the blood pressure should be the same in the upper and lower extremities. If the blood pressure is higher in the arms than in the legs by 20 mm Hg or more, this difference is considered significant and may be the diagnostic indicator of coarctation of the aorta. The use of an inadequate-size leg cuff can artifactually increase the leg pressures, leading to failure to detect a significant systolic pressure difference when one exists.

In infants with congestive cardiac failure secondary to severe coarctation of the aorta, the blood pressure values may be similar in the arms and legs, but at extremely low levels at both sites, because cardiac output is so reduced. Following stabilization of such infants however, the pressure difference between the upper and lower extremities usually becomes apparent.

An open ductus, either native or one due to pharmacotherapy with prostaglandin, will palliate a neonate with coarctation and will equalize upper- and lower-extremity pulses because the aortic end of the ductus provides a bypass around the coarctation.

The examination of the heart may reveal cardiac enlargement. Palpation in the suprasternal notch reveals a prominent aortic pulsation and perhaps a thrill in patients with a coexistent bicuspid aortic valve. An ejection-type murmur is present along the sternal border, at the apex, and over the back between the left scapulae and the spine in the fourth interspace. The murmur is generally grade 2/6–3/6.

> It is rare for a patient with coarctation not to have a murmur over the left back along the spine. This is a valuable diagnostic clue.

An aortic systolic ejection click is often heard, indicating dilation of the ascending aorta from the coexistent bicuspid aortic valve. The aortic component of the second heart sound may be increased in loudness. In the infant with congestive cardiac failure, auscultatory findings may be muffled until after pharmacologic support to improve cardiac performance.

Electrocardiogram
The electrocardiographic findings vary with the age of the patient.

Neonate
In the neonatal and early infancy periods, the electrocardiogram usually reveals right ventricular hypertrophy.

Several explanations have been offered for this seemingly paradoxical finding. If the ductus arteriosus remains patent, the right ventricle, because of its communication through the pulmonary artery and ductus arteriosus, continues working against the resistance imposed by the systemic circulation. In other patients with coarctation of the aorta and patent ductus arteriosus, the left ventricle is hypoplastic, so the electrocardiogram shows a pattern of right ventricular hypertrophy. Right ventricular hypertrophy has also been explained by the development of pulmonary hypertension secondary to left ventricular failure. The load placed on the fetal right ventricle, normally about 60% of the combined output from both fetal ventricles, may increase because less blood is able to traverse the left ventricle and to pass through the narrowed aortic isthmus.

> Regardless of its origin, the typical pattern of coarctation of the aorta in a symptomatic infant is right ventricular hypertrophy and inverted T waves in the left precordial leads.

Subsequently, the electrocardiogram shifts to a pattern of left ventricular hypertrophy.

Older infants
In older infants with severe coarctation of the aorta or in those with coexistent aortic outflow obstruction and endocardial fibroelastosis (representing subendocardial scarring) of the left ventricle, a pattern of left ventricular hypertrophy, inverted T waves, and ST depression in the left precordial leads is present. These ventricular repolarization abnormalities are often signs of a poor prognosis.

Older patient
In the older patient with coarctation of the aorta, the precordial leads show either left ventricular hypertrophy or a normal pattern.

Chest X-ray
In symptomatic infants, significant cardiac enlargement is present, with the cardiomegaly consisting primarily of left ventricular and left atrial enlargement. The lung fields show a diffuse reticular pattern of pulmonary edema and pulmonary venous congestion.

In older children cardiac size and pulmonary vasculature are normal.

The roentgenographic appearance of the descending aorta is often diagnostic of coarctation of the aorta by showing poststenotic dilation. The barium swallow shows an E sign. The upper portion of the E is formed by the segment of the aorta proximal to the coarctation, and the lower portion of the E is formed by the deviation of the barium from the poststenotic dilation. On plain chest X-rays, often the left side of the thoracic aorta shows soft-tissue densities in the form of the number 3 that mirror the barium sign. The upper portion of the 3 sign represents the aortic knob, and the lower portion represents the poststenotic dilation. These findings help identify the extent of the coarctation.

The ascending aorta may be prominent if a bicuspid aortic valve coexists.

Rib notching (Fig. 5.2) may be apparent in older children and adolescents, but its absence does not rule out the diagnosis of coarctation. The inferior margins of the upper ribs show scalloping caused by pressure from enlarged intercostal arteries that are serving as collaterals.

Summary of clinical findings. Whether the patient is an infant in congestive cardiac failure or is asymptomatic, the clinical diagnosis rests upon the demonstration of a blood pressure difference between the arms and leg. Other findings, such as those on the electrocardiogram and chest X-ray, reflect the severity of the condition. Prominence of the ascending aorta on chest X-ray and an apical systolic ejection click indicate a coexistent bicuspid aortic valve.

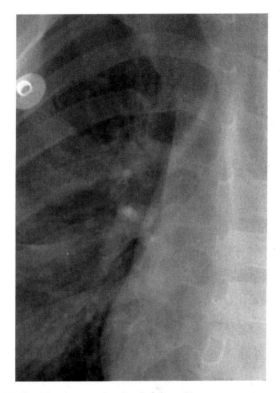

Figure 5.2 Chest X-ray in coarctation. Detail of rib notching.

Echocardiogram

Cross-sectional images of the aortic arch, usually best obtained with the transducer positioned near the suprasternal notch, reveal narrowing at the site of coarctation and, in some patients, relative hypoplasia of the transverse segment of the aortic arch, extending from the ascending aorta to the coarctation. The proximal thoracic descending aorta just distal to the coarctation may be normal in size or may be slightly dilated, representing poststenotic dilation.

Color Doppler shows a disturbed (turbulent) signal at the stenosis, and spectral Doppler shows high-velocity flow from the transverse aortic arch to the descending aorta with a continuous pattern (extending from systole into diastole).

In neonates, the diagnosis may be difficult as long as the ductus arteriosus remains large. The flow through a ductus in a neonate with coarctation is bidirectional, often predominantly right to left (pulmonary artery to aorta), which is an important echocardiographic clue to the diagnosis.

The echocardiogram provides rapid assessment of left ventricular hypertrophy, size, and function and also allows diagnosis of possible associated lesions, such as bicuspid aortic valve, mitral valve malformations, and ventricular septal defect.

Cardiac catheterization and angiography

Usually, the clinical findings and echocardiogram are sufficient to diagnose coarctation of the aorta, so diagnostic catheterization and angiography are unnecessary, unless performed in conjunction with balloon dilation.

Oximetry data are usually normal, except in neonates with a large ductus. Pressure measurements demonstrate systolic hypertension proximal to the coarctation and a gradient at the site of the coarctation, often dramatically shown by pullback of the catheter across the lesion during pressure recording.

Treatment
Medical management prior to gradient relief

Infants with a coarctation of the aorta who develop congestive cardiac failure usually respond to medical management within a few hours and then undergo successful repair. Infants who fail to respond promptly to medical management or to reopening of the ductus with prostaglandin may require emergency repair. The operative risk is higher in this group.

Assessment in preparation for gradient relief

To make operative decisions, one must know the exact location of the coarctation of the aorta. This is done by integrating information from the physical examination, and by directly imaging the lesion by echocardiography, angiography/arteriography, MRI/MRA, or CTA.

The distal extent of the coarctation can be recognized by the roentgenographic identification of poststenotic dilation, and the proximal extent, by the blood pressure in the two arms. Usually, the recordings are similar in both arms, indicating that the coarctation is located distal to the left subclavian artery. Occasionally, the blood pressure of the left arm is lower than that of the right arm, indicating that the coarctation of the aorta involves the origin of the left subclavian artery and therefore a longer segment of the aorta.

Echocardiographic images are often limited by the size of older patients. MRI/MRA or CTA are particularly useful imaging techniques in adolescents and adults with coarctation, since the coarcted segment of aorta has little motion throughout the cardiac cycle.

In an infant in cardiac failure, the diagnosis may be difficult, in which case aortography, MRI/MRA, or CTA may be helpful.

Surgery

Two major types of operation for coarctation are widely used.

Excision and end-to-end anastomosis. A discrete coarctation can be excised the two ends of the aorta reanastomosed. An elliptical incision is made to minimize narrowing that may accompany growth of the patient and/or shrinkage of the anastomotic scar.

Subclavian flap repair. In patients with a very hypoplastic aorta or long-segment stenosis, the repair site can be augmented by transecting the left subclavian artery distally and opening it linearly to create a flap of living tissue. Early attempts to augment the arch repair with synthetic or pericardial patch material often led to late aneurysm formation.

Although long-term surgical results are very good, no operative technique is free from the risk of late restenosis.

Operation should be performed on most patients with coarctation of the aorta when the defect is diagnosed, except perhaps in a small premature infant who can often be palliated with prostaglandin infusion and allowed to grow to near-term weight. Doing this improves the efficacy of repair and minimizes the risk of late restenosis. The operative mortality risk is low (less than 1 in 400) in patients with an uncomplicated coarctation.

Infants with severe associated anomalies, such as a very large ventricular septal defect, small left ventricular outflow tract, and associated left ventricular failure from volume and pressure overload, may benefit from a staged repair, with repair of coarctation and pulmonary artery banding first, which often leads to rapid improvement in the left ventricular dysfunction and eventual growth of the outflow tract. Several weeks or months later, debanding of the pulmonary artery and closure of the ventricular septal defect follow. The operative mortality for one-stage neonatal repair of such infants can be higher than that of a staged approach.

Interventional catheterization

Balloon dilation of coarctation at the time of cardiac catheterization has been successfully employed for native (previously unoperated) coarctation and for postoperative restenosis.

In postoperative restenosis, the results of gradient relief are good; and the risk of balloon dilation is low, possibly due to the external buttressing of the dilated region by the old operative scar. In this same group of patients, reoperation for restenosis carries increased risk in comparison to balloon dilation, partly because of the same scarring, which must be dissected to achieve exposure.

Balloon dilation of native coarctation avoids some operative disadvantages but, compared with operative repair, it appears to involve a greater chance of immediate complications like extravasation and increased risk of late complications like aneurysm and restenosis. The age and size of the patient at the time of balloon dilation influence the risks and long-term outcomes: younger and smaller patients have higher risk.

Implantation of a metallic stent at the time of balloon dilation may lessen the risk of aneurysm formation but in small patients, the stents do not allow for growth, thus, repeat balloon dilation of the stented region is usually needed.

Natural history

The anastomotic site following coarctation repair may not grow in proportion to the growth of the aortic diameter. Therefore recoarctation may develop, often necessitating a second operation when the patient is older. This need occurs more frequently among children with a very hypoplastic aorta who were operated upon in infancy. Follow-up of all operated patients includes periodic determination of blood pressure in both the upper and lower extremities.

Since half of the patients with coarctation of the aorta have a bicuspid aortic valve, they are at some increased risk for development of endocarditis compared to persons with a normal aortic valve. The long-term course of patients with bicuspid aortic valve is variable as the valve may become slowly insufficient or stenotic with age, and at a future time they may require valvar surgery.

Following operation, some patients have persistent hypertension in both the arms and the legs. The reasons are not well understood, but it does not seem related to elevated levels of renin and angiotensin. Abnormal reactivity has been demonstrated in the systemic vascular bed of well-repaired coarctation patients. Some repaired patients who have normal blood pressure at rest have an exaggerated hypertensive response to exercise. This hypertension requires management. Delay in diagnosis and corrective surgery until an older age in childhood increases the risk of permanent systemic hypertension.

Summary. Coarctation of the aorta is usually an easily diagnosed condition. In most patients it requires treatment, as it can lead to several problems: congestive cardiac failure, hypertension, and left ventricular dysfunction. In most patients, either operation or balloon dilation is used to relieve the obstruction. Despite the apparent anatomic success of intervention, recoarctation, persistent hypertension, and a coexistent bicuspid aortic valve are long-term problems following successful gradient relief.

AORTIC STENOSIS

Aortic stenosis can occur at one of three anatomic locations (Fig. 5.3). Most frequently, aortic stenosis is caused by a stenotic congenital bicuspid or unicuspid valve. Obstruction to left ventricular outflow may also occur below the aortic valve, either as an isolated fibrous ring (discrete membranous subaortic stenosis) or as septal hypertrophy (idiopathic hypertrophic subaortic stenosis [i.e., hypertrophic cardiomyopathy]) (see Chapter 9). Rarely, aortic stenosis is located in the proximal ascending aorta (supravalvar aortic stenosis).

Regardless of the site of obstruction, the effect upon the left ventricle is similar. Because of the stenosis, the left ventricular systolic pressure rises to maintain a normal cardiac output.

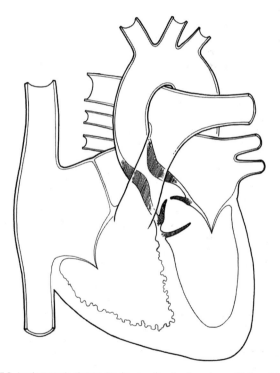

Figure 5.3 Aortic stenosis. Composite drawing showing three types of left ventricular outflow obstruction: subvalvar (fibromuscular ridge or membrane), valvar, and supravalvar aortic stenosis.

This relationship can be illustrated by the formula used to calculate the severity of valvar aortic stenosis:

$$AVA = \frac{AVF}{K\sqrt{LV - AO}},$$

where AVA is aortic valve area (area of stenotic orifice; cm^2); AVF is aortic valve flow (blood flow occurring during the systolic ejection period; mL/s); LV is mean left ventricular pressure during ejection (mm Hg); AO is mean aortic pressure during ejection (mm Hg); and K is a constant.

This equation uses data obtained at catheterization, specifically the mean pressure difference between the left ventricle and aorta, to essentially derive velocities.

The aortic valve area may also be calculated by Doppler echocardiography in a more direct fashion, since velocity is directly measured.

The mean velocities both proximal and distal to the aortic valve are measured by integrating the area under the respective Doppler curves (the velocity time integral, or VTI).

By measuring the diameter of the left ventricular outflow tract the cross-sectional area proximal to the stenosis can be easily calculated.

Volume (V) in cm^3 can be found when the VTI (in cm) is multiplied by area (in cm^2).

As flow (volume/time) is the same through the normal left ventricular outflow tract as via the stenotic aortic valve, in the same amount of time, one systolic ejection period, the following formula can be derived:

$$AVA = \frac{(\pi d^2 / 4) \times VTI_{LVOT}}{VTI_{Ao}},$$

where AVA is aortic valve area (cm^2); d is left ventricular outflow tract diameter (cm); VTI_{LVOT} is velocity time integral of the left ventricular outflow tract flow, mean velocity (cm); and VTI_{Ao} is velocity time integral of the aortic valve flow, mean velocity (cm).

In practice, the Doppler maximum velocities in the left ventricular outflow tract and in the aorta are sometimes substituted for the mean velocities.

In patients with more severe aortic stenosis (smaller aortic valve area) for a given cardiac output (CO), left ventricular systolic pressure is higher. Similarly, when the patient exercises, since the aortic valve area is fixed, as the cardiac output rises, the left ventricular systolic pressure increases as a squared function (Fig. 5.4).

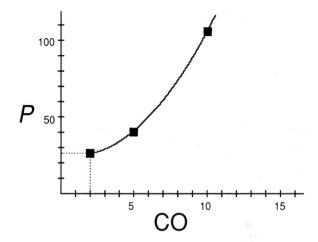

Figure 5.4 Effect of exercise on the gradient in aortic stenosis. Hypothetical values are shown. At rest, cardiac output is 2 L/min, and the systolic gradient is 25 mm Hg. Two levels of exercise are shown. At moderate exercise, cardiac output is 5 L/min, and the gradient is 40 mm Hg; but at maximal exercise, the cardiac output is 10 L/min, and the gradient exceeds 100 mm Hg. (Abbreviations: P, pressure; CO, cardiac output.)

The primary effect upon the heart of each type of aortic stenosis is elevation of left ventricular systolic pressure, resulting in left ventricular hypertrophy. Many of the clinical and laboratory features of aortic stenosis are related to the left ventricular hypertrophy and its effects. Because of the elevated left ventricular systolic pressure, the myocardial oxygen demands are increased. During exercise the oxygen demands are further increased because both heart rate and left ventricular systolic pressure increase. If these oxygen needs are unmet, myocardial ischemia may occur and lead to syncope, chest pain, or electrocardiogram changes. Recurrent myocardial ischemic episodes can lead to left ventricular fibrosis, which can ultimately progress to cardiac failure and cardiomegaly.

Other clinical features of aortic stenosis are related to the turbulence of blood flow through the stenotic area, manifested by a systolic ejection murmur, and in valvar aortic stenosis, by poststenotic dilation of the ascending aorta.

Aortic valvar stenosis

Aortic valvar stenosis is related to either a unicuspid valve (most often presenting in infants) or a congenitally bicuspid valve (usually presenting in older children and adults; Fig. 5.3). The orifices of these abnormal valves are narrowed, accompanied by various degrees of aortic insufficiency in some patients.

History

Aortic stenosis is commonly associated with a significant murmur at birth. In most other congenital cardiac conditions, the murmur is often first recognized later in infancy or childhood. Aortic stenosis occurs three times more frequently in males.

Patients with aortic stenosis are usually asymptomatic throughout childhood, even when stenosis is severe. Only 5% of children with aortic stenosis develop congestive cardiac failure in the neonatal period, but it can develop later in childhood in patients who do not receive gradient-relief. Exercise intolerance may occur so gradually that it is unnoticed by parents and teachers. Some asymptomatic children, as they approach adolescence, may develop episodes of chest pain that have the characteristics of angina. These episodes signify myocardial ischemia and may precede sudden death.

Syncope is another serious symptom of patients with aortic stenosis and may occur upon exercise. This symptom has also been associated with sudden death.

Physical examination

Several clinical findings suggest the diagnosis of aortic valvar stenosis. With severe stenotic lesions the pulse pressure is narrow and the peripheral pulses feel weak; but in most patients the pulses are normal. A thrill may be present in the aortic area along the upper right sternal border and in the suprasternal notch.

The aortic systolic ejection murmur that is present begins after the first heart sound and extends to the aortic component of the second sound. In older children the murmur is located in the aortic area, but in infancy it is most prominent along the left sternal border; because of its location it may be confused with the murmur of ventricular septal defect. The murmur of aortic stenosis characteristically transmits into the carotid arteries. However, in normal children a functional systolic carotid arterial bruit may be heard; therefore a murmur in the neck does not, by itself, prove the diagnosis of aortic valvar stenosis.

The murmur usually follows a systolic ejection click that reflects poststenotic dilation of the aorta. Aortic ejection clicks are heard best at the apex of the heart when the patient is reclining and may also be heard over the left lower back. The click is generally present in milder degrees of aortic stenosis but may be absent in patients with severe stenosis.

In about 30% of children with aortic stenosis, a soft, early diastolic murmur of aortic insufficiency is heard along the mid-left sternal border.

Electrocardiogram

The electrocardiogram (Fig. 5.5) generally reveals a normal axis; but in a few patients left axis deviation, suggesting severe left ventricular hypertrophy, is observed. Occasionally in infants and less frequently in older children, left atrial enlargement occurs. The prominent findings are those of left ventricular hypertrophy, usually manifested by deep S waves in lead V_1 and normal or tall R waves in lead V_6.

Attention should be directed to changes in the ST segment and T waves in precordial leads V_5 and V_6. The development of T wave inversion and ST segment depression indicates increasing left ventricular hypertrophy and strain. The presence of left ventricular strain is a warning; the few children with aortic stenosis who die suddenly usually manifest these electrocardiographic changes of abnormal ventricular repolarization.

Chest X-ray

The cardiac size is normal in most children with aortic stenosis because the volume of blood in the heart is normal. Cardiomegaly occurs in infants with severe stenosis and congestive cardiac failure, but it rarely occurs in older children; when present, it indicates fibrotic changes in the left ventricular myocardium. Severe stenosis may be present with a normal cardiac size. The ascending aorta is prominent because of poststenotic dilation. The pulmonary vasculature is normal, unless marked left ventricular dysfunction has occurred, at which point pulmonary venous markings appear increased.

> Summary of clinical findings. An aortic ejection murmur, often associated with a thrill in the suprasternal notch, indicates that the site of the obstruction is in the left ventricular outflow area. Prominent ascending aorta on chest X-ray and the presence of a systolic ejection click reflect poststenotic dilation of the ascending aorta. The electrocardiogram shows left ventricular hypertrophy. Chest pain, syncope, ST and T wave changes, and cardiomegaly are serious findings, indicating inadequate myocardial oxygen supply, and should prompt relief of the stenosis.

Natural history

Aortic valvar stenosis is progressive. Two processes probably account for this: the development of myocardial fibrosis and the absolute or relative (because of differential growth) decrease in size of the stenotic aortic valvar orifice by cartilaginous changes and ultimately by calcification of the valve.

Patients with mild congenital aortic stenosis may live 50 years before they develop symptoms. Such cases represent the calcific aortic stenosis syndrome of adulthood.

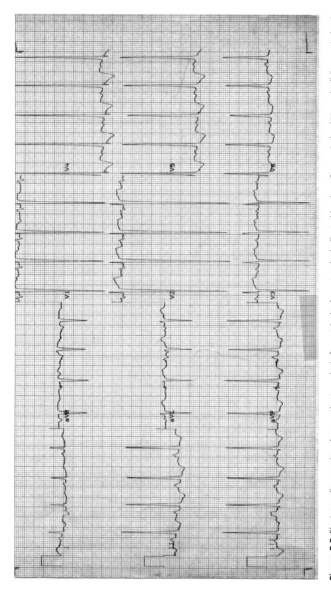

Figure 5.5 Electrocardiogram in valvar aortic stenosis. Left ventricular hypertrophy indicated by deep S wave in lead V$_1$ and tall R wave in lead V$_5$. Inverted T waves in left precordial leads. Biphasic P waves in V$_1$ indicate left atrial enlargement.

Echocardiogram

The architecture of the aortic valve can usually be determined with great accuracy by cross-sectional echocardiography. A normal aortic valve has three leaflets that appear thin, open completely in systole, and close (coapt) fully, without prolapse, in diastole. In contrast, stenotic aortic valves are often bicuspid or unicuspid with thick-appearing, highly echo-reflective leaflets that do not open fully in systole, producing the appearance of a dome at their maximal excursion. These stenotic valves rarely show prolapse.

Color Doppler provides a highly sensitive means for detecting aortic insufficiency, often when it cannot be detected by auscultation.

Spectral Doppler allows highly accurate estimation of the pressure gradient across a stenotic valve, although the gradient estimated using the maximum velocity represents a peak instantaneous systolic gradient that is usually 25–30% greater than the peak-to-peak systolic gradient derived from direct measurement of left ventricular and ascending aortic pressure at catheterization. A Doppler mean gradient may more closely approximate the values obtained by catheterization.

Aortic valve area can be estimated using Doppler, and 2D measurements of the area of the normal outflow tract proximal to the obstructed valve.

Echocardiography allows precise measurement of left ventricular function, enlargement, and hypertrophy. The presence of mitral valve regurgitation, even in the absence of a holosystolic murmur, suggests left ventricular dysfunction.

Neonates with severe aortic obstruction may have highly echo-reflective endocardium (so-called endocardial fibroelastosis) representing scarring from intrauterine subendocardial ischemia.

Cardiac catheterization

Cardiac catheterization may be indicated when children become symptomatic or develop electrocardiographic or echocardiographic changes. Catheterization is often integral with balloon dilation of the aortic valve stenosis.

The oxygen data are usually normal. The important finding is a systolic pressure difference across the aortic valve (Fig. 5.6). This gradient reflects the degree of obstruction, but to assess the severity adequately, cardiac output must also be considered, as the gradient depends upon it also.

During cardiac catheterization, the measurements of both the pressures and of the cardiac output can be made simultaneously; with this information the size of the stenotic orifice can be calculated according to the previously shown formula.

Aortography or left ventriculography is routinely performed to show the details of the aortic valve and the surrounding vascular and cardiac structures. The aortogram may be used to grade any coexistent aortic valvar insufficiency.

Balloon dilation is commonly performed to improve the gradient. A fluid-filled catheter-mounted balloon with inflated diameter similar to that of the

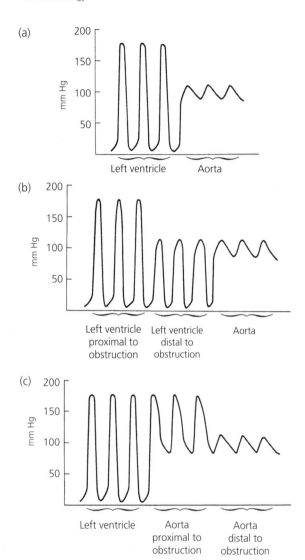

Figure 5.6 Pressure tracings in different types of aortic stenosis as the catheter is withdrawn from the left ventricle to the aorta. (a) Valvar aortic stenosis; (b) subvalvar aortic stenosis; (c) supravalvar aortic stenosis.

measured aortic valve annulus diameter is positioned across the aortic valve and then rapidly inflated and deflated. Balloon dilation may result in valvar insufficiency, but as long as predilation aortic insufficiency is not severe, any increase in insufficiency is usually well tolerated.

Operative considerations

Relief of the aortic stenosis gradient, either by balloon dilation or cardiac surgery, is indicated for patients with significant symptoms or for those whose catheterization data or echocardiogram indicates moderate or severe stenosis.

Aortic stenosis gradient—indications for intervention
  Echocardiogram—Doppler
    Peak instantaneous systolic gradient (PISG) = 70–80 mm Hg
    Mean gradient = 45–50 mm Hg
  Catheterization
    Peak-to-peak systolic pressure gradient = 50–60 mm Hg
  Catheterization or echocardiogram—Doppler
    Aortic valve area (AVA) $\leq$0.5–0.7 cm^2/m^2

These criteria are not absolute; the decision to intervene varies between cardiac centers, with the diagnostic modality used, and depend on the age and condition of the patient.

In children, the stenotic valve is usually pliable enough for valvotomy or valvuloplasty so that an aortic valve replacement with a prosthesis, or homograft (cadaveric human valve) is not required. Ultimately, children who have undergone aortic valvotomy may require a prosthesis or homograft in adulthood if the valve becomes calcified or rigid, or sooner, if the valve develops important insufficiency.

No currently available replacement valve is perfect: mechanical prostheses are long-lived but thrombogenic, so anticoagulation is required; homograft valves, although free from thrombogenic complications, are often shorter-lived because of destruction by calcification at an unpredictable rate.

An alternative is the Ross autograft procedure, in which the patient's normal pulmonary valve is excised and placed in the aortic position. A homograft valve is placed in the pulmonary position, where performing balloon dilation or future surgical revision is less risky because of its more accessible anterior location and presence on the pulmonary side of the circulation. Higher operative risk and longevity of the patient's native pulmonary valve functioning in the aortic position have been limitations with the Ross operation.

Summary. In aortic valvar stenosis, a suprasternal notch thrill is present, associated with a systolic ejection murmur in the aortic area and with an aortic systolic ejection click. Chest X-ray may show cardiomegaly but usually appears normal. The electrocardiogram may show left ventricular hypertrophy and repolarization abnormalities. The echocardiogram is the most crucial laboratory examination for following the course of the patient. The echocardiographic estimate of the degree of obstruction or symptoms, such as chest pain or syncope, alerts the provider that further diagnostic studies and intervention are warranted. Relief of the obstruction by valvotomy or valvuloplasty can be done at low risk in children with moderate or severe stenosis.

Discrete membranous subaortic stenosis

This is the second most common form of left ventricular outflow obstruction. This obstruction is a fibromuscular membrane with a small central orifice located in the left ventricle, usually within 1 cm of the aortic valve (Fig. 5.3). A jet of blood passes through the orifice and strikes the aortic valve. Because the jet strikes the aortic valve, the energy of the jet is dissipated so that poststenotic dilation of the ascending aorta rarely occurs; however, problems with aortic valve insufficiency frequently result from alterations in the aortic valve.

History

The murmur is usually recognized in infancy. Congestive cardiac failure is rare. The symptoms of chest pain and syncope may occur in patients with severe obstruction, but most patients are asymptomatic.

Physical examination

The prominent physical finding is an aortic systolic ejection murmur that is heard best along the left sternal border, often lower than in patients with valvar aortic stenosis. A suprasternal notch thrill is present infrequently. Systolic ejection clicks rarely occur because the ascending aorta is usually normal in size.

An aortic early diastolic murmur of aortic insufficiency is present in about 70% of the patients.

Electrocardiogram

The electrocardiogram shows findings similar to those of valvar aortic stenosis: left ventricular hypertrophy and ST and T wave changes that may indicate ischemia. Some patients have an rSr' pattern in lead V_1 and an Rs in lead V_6. The reason for these findings is unknown.

Chest X-ray

Heart size is normal without enlargement of the ascending aorta. Pulmonary vasculature is normal.

Natural history

Discrete membranous subaortic stenosis is considered a progressive lesion, not usually because of increasing subaortic stenosis but because of aortic valvar insufficiency. The aortic insufficiency that develops and progresses is probably secondary to the trauma of the jet upon the aortic valve.

Echocardiogram

A discrete subaortic ridge can usually be seen projecting from the septum into the left ventricular outflow tract. In contrast to valvar aortic stenosis, the disturbed color Doppler signals indicating turbulent flow begin at the site of the membrane, proximal to the valve itself. The maximum velocity of flow through the outflow tract is used to estimate the gradient. Some patients with a relatively unimportant gradient, less than 40 mm Hg, have important aortic valvar insufficiency.

Cardiac catheterization

Cardiac catheterization is not needed for making a decision to treat surgically if echocardiography indicates important progressive obstruction and/or insufficiency.

Oxygen data are normal. A systolic pressure gradient is found below the level of the aortic valve within the left ventricle (Fig. 5.6). Aortic insufficiency, if severe, causes a wide aortic pulse pressure and an elevated left ventricular end-diastolic pressure. Left ventriculography may identify the location of the membrane but is less helpful than echocardiography. If aortic insufficiency is present, it is best observed by contrast injection into the aorta.

Operative considerations

Excision of the membrane is indicated in all patients in whom it is found, unless a small gradient is discovered with cardiac catheterization or by echocardiography. Balloon dilation of subaortic membrane has been generally unsuccessful in reducing the gradient. The purposes of operation are relief of the elevated left ventricular systolic pressure and reduction of the trauma to the aortic valve.

The operative risk, which is minimal, approaches that of operation for valvar aortic stenosis. The major hazard of the operation is the possibility of damage to the septal leaflet of the mitral valve, since the membrane is often attached to this leaflet. The results are generally very good, with near normal left ventricular systolic pressure postoperatively. The degree of aortic valve insufficiency is usually less and progression of insufficiency is generally halted by successful resection of the membrane. Regrowth of the subaortic membrane can occur, but this risk is virtually eliminated by removal of a shallow layer of myocardium forming the base of the membrane's attachment to the left ventricular walls.

Summary. Discrete membranous subaortic stenosis clinically resembles valvar aortic stenosis in many respects, but it lacks the clinical and roentgenographic findings of poststenotic dilation of the aorta.

Supravalvar aortic stenosis

Obstruction to left ventricular outflow can also result from supravalvar stenosis. In most of these patients, the ascending aorta narrows in an hourglass deformity (Fig. 5.3). Although the abnormality is usually limited to the ascending aorta, other arteries, such as the brachiocephalic and even the renal arteries, may also be narrowed. Peripheral pulmonary arterial stenosis and hypoplasia may coexist and indeed represent the most important problem.

The systolic pressure is elevated in the ascending aorta proximal to the obstruction, therefore, the coronary arteries are submitted to an elevated systolic pressure. The elevation can lead to tortuosity of the coronary arteries and to premature atherosclerosis. Involvement of the coronary artery ostia by the same obstructive process operating in the aorta and other large vessels occurs occasionally and carries a poor prognosis.

Two factors have been implicated in the etiology of this condition. The first is Williams syndrome, in which a defect in the elastin gene is present. The second is familial supravalvar aortic stenosis, which occurs in patients who do not have Williams syndrome; they probably carry a mutated elastin gene (see Chapter 2).

History

Most patients are asymptomatic; cardiac disease has been identified by the presence of a murmur or by the facial characteristics associated with Williams syndrome. Congestive cardiac failure or growth retardation is rare, as in other forms of aortic stenosis, but sudden death can occur. The risk might even be higher because of acquired abnormalities of the coronary arteries.

Physical examination

The general physical characteristics of the child, particularly the facies, suggest the diagnosis of supravalvar aortic stenosis (see Chapter 2). However, many children appear normal.

Careful blood pressure recording in both arms and legs can lead to suspicion of supravalvar aortic stenosis if a blood pressure discrepancy of at least 20 mm Hg is found between the arms (Coanda effect). This effect is related to a narrowing of a subclavian artery or to the pressure effect of the jet from the supravalvar aortic stenosis that is directed into the origin of the right subclavian artery. In the latter circumstance, the blood pressure is higher in the right arm.

An aortic systolic ejection murmur is the prominent cardiac finding and, in contrast to valvar stenosis, is located maximally beneath the right clavicle, not along the left sternal border. A systolic ejection click is not present because poststenotic dilation does not occur. Diastole is silent, as valvar insufficiency does not occur.

Electrocardiogram

The electrocardiogram usually shows features similar to those of valvar aortic stenosis, including left ventricular hypertrophy. Some patients, for unknown reasons, show an rSr' pattern in lead V_1 and an Rs in lead V_6, and no voltage criteria of left ventricular hypertrophy. ST segment and T wave changes may be present, reflecting myocardial ischemia that is possibly accentuated by coronary arterial abnormalities.

Chest X-ray

The cardiac size is normal, with the absence of poststenotic dilation.

Natural history

The arterial narrowing in all affected vessels may progress. The major change over the course of this disease is the development of myocardial ischemia and fibrosis and its consequences, although findings of right heart hypertension predominate in some individuals. In following the patient, attention must be directed to the history of syncope or chest pain and to electrocardiographic changes in the ST segment and T waves.

Echocardiogram

Cross-sectional views of the ascending aorta parallel to its long axis show discrete and often severe narrowing at the sinotubular junction and, at times, more diffuse narrowing of the distal ascending aorta. Unlike valvar aortic stenosis, flow acceleration and turbulence begin at the supravalvar narrowing. The gradient is estimated using spectral Doppler. Associated lesions, such as branch pulmonary artery hypoplasia and stenosis, are readily detectable by cross-sectional echo; the presence of tricuspid and pulmonary valve regurgitation allows estimation of right-sided cardiac pressures.

Cardiac catheterization

The oxygen data are normal. The diagnosis is established by measuring a systolic pressure difference within the ascending aorta (Fig. 5.6) and/or the pulmonary arteries. Angiography demonstrates the anatomic details of the obstruction and, more importantly, identifies associated lesions-involvement of coronary, brachiocephalic, and peripheral pulmonary arteries—which is usually difficult by echocardiography. Because a greater risk of coronary artery compromise exists, contrast injection into individual coronary arteries is usually avoided in favor of aortography.

Operative considerations

Operative relief of the obstruction may be indicated for a lesser gradient, 30 or 40 mm Hg, compared with aortic valvar stenosis, or if symptoms related to myocardial ischemia are present. A longitudinal incision is made across the stenotic area, which is widened by placement of a diamond-shaped patch. During the operation, the coronary ostia are inspected; but rarely is coronary arterial bypass indicated. The operative risk for supravalvar aortic stenosis is higher than that for valvar aortic stenosis. Over the long term, reobstruction can occur because of progressive medial thickening of affected vessels.

Summary. Supravalvar aortic stenosis differs from valvar aortic stenosis since findings of poststenotic dilation are absent. The lesion can progress and may involve multiple arteries. Characteristic facies and abnormal chromosome probe is seen in Williams syndrome, which occurs sporadically, whereas other patients appear normal and have a normal chromosome probe but usually have multiple family members who are affected. Relief of the obstruction in the ascending aorta can be accomplished by surgical widening of the narrowing with a patch.

PULMONARY STENOSIS

Pulmonary stenosis (Fig. 5.7) occurs at three sites in the right heart outflow area: below the pulmonary valve (infundibular), at the level of the valve (valvar), or above the valve (supravalvar). Infundibular pulmonary stenosis rarely occurs as an isolated lesion. Supravalvar stenosis or stenosis of the individual pulmonary arteries is also uncommon. In most patients, obstruction occurs at the level of the pulmonary valve.

Regardless of the anatomic type of stenosis, the results are similar. Blood flow through the stenotic area is turbulent and leads to murmurs. The other major effect is an increase in right ventricular systolic pressure. This effect is illustrated best by the formula used to calculate the area of the stenotic pulmonary valve orifice in pulmonary stenosis:

$$PVA = \frac{PVF}{K\sqrt{RV - PA}},$$

where PVA is pulmonary valve area (area of stenotic orifice; cm^2); PVF is pulmonary valve flow (blood flow occurring during the systolic ejection period; mL/s); RV is mean right ventricular pressure during ejection (mm Hg);

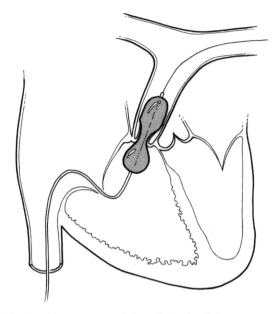

Figure 5.7 Valvar pulmonary stenosis. Balloon dilation via catheter.

PA is mean pulmonary artery pressure during ejection (mm Hg); and K is a constant.

Because of the restricted orifice, the level of right ventricular systolic pressure increases to maintain a normal cardiac output. With the elevation of right ventricular systolic pressure, right ventricular hypertrophy develops, the degree of which parallels the level of pressure elevation. As a consequence of the hypertrophy, right ventricular compliance is reduced, elevating right atrial pressure and causing right atrial enlargement. As a result of the right atrial changes, the foramen ovale is stretched open, leading to a right-to-left shunt at the atrial level. Right ventricular compliance may be reduced by the development of myocardial fibrosis, secondary to the inability to meet augmented myocardial oxygen requirements.

A second complication of right ventricular hypertrophy is the development of infundibular stenosis that may become significant enough to pose a secondary area of obstruction.

The clinical and laboratory manifestations of right ventricular hypertrophy serve as indicators of the severity of the pulmonary stenosis.

Valvar pulmonary stenosis

In the usual form of pulmonary stenosis, the valve cusps are fused; and the valve appears domed in systole. A small central orifice and poststenotic dilation are found.

History

No gender predominance in pulmonary stenosis exists. The murmur of pulmonary stenosis is frequently heard in the neonatal period; critical pulmonary stenosis may present with cyanosis. Rare older patients may present with cyanosis and cardiac failure. This combination of cyanosis and failure in pulmonary stenosis with intact ventricular septum is most frequently seen early in the first year of life, although it may occur at any age, and indicates severe stenosis and decompensation of the right ventricle. Many of the patients are completely asymptomatic throughout childhood, but those with more severe degrees of pulmonary stenosis complain of fatigue on exercise.

Physical examination

Most of the children appear normal, although cyanosis and clubbing exist in the few with right-to-left atrial shunt. In most patients the cardiac apex is not displaced. Typically, a systolic thrill is present below the left clavicle and upper left sternal border and, occasionally, in the suprasternal notch.

A systolic ejection murmur, heard along the upper left sternal border and below the clavicle, transmits to the left upper back. Usually, the murmurs are loud (grade 4/6) because the volume of flow across the valve is normal; but in patients with severe stenosis, particularly with cyanosis or cardiac failure, the murmur is softer because of reduced cardiac output.

The quality and characteristics of the second heart sound give an indication of the severity of the stenosis. In severe stenosis the pulmonary valve closure sound is delayed and soft (i.e., it can be so soft that the second heart sound seems single).

If a pulmonary systolic ejection click is present, it indicates poststenotic dilation of the pulmonary artery. This finding is generally present in mild to moderate pulmonary stenosis, but it may be absent in severe pulmonary stenosis.

Electrocardiogram

The electrocardiogram (Fig. 5.8) is useful in estimating the severity of the pulmonary stenosis. In mild pulmonary stenosis the electrocardiogram may appear normal. With more severe degrees of stenosis, right axis deviation and right ventricular hypertrophy are found, with a tall R wave in lead V_1 and a prominent S wave in lead V_6. The height of the R wave roughly correlates with the level of right ventricular systolic pressure.

Right atrial enlargement commonly occurs, reflecting elevated right ventricular filling pressure.

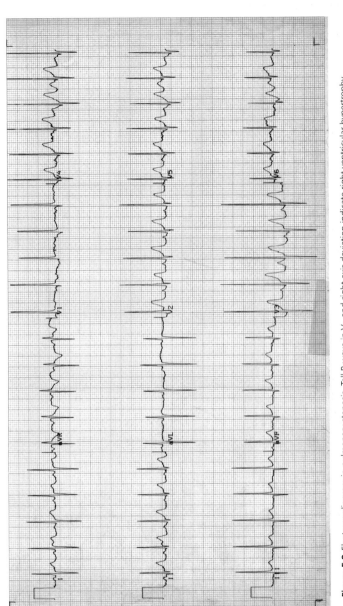

Figure 5.8 Electrocardiogram in pulmonary stenosis. Tall R wave in V₁ and right axis deviation indicate right ventricular hypertrophy.

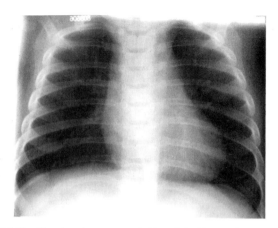

Figure 5.9 Chest X-ray in pulmonary stenosis. Normal-sized heart and pulmonary vasculature. Poststenotic dilation of pulmonary artery.

In patients with severe stenosis, a pattern of right ventricular strain develops, manifested by deep inversion of T waves from the right precordial leads and accompanied by ST segment depression. Inverted T waves in leads $V_1–V_4$ do not indicate strain in and of themselves because this pattern is normal in younger children.

Chest X-ray

Usually, cardiac size is normal because the right heart volume is normal. However, those with congestive cardiac failure or cyanosis show cardiac enlargement because of increased volume in the right atrium and right ventricle. Except in patients with cyanosis, the pulmonary vascularity appears normal, not decreased, because most patients with pulmonary stenosis have normal systemic output and a normal quantity of blood passes through the pulmonary valve.

A distinctive feature of pulmonary valvar stenosis is poststenotic dilation of the pulmonary trunk and the left pulmonary artery (Fig. 5.9). This distinction appears as a prominent bulge along the upper left cardiac border. In patients with severe stenosis, this finding can be absent.

Summary of clinical findings. The systolic ejection murmur indicates the turbulence of flow through the stenotic pulmonary valve. Poststenotic dilation is indicated by the pulmonary systolic ejection click and the roentgenographic findings of an enlarged pulmonary trunk. The electrocardiogram is the best indicator of the degree of right ventricular hypertrophy. Right atrial enlargement, cyanosis, and congestive cardiac failure are indicators of altered right ventricular compliance resulting from severe right ventricular hypertrophy and/or fibrosis.

Natural history

The orifice of the stenotic pulmonary valve increases as the child grows, meaning the degree of obstruction usually does not increase with age. The deterioration of the clinical status that occurs in some patients appears to result from altered right ventricular myocardial performance related to fibrosis. This complication occurs in infancy and in adulthood, but rarely in the mid-childhood years. Occasionally, an infant or toddler has progression of infundibular stenosis without apparent change in the degree of valvar stenosis.

Echocardiography

Similar to aortic valvar stenosis, cross-sectional echocardiography shows thickened and doming pulmonary valve leaflets. Poststenotic dilation of the main pulmonary artery and ductus "diverticulum" is potentially dramatic. Doppler reveals turbulent high-velocity flow through the pulmonary valve; the maximum velocity allows estimation of the pressure gradient between the right ventricle and the pulmonary artery. Right ventricular hypertrophy may occur, but quantitation is more difficult than in left ventricular hypertrophy, partly because of the geometry of the right ventricle and of the opposition between the right ventricular wall and the chest wall, making differentiation of the boundary between the two structures problematic. However, hypertrophy of the infundibulum, the tubular right ventricular outflow tract, can become severe and is easily demonstrated by cross-sectional echocardiography as the muscular walls squeeze the pathway virtually closed by the end of each systole.

Cardiac catheterization

Oximetry data are normal except in an occasional patient with a right-to-left shunt at the atrial level. The right ventricular systolic pressure is elevated, whereas pulmonary arterial pressure is normal or low. Both the pressure data and the cardiac output data may be needed to assess accurately the severity of the stenosis, which is done by calculating the pulmonary valve area. Right ventricular angiography outlines the details of the pulmonary valve and associated infundibular narrowing.

Balloon dilation is the procedure of choice for gradient relief. Any patient with dome-shaped pulmonary valvar stenosis and a right ventricular systolic pressure gradient greater than 35 mm Hg should undergo a balloon valvotomy. This low-risk procedure almost always results in a favorable outcome and reduction of right ventricular systolic pressure to normal or near normal. Even though pulmonary valvar insufficiency regularly results from valvuloplasty, it is well tolerated because pulmonary arterial pressure is low.

In patients with a significant infundibular component, this procedure may not produce an immediate fall in right ventricular pressure; the infundibular stenosis usually resolves over several weeks.

Operative considerations

Since the development of catheter balloon dilation, operative valvotomy is indicated for those patients who have failed dilation (e.g., Noonan syndrome patients with dysplastic valves) or who are not candidates for balloon dilation (e.g., the neonate with critical stenosis and an extremely hypoplastic pulmonary annulus instead requires outflow tract widening by use of a patch). Infundibular narrowing may require excision in some patients.

> Summary. Pulmonary stenosis can usually be diagnosed on the basis of clinical and laboratory findings. Cardiac catheterization is required to determine precisely the severity and to perform balloon valvotomy in patients with moderate or severe stenosis; it can be performed at low risk and with excellent results.

Pulmonary stenosis secondary to dysplastic pulmonary valve

This distinctive form of pulmonary stenosis accounts for less than 10% of valvar pulmonary stenosis. Anatomically, the pulmonary valve leaflets do not show commissural fusion as in most examples of stenotic valves. Rather, the commissures are open; but each leaflet is greatly thickened and redundant. The valvar obstruction is caused by the bulk of valvar tissue located in the pulmonary annulus. The pulmonary annulus can be reduced in diameter. Poststenotic dilation usually does not occur.

History

The history is similar to that of patients with pulmonary stenosis secondary to a dome-shaped pulmonary valve.

Physical examination

In most patients, dysplastic pulmonary valve is associated with various noncardiac abnormalities of Noonan and similar syndromes (see Chapter 2). Auscultation shows a pulmonary systolic ejection murmur, usually grades 2/6–4/6. Poststenotic dilation and a systolic ejection click are not found. The P_2 is soft and delayed.

Electrocardiogram

The electrocardiogram is distinctive. The QRS axis is almost always superiorly directed ($-60°$ to $-150°$) and distinguishes the dysplastic from dome-shaped pulmonary stenosis, in which the QRS axis rarely exceeds $+180°$. The reason for this alteration of the QRS axis is not known but is thought to represent an abnormality in the location of the conduction system.

Right ventricular hypertrophy is present, its degree reflecting the level of right ventricular systolic pressure. Right atrial enlargement may appear.

Chest X-ray

The heart size is normal, as is the vascularity. The pulmonary arterial segment is of normal size as compared with dome-shaped valvar pulmonary stenosis.

Natural history

In this form of pulmonary stenosis the stenotic valve orifice probably grows in relation to the growth of the child. Changes that occur with age are related to the effects of the elevated right ventricular systolic pressure and right ventricular hypertrophy upon the right ventricle, to the frequent development of severe infundibular stenosis, and perhaps to changes in the pliability of the thickened valve leaflets themselves.

Echocardiogram

In patients with a so-called dysplastic valve, the leaflets may be so thick that they appear globular, with very little motion or opening during systole. Some patients have biventricular hypertrophy disproportionate to the degree of outflow obstruction. Although this finding may represent a form of hypertrophic cardiomyopathy for Noonan syndrome patients, it has a more benign natural history than in idiopathic forms.

Cardiac catheterization

The data are similar to those obtained in dome-shaped pulmonary stenosis. However, angiography confirms the dysplastic nature of the valve because the valve leaflets appear thickened and immobile. The pulmonary artery is only slightly enlarged. Balloon dilation is not effective in most patients.

Operative considerations

The indications for operation are similar to those for dome-shaped pulmonary stenosis; however, the operative approach is different. Valvotomy cannot be performed because commissural fusion is not present. One or two leaflets must be excised, and in some patients a patch must be placed across the annulus to widen this area of right ventricular outflow. Resection of infundibular muscle often accompanies valvotomy.

Peripheral pulmonary artery stenosis

Stenosis also occurs above the pulmonary valve and in the branches of the pulmonary arteries. One or more major branches may be involved, showing either a long area of narrowing or a discrete narrowing. In the other examples, the entire pulmonary arterial tree may be hypoplastic.

Peripheral pulmonary artery stenosis results from the congenital rubella syndrome; occurs in children with supravalvar aortic stenosis, particularly those with Williams syndrome; occurs with Alagille syndrome (with a clinical presentation similar to biliary atresia); or appears without apparent cause. Hypoplastic pulmonary arteries frequently accompany tetralogy of Fallot with pulmonary valve atresia; these patients often have DiGeorge syndrome.

History

Most patients with this condition are asymptomatic unless other conditions such as Williams syndrome are present.

Physical examination

Features of one of the syndromes mentioned above may be discovered. Occasionally, normal neonates have auscultatory findings of peripheral pulmonary artery "stenosis," but this type of innocent murmur disappears with time (see Chapter 1); and the pulmonary arteries are, in fact, normal.

The classic finding is a systolic ejection murmur present under the left clavicle that is well heard throughout both the lung fields and the axillae. Typically, either no murmur, or only a soft murmur is heard over the precordium. The second heart sound is normal, and a systolic ejection click is not heard because the pulmonary artery is not dilated.

Electrocardiogram

No features distinguish peripheral pulmonary artery stenosis from valvar pulmonary stenosis. Right ventricular hypertrophy exists proportional to the degree of hypertrophy.

Chest X-ray

This usually appears normal. Pulmonary blood flow appears symmetric because most children have symmetric stenoses.

Natural history

The prognosis is extremely variable. Since the degree of stenosis is often mild and does not increase with age in most patients, it has been considered a benign condition. Apparent growth of the pulmonary arteries does occur in some and results in clinical and laboratory features becoming more normal with age. Rarely, especially in Williams syndrome patients, stenosis may progress in

Table 5.1 Summary of Obstructive Lesions.

		History			Physical Examination				
Malformation	Sex	Major Syndrome	Age Murmur	Congestive Cardiac Failure	Symptoms	Blood Pressure	Thrill	Murmur	Systolic Ejection Click
Coarctation of aorta	M > F	Turner	Infancy	±	None, or headache	Diminished in legs	Suprasternal notch	Systolic, precordium and back	Aortic (if bicuspid valve present)
Aortic stenosis	M > F	Williams (supravalvar AS)	Birth	±	None, or chest pain, syncope, sudden death	Normal, or narrow pulse pressure	Suprasternal notch and/or aortic area	Systolic ejection, aortic area and left sternal border	Aortic
Pulmonary stenosis	M = F	Noonan	Birth	±	None, or exercise intolerance, variable cyanosis (neonates)	Normal	Pulmonic area	Systolic ejection, pulmonic area and left back	Pulmonic

		Electrocardiogram			Chest X-ray			
Malformation	Axis (QRS)	Atrial Enlargement	Ventricular Hypertrophy/Enlargement	Other	Aortic Enlargement	Pulmonary Artery Enlargement	Chamber Enlargement	Other
Coarctation of aorta	Normal	None or left	Right (neonate and infant), left (older child)	Strain pattern if severe	Absent unless bicuspid valve	Absent	± Left ventricle	Poststenotic dilatation descending aorta
Aortic stenosis	Normal	None or left	Left	Strain pattern if severe	Present	Absent	± Left ventricle	None
Pulmonary stenosis	Normal or right	Normal or right	Right	Strain pattern if severe	Absent	Present	± Right ventricle	None

F, female; M, male; htn, hypertension; ± may be present or absent.

severity and can cause suprasystemic right ventricular pressure and eventual right heart failure.

Echocardiogram

The proximal several centimeters of each branch pulmonary artery are easily seen by cross-sectional echocardiogram, particularly in young infants; and precise diameter measurements can be made. Doppler is used to estimate pressure gradients within the branch pulmonary arteries; however, the Bernoulli equation is more applicable to discrete stenoses, so gradient estimates of long tubular (or serial) stenoses are often inaccurate.

Cardiac catheterization

Oxygen data are normal. Pressure tracings show a systolic gradient within the pulmonary arteries. Diastolic pressures are identical proximal and distal to the obstruction. The anatomic details are shown by pulmonary arteriography.

Catheter balloon dilation, sometimes with placement of endovascular metal stents, is widely used, although with variable results that depend greatly on the etiology and severity of the stenosis.

Operative considerations

Most patients do not require operation as the degree of stenosis is not severe. In patients with severe obstruction, operation often cannot be performed because anatomic features, such as diffuse hypoplasia of the pulmonary arteries or multiple areas of stenosis, preclude an operative approach and are best served by having catheter balloon dilation.

SUMMARY OF OBSTRUCTIVE LESIONS
In each of the conditions discussed, turbulence occurs through a narrowed orifice, causing a systolic ejection murmur. Beyond the obstruction, poststenotic dilation occurs; this is evidenced either by roentgenographic findings or by an ejection click. The restricted orifice leads to elevation of systolic pressures proximally and to ventricular hypertrophy. The clinical and laboratory findings reflecting this hypertrophy permit assessment of the severity of the condition (Table 5.1). In patients with moderate or severe obstruction gradient relief can be performed successfully by operative and catheterization means.

Chapter 6
Cardiac conditions associated with right-to-left shunt (cyanotic lesions)

Admixture lesions
    Complete transposition of the great arteries (d-TGA or d-TGV)
    Total anomalous pulmonary venous connection (TAPVC or TAPVR)
    Truncus arteriosus
Cyanosis and diminished pulmonary blood flow
    Tetralogy of Fallot
    Tricuspid atresia
    Pulmonary atresia with intact ventricular septum
    Ebstein's malformation of the tricuspid valve

In most patients with cyanosis related to congenital cardiac abnormalities, an abnormality permits a portion of the systemic venous return to bypass the lungs and to enter the systemic circulation directly. Right-to-left shunt results from two general types of cardiac malformations: (a) admixture of the systemic and pulmonary venous returns or (b) an intracardiac defect and obstruction to pulmonary blood flow. The first group shows increased pulmonary vascularity, but the second shows diminished pulmonary vascularity. Therefore, the most common conditions resulting in cyanosis are divided between these two categories (Table 6.1).

Regardless of the type of cardiac malformation leading to cyanosis, a risk of polycythemia, clubbing, slow growth, and brain abscess exists. The first three findings related to tissue hypoxia have been discussed previously. Brain abscess results from the direct access of bacteria to the systemic circuit as a result of the right-to-left shunt.

ADMIXTURE LESIONS

The combination of cyanosis and increased pulmonary vascular markings on a chest X-ray indicates an admixture lesion. In most cardiac malformations

Pediatric Cardiology, by W Johnson, J Moller © 2008 Blackwell Publishing, ISBN: 978-1-4051-7818-1.

Table 6.1 Physiologic Classification of Cyanotic Malformations.

Admixture lesions (increased pulmonary vascularity):
  Complete transposition of the great arteries
  Total anomalous pulmonary venous connection
  Persistent truncus arteriosus
Obstruction to pulmonary blood flow and an intracardiac defect (decreased pulmonary vascularity):
  Tetralogy of Fallot
  Tricuspid atresia*
  Pulmonary atresia*
  Ebstein's malformation

---

*The physiology of these lesions can be considered complete admixture, although the pulmonary vascularity is usually decreased.

classified in this group, a single chamber receives the total systemic and pulmonary venous returns and from that point an admixture of blood flows to both systemic and pulmonary circuits. The admixture lesion can occur at any cardiac level: venous (e.g., total anomalous pulmonary venous connection), atrial (e.g., single atrium), ventricular (e.g., single ventricle), or great vessel (e.g., persistent truncus arteriosus).

Near-uniform mixing of the two venous returns occurs. Complete transposition is included in the admixture group because the patients are cyanotic with increased pulmonary blood flow. They usually have partial admixture of the two venous returns; this incomplete mixing leads to symptoms of severe hypoxia.

> The hemodynamics of the admixture lesions resemble those of the left-to-right shunts occurring at the same level. The direction and magnitude of blood flow in total anomalous pulmonary venous connection and single atrium are governed, as in isolated atrial septal defect, by the relative ventricular compliances. Relative resistances to systemic and pulmonary flow determine the distribution of blood in patients with single ventricle and persistent truncus arteriosus, similar to ventricular septal defect. Thus, the natural history and many of the clinical and laboratory findings of the admixture lesions are identical to those of similar left-to-right shunts, including the development of pulmonary vascular disease.

In admixture lesions the systemic arterial oxygen saturation or the hemoglobin and hematocrit values are valuable indicators of the volume of pulmonary blood flow, since the degree of cyanosis is inversely related to the volume of pulmonary blood flow.

In patients with large pulmonary blood flow, the degree of cyanosis is slight because large amounts of fully saturated blood return from the lungs and mix with a relatively smaller volume of systemic venous return (Fig. 6.1). If the patient develops pulmonary vascular disease or another factor that limits pulmonary blood flow, the amount of fully oxygenated blood returning from the lungs and mixing with the systemic venous return is reduced; so the patient becomes more cyanotic, and the hemoglobin and hematocrit values rise.

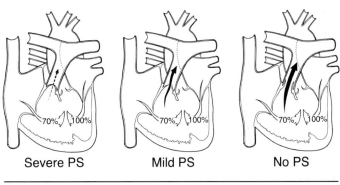

	Severe PS	Mild PS	No PS
	$\frac{Q_P}{Q_S} = \frac{0.5}{1} = 0.5$	$\frac{Q_P}{Q_S} = \frac{1}{1} = 1$	$\frac{Q_P}{Q_S} = \frac{4}{1} = 4$
Pulmonary venous blood (100% saturation)	0.5 part	1 part	4 parts
Plus			
Systemic venous blood (70% saturation)	1 part	1 part	1 part
Equals			
Systemic artery saturation	80%	85%	94%

PS, pulmonary stenosis; Q_P/Q_S, ratio of pulmonary blood flow to systemic blood flow.

Figure 6.1 Estimation of the pulmonary blood flow in admixture lesions. Using a single ventricle, three clinical examples are shown, each with different degrees of pulmonary stenosis and pulmonary blood flow. Cyanosis is inversely related to the pulmonary blood flow. Assuming healthy lungs and complete mixture of the systemic and pulmonary venous return, the systemic arterial oxygen saturation represents the average of the contribution of the pulmonary blood flow (Q_P), represented by the pulmonary venous return, and the systemic blood flow (Q_S), represented by the systemic venous return. A Q_P/Q_S can be estimated from the pulse oximetry value. (Abbreviations: PS, pulmonary stenosis; Q_P/Q_S, ratio of pulmonary blood flow to systemic blood flow.)

Complete transposition of the great arteries (d-TGA or d-TGV)

The term *transposition* indicates an anatomic reversal in anteroposterior relationships, not in left–right relationships as commonly thought. Normally, the pulmonary artery lies anterior to and slightly to the left of the aorta. In complete transposition of the great arteries (Fig. 6.2), the aorta lies anteriorly to the pulmonary artery. Normally, the anterior blood vessel arises from the infundibulum, which is the conus portion of the right ventricle. The aorta in complete transposition arises from the right ventricle. The pulmonary trunk, on the other hand, originates from the left ventricle.

Because of the transposition of the great vessels and their anomalous anatomic relationship to the ventricles, two more or less independent circulations exist. The systemic venous blood returns to the right atrium, enters the right ventricle, and is ejected into the aorta, while the pulmonary venous blood flows through the left side of the heart into the pulmonary artery and returns to the lungs.

A communication must exist between the left and right sides of the heart to allow some mixing of the pulmonary and systemic venous returns. The communication is found in one or more of the following: patent foramen ovale, atrial septal defect, ventricular septal defect, or patent ductus arteriosus. In half of the patients, the ventricular septum is intact and the shunt occurs at the atrial level. In the other half, a ventricular septal defect is present. Pulmonary stenosis, often valvar and subpulmonic, may coexist.

In patients with an intact ventricular septum, the communication (either a patent foramen ovale or a patent ductus arteriosus) between the two sides of the circulation is often narrow. As these communications follow the normal neonatal course and close, neonates with transposition and an intact septum develop profound cyanosis. Because a greater degree of mixing usually occurs in patients with a coexistent ventricular septal defect, cyanosis is mild in such infants with transposition and diagnosis is sometimes delayed.

History

Complete transposition of the great arteries occurs more frequently in males. Cyanosis becomes evident shortly after birth. Without intervention, almost all infants exhibit dyspnea and other signs of cardiac failure in the first month of life; infants with intact ventricular septum develop cardiac symptoms earlier and are more intensely cyanotic than those with coexistent ventricular septal defect. In the absence of operation, death occurs, usually in neonates, and in nearly every patient by 6 months of age. Patients with ventricular septal defect and pulmonary stenosis are often the least symptomatic because the pulmonary stenosis prevents excessive pulmonary blood flow and enhances

(a)

(b)

(c)

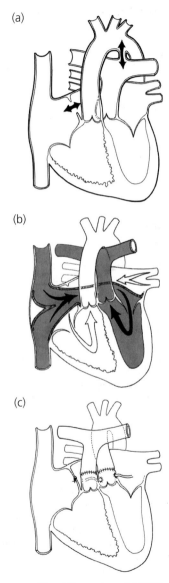

Figure 6.2 Complete transposition of the great vessels (d-TGV). (a) Central circulation. Surgical options: (b) venous switch; (c) arterial switch.

flow of fully saturated blood through the ventricular septal defect into the aorta; these patients resemble those with tetralogy of Fallot.

Physical examination

Infants are often large for gestational age. Setting aside cyanosis and congestive cardiac failure, physical findings vary with the defect associated with complete transposition of the great vessels. Newborns are often asymptomatic, except for cyanosis, but quickly develop tachypnea.

With an intact ventricular septum, the intracardiac shunt is found at the atrial level. In these cases, either no murmur is present; or a soft, nonspecific murmur is audible. With an associated ventricular septal defect, a louder murmur is present. The second heart sound is single and loud along the upper left sternal border, representing closure of the anteriorly placed aortic valve. Thus, the murmur does not help diagnose transposition of the great vessels, although it does indicate the type of associated defect. If pulmonary stenosis coexists, the murmur often radiates to the right side of the back.

Electrocardiogram

Since the aorta arises from the right ventricle, the pressure in the right ventricle is elevated to systemic levels and is associated with a thick-walled right ventricle. The electrocardiogram reflects this by a pattern of right axis deviation and right ventricular hypertrophy. The latter is manifested by tall R waves in the right precordial leads. Right atrial enlargement is also possible.

Patients with a large volume of pulmonary blood flow, as with coexistent ventricular septal defect, also may have left ventricular enlargement/hypertrophy because of the volume load on the left ventricle.

Chest X-ray

Cardiomegaly is generally present. The cardiac silhouette has a characteristic egg-shaped appearance (Fig. 6.3); the superior mediastinum is narrow because the great vessels lie one in front of the other; the thymus is usually small. Left atrial enlargement exists in the unoperated patient.

Summary of clinical findings. The diagnosis of complete transposition is usually indicated by a combination of rather intense cyanosis in the neonatal period, roentgenographic findings of increased pulmonary vasculature, and characteristic cardiac contour.

Echocardiogram

The key to the echocardiographic diagnosis of complete transposition is the recognition of an anteriorly arising aorta and a posteriorly arising pulmonary

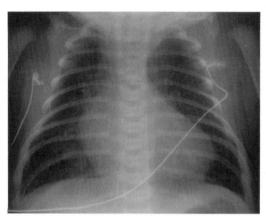

Figure 6.3 Chest X-ray in complete transposition of the great vessels: cardiomegaly, narrow mediastinum, and increased pulmonary vasculature.

artery. In views parallel to the long axis of the left ventricle, both great vessels may appear to course parallel to each other for a short distance, which is not seen in normal hearts, where the great vessels cross each other at an acute angle. In views profiling the short axis of the left ventricle, the aorta is seen arising anterior and rightward of the central and posterior pulmonary artery (hence the term d-transposition, or dextro-transposition). A cross-sectional view of the aortic root allows demonstration of the origins, branching, and proximal courses of the coronary arteries.

In neonates with transposition, the interventricular septum usually has a flat contour when viewed in cross section; however, as the infant ages, the septum gradually bows away from the right (systemic) ventricle and bulges into the left (pulmonary) ventricle.

Ventricular septal defect represents the most important associated lesion diagnosed by echocardiography; the shunt through it and any atrial septal defect or ductus is bidirectional, consistent with the physiology of transposition described earlier. The atrial septal defect may be small and restrictive (Doppler signals are high velocity) before balloon septostomy; after, it is typically large and unrestrictive, with a mobile flap of the torn fossa ovalis waving to and fro across the defect. Balloon septostomy may be performed under echocardiographic guidance.

Cardiac catheterization
In patients with an intact septum, oximetry data show little increase in oxygen saturation values through the right side of the heart, and little decrease

through the left side. Among those with coexistent ventricular septal defect, larger changes in oxygen values are found. The oxygen saturation values in the pulmonary artery are higher than those in the aorta, a finding virtually diagnostic of transposition of the great vessels.

In all patients, right ventricular systolic pressure is elevated. When the ventricular septum is intact, left ventricular pressure may be low; but in most patients with coexistent ventricular septal defect or in those who have a large patent ductus arteriosus, the left ventricular pressure is elevated to levels similar to those of the right (systemic) ventricle.

Angiography confirms the diagnosis by showing the aorta arising from the right ventricle and the pulmonary artery arising from the left ventricle, and it identifies coexistent malformations. Aortic root injection demonstrates coronary artery anatomy in preparation for surgery. A left ventricular injection is indicated to demonstrate ventricular septal defect(s) and pulmonic stenosis.

Operative considerations
Palliation. Hypoxia, one of the major symptoms of infants with transposition of the great vessels, results from inadequate mixing of the two venous returns, and palliation is directed toward improvement of mixing by two means.

Intravenous prostaglandin. This substance opens and/or maintains patency of the ductus arteriosus and improves mixing.

Rashkind balloon atrial septostomy procedure. Patients with inadequate mixing benefit from the creation of an atrial septal defect (enlargement of the foramen ovale). At cardiac catheterization or by echocardiographic guidance, a balloon catheter is inserted via a systemic vein and is advanced into the left atrium through the foramen ovale. The balloon is inflated and then is rapidly and forcefully withdrawn across the septum, creating a larger defect and often improving the hypoxia.

Infants who do not experience adequate improvement of cyanosis despite a large atrial defect and patent ductus are rare. Multiple factors may be responsible, including nearly identical ventricular compliances, which do not favor mixing across the atrial defect, and an element of elevated pulmonary vascular resistance, which may limit the shunt at the ductus and result in inadequate pulmonary blood flow. Increased central volume via increased intravenous fluids may benefit the patient.

Rarely, the atrial defect is created surgically by atrial septectomy, an open-heart procedure. A closed heart technique, the Blalock–Hanlon procedure, was used previously but frequently resulted in scarring of the pulmonary veins.

Corrective operation

Atrial (venous) switch (see Fig. 6.2). The first successful procedure was performed by Senning in the late 1950s and later modified by Mustard. This procedure involves removal of the atrial septum and creation of an intratrial baffle
to divert the systemic venous return into the left ventricle and thus to the lungs,
whereas the pulmonary venous return is directed to the right ventricle and thus
to the aorta.

It can be performed at low risk in patients with an intact ventricular septum
and at a higher risk in patients with ventricular septal defect. Serious complications, stroke, or death can occur in infants prior to atrial (venous) switch
procedures, which are usually done no earlier than 3 months of age.

The long-term results of the atrial switch procedure are well known. Arrhythmias, the most frequent long-term complication, are often related to abnormalities of the sinoatrial node and of the atrial surgical scar. Sometimes these
are life-threatening, although the exact mechanism of sudden death in the rare
child who succumbs is not usually known. Scarring can also cause systemic or
pulmonary obstruction of the venous return. The most common severe complication is not sudden death but is progressive dysfunction of the right ventricle,
leading to death from chronic heart failure. This complication is undoubtedly
related to the right ventricle performing as a systemic ventricle (i.e., at higher
systolic pressures than normal). Predicting which patients will have failure and
at what age postoperatively is not possible.

Arterial switch (Jatene) (see Fig. 6.2). This operation, developed in the 1970s,
avoids the complications inherent with the atrial (venous) switch. The great
vessels are transected and reanastomosed, so blood flows from left ventricle to aorta and from right ventricle to pulmonary arteries. Since the coronary arteries arise from the aortic root, they have to be transferred to the
pulmonary (neoaortic) root. Certain variations of coronary artery origins or
branching make transfer more risky. The arterial switch operation must occur
early in life (within the first 2 weeks) before the pulmonary resistance falls;
the left ventricle will then become "deconditioned" to a systemic pressure
load.

Arterial switch is not free from complications: coronary artery compromise
may result in left ventricular infarct or failure; pulmonary artery stenosis can
result from stretching or kinking during the surgical repositioning of the great
vessels; and the operative mortality may be higher, partly because of the risks
of neonatal open-heart surgery.

The short- and long-term outcomes favor those receiving the arterial switch
procedure.

Summary. Complete transposition of the great arteries is a common cardiac anomaly that results in neonatal cyanosis and ultimately in cardiac failure. Many neonates are asymptomatic. The physical findings and electrocardiogram vary with associated malformations. The chest X-ray reveals cardiomegaly and increased pulmonary vascularity. Palliative and corrective procedures are available.

Total anomalous pulmonary venous connection (TAPVC or TAPVR) (see Fig. 6.4)

The pulmonary veins, instead of entering the left atrium, connect with a systemic venous channel that delivers pulmonary venous blood to the right side of the heart. Developmentally, this anomaly results from failure of incorporation of the pulmonary veins into the left atrium, so that the pulmonary venous system retains an earlier embryologic communication to the systemic venous system.

In the embryo, the pulmonary veins communicate with both the left and right anterior cardinal veins and the umbilical vitelline system, both precursors of systemic veins. If the pulmonary veins, which form with the lungs as outpouchings of the foregut, are not incorporated into the left atrium, the result is anomalous pulmonary venous connection to one of the following structures: right superior vena cava (right anterior cardinal vein), left superior vena cava (distal left anterior cardinal vein), coronary sinus (proximal left anterior cardinal vein), or infradiaphragmatic site (umbilical–vitelline system), usually a tributary of the portal system.

Therefore, the right atrium receives not only the entire systemic venous return, but also the entire pulmonary venous return. The left atrium has no direct venous supply. An obligatory right-to-left shunt exists at the atrial level through either a patent foramen ovale or an atrial septal defect.

The volume of blood shunted from the right to the left atrium and the volume of blood that enters each ventricle depends upon their relative compliances. Ventricular compliance is influenced by ventricular pressures and vascular resistances. Right ventricular compliance normally falls following birth as a result of the normal neonatal decrease in pulmonary vascular resistance and pulmonary arterial pressure. Therefore, in most patients with total anomalous pulmonary venous connection, pulmonary blood flow is considerably greater than normal; systemic blood flow is usually normal. Since a disparity exists between the volume of blood being carried by the right and left sides of the heart, the right side is dilated and hypertrophied, whereas the left side is relatively smaller but near-normal size.

In patients with total anomalous pulmonary venous connection, the degree of cyanosis inversely relates to the volume of pulmonary blood flow. When the

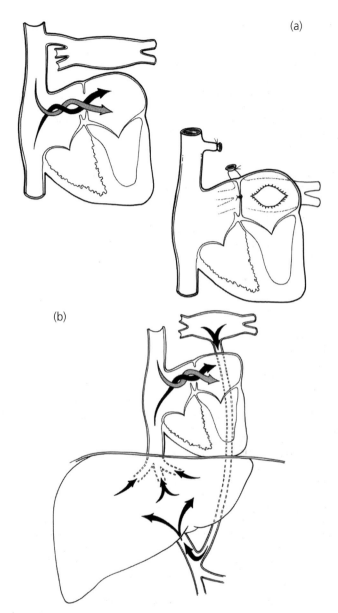

Figure 6.4 Total anomalous pulmonary venous connection. (a) Central circulation and surgical repair of unobstructed type; (b) central circulation in obstructed type.

volume of pulmonary blood flow is larger, the proportion of the pulmonary venous blood to total venous blood returning to the right atrium is greater. As a result, the saturation of blood shunted to the left side of the heart may be only slightly reduced from normal.

On the other hand, in hemodynamic situations in which the resistance to flow through the lungs is increased (e.g., the neonatal period), the volume of blood flow through the lungs is nearly normal (i.e., equal to systemic blood flow). Therefore, the pulmonary and systemic venous systems contribute nearly equal volumes of blood to the right atrium, and these patients exhibit noticeable cyanosis.

Total anomalous pulmonary venous connection is an example of bidirectional shunting: a right-to-left shunt at the venous level and a left-to-right shunt at the atrial level exist since all the pulmonary venous blood returns to the right atrium.

Total anomalous pulmonary venous connection presents two clinical pictures. One resembles atrial septal defect, and the other shows intense cyanosis and a radiographic pattern of pulmonary venous obstruction. In the second, the connecting venous channel is narrowed and obstructed, whereas in the first, the venous channel has no obstruction.

Total anomalous pulmonary venous connection without obstruction (see Fig. 6.4)

History. The clinical manifestations of patients with total anomalous pulmonary venous connection vary considerably. Usually, total anomalous pulmonary venous connection is recognized in the neonatal period or with fetal echocardiography. If not operated upon in early infancy, most patients develop congestive cardiac failure, grow slowly, and have frequent respiratory infections, but a few may be asymptomatic into later childhood.

Physical examination. The degree of cyanosis varies as previously described because of differences in the amount of pulmonary blood flow. Although systemic arterial desaturation is always present, children with greatly increased pulmonary blood flow appear acyanotic or show only slight cyanosis.

The physical findings mimic isolated atrial septal defect. Cardiomegaly, precordial bulge, and right ventricular heave are found in older unoperated infants. A grade 2/6–3/6 pulmonary systolic ejection murmur due to excess flow across the pulmonary valve is present along the upper left sternal border. Wide, fixed splitting of the second heart sound is heard and the pulmonary component may be accentuated, reflecting pulmonary hypertension. A mid-diastolic murmur caused by increased blood flow across the tricuspid valve is found along the lower left sternal border and is associated with greatly increased pulmonary blood flow. In total anomalous pulmonary venous connection to the superior vena cava, a venous hum may exist along the upper right sternal border.

Electrocardiogram. Electrocardiogram reveals enlargement of the right-sided cardiac chambers with right axis deviation, right atrial enlargement, and right ventricular enlargement/hypertrophy. Usually, the pattern is of the type reflecting volume overload, an rSR' pattern in lead V_1.

Chest X-ray. Chest X-ray findings also resemble isolated atrial septal defect. Cardiomegaly, primarily of right-sided chambers, and increased pulmonary blood flow are found. In contrast to most other admixture lesions, the left atrium is not enlarged because blood flow through this chamber is normal.

Except for total anomalous pulmonary venous connection to a left superior vena cava ("vertical vein"), the roentgenographic contour is not characteristic. In this form the cardiac silhouette can be described as a figure eight or as a "snowman heart" (Fig. 6.5a). The upper portion of the cardiac contour is formed by the left and right superior venae cavae, which are enlarged since both carry the pulmonary venous return. The lower portion of the contour is formed by the cardiac chambers.

> **Summary of clinical findings.** The clinical, electrocardiographic, and roentgenographic findings resemble those of atrial septal defect because the effects upon the heart are similar. Cyanosis distinguishes the conditions; although it may be minimal or not clinically evident, it is easily detectable by pulse oximetry. Unlike uncomplicated atrial septal defect, congestive cardiac failure and elevated pulmonary arterial pressure may be found in total anomalous pulmonary venous connection.

Echocardiogram. Cross-sectional echocardiography reveals an atrial septal defect and an enlarged right atrium, right ventricle, and pulmonary arteries. The left atrium and left ventricle appear smaller than normal. In contrast to most normal neonates with an atrial septal defect the shunt is from right atrium to left atrium. Doppler demonstrates a right-to-left atrial septal defect shunt because the entire pulmonary venous return mixes with the entire systemic venous return at or proximal to the right atrium. The only blood entering the left atrium is via the atrial septal defect. The individual pulmonary veins are seen joining a common pulmonary vein, which then joins the coronary sinus or the superior vena cava via a vertical vein (the left-sided superior vena cava), or the hepatic portal venous system after a descent into the abdomen.

Cardiac catheterization. Oxygen saturation values in each cardiac chamber and in both great vessels are virtually identical. An increase in oxygen saturation is found in the vena cava, coronary sinus, or other systemic venous sites into which the pulmonary venous blood flows. The saturation of blood in the left

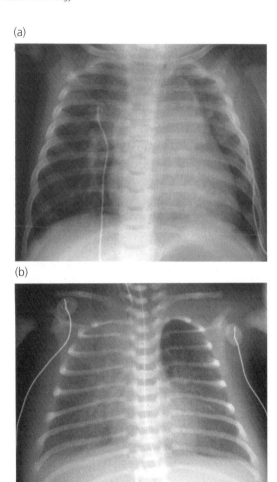

Figure 6.5 Chest X-ray in total anomalous pulmonary venous connection. (a) Unobstructed (supracardiac) connection to the left superior vena cava ("snowman" heart). Upper portion of cardiac silhouette formed by dilated right and left superior venae cavae. (b) Obstructed (infradiaphragmatic) type. Pulmonary vascular congestion, a pleural effusion, and a small heart shadow.

atrium and left ventricle is reduced because of the obligatory right-to-left atrial shunt.

Pulmonary hypertension may be found in infants, but some patients, particularly older ones, show near-normal levels of pulmonary arterial pressures.

Pulmonary angiography is indicated in these patients. During the later phases of the angiogram (the so-called levophase), the pulmonary veins opacify and subsequently fill the connecting venous channel, delineating the anatomic form of anomalous pulmonary venous connection.

Operative considerations. Under cardiopulmonary bypass, the confluence of pulmonary veins is connected to the left atrium. At the same time, the atrial communication is closed, and the connecting vessel is divided. This operation can be performed with low risk, even in neonates and younger infants.

> Summary. Each of the anatomic types of total anomalous pulmonary venous connection is associated with cyanosis of variable degree. The physical findings are those of atrial septal defect; pulmonary hypertension may also be found. Both the electrocardiogram and the chest X-ray reveal enlargement of the right-sided cardiac chambers. Corrective operations can be performed successfully for each of the forms of total anomalous pulmonary venous connection.

Total anomalous pulmonary venous connection with obstruction (see Fig. 6.4b)

In total anomalous pulmonary venous connection, an obstruction can be present in the channel returning pulmonary venous blood to the right side of the heart. Obstruction is always present in patients with an infradiaphragmatic connection and occasionally in patients with a supradiaphragmatic connection. In the latter, obstruction may occur intrinsically from narrowing of the channel or extrinsically as the channel passes between the bronchus and the branch pulmonary artery.

In infradiaphragmatic connection, four mechanisms contribute to obstruction in pulmonary venous flow: (1) the venous channel is long; (2) the channel traverses the diaphragm through the esophageal hiatus and is compressed by either esophageal or diaphragmatic action; (3) the channel narrows at its junction with the portal venous system; and (4) the pulmonary venous blood must traverse the hepatic capillary system before returning to the right atrium by way of the hepatic veins.

The obstruction elevates pulmonary venous pressure. Consequently, pulmonary capillary pressure is raised, leading to pulmonary edema and a dilated pulmonary lymphatic system which removes the pulmonary edema. Pulmonary arterial pressure is elevated because of both elevated pulmonary capillary pressure and reflex pulmonary vasoconstriction. As a result of the pulmonary hypertension, the right ventricle remains thick-walled, does not undergo its normal evolution following birth, and stays relatively noncompliant. As a result the volume of flow into the right ventricle is limited. Because of this reduced pulmonary blood flow, these patients show more intense cyanosis than do patients with total anomalous pulmonary venous connection without obstruction.

The clinical features of total anomalous pulmonary venous connection with obstruction relate to the consequences of pulmonary venous obstruction and to the limited pulmonary blood flow.

History. Patients with total anomalous pulmonary venous connection with obstruction present in the neonatal period with significant cyanosis and respiratory distress. Cyanosis is often intense because of the limited volume of pulmonary flow caused by the obstruction in the venous channel and by the effect of pulmonary hypertension on reducing right ventricular compliance. The cyanosis is accentuated by the pulmonary edema that interferes with oxygen transport from the alveolus to the pulmonary capillary. Respiratory symptoms of tachypnea and dyspnea result from the altered pulmonary compliance produced by pulmonary edema and hypertensive pulmonary arteries.

Physical examination. Cyanosis is present, and increased respiratory effort is manifested by intercostal retractions and tachypnea. On clinical examination the heart size is normal. In unobstructed total anomalous venous connection, systolic and diastolic murmurs originate from increased blood flow across the tricuspid and pulmonary valves, respectively. In patients with obstruction to pulmonary venous flow, however, the volume of flow through the right side of the heart is normal so that no murmurs appear. The accentuated pulmonic component of the second heart sound reflects pulmonary hypertension.

Beyond the immediate neonatal period, the infants appear scrawny and malnourished.

Electrocardiogram. Right ventricular hypertrophy, right axis deviation, and right atrial enlargement are found. In a normal neonate, however, the QRS axis is usually directed toward the right; the P waves may approach 3 mm in amplitude; and the R waves are tall in the right precordial leads. Therefore, the electrocardiograms of neonates with total anomalous pulmonary venous connection can appear similar to those of normal neonates. Such a pattern, however, is compatible with the diagnosis.

Chest X-ray (see Fig. 6.5b). Cardiac size is normal because the volume of systemic and pulmonary blood flows is normal. The pulmonary vasculature shows a diffuse reticular pattern of pulmonary edema. Even in young children,

Kerley B lines, which are small horizontal lines at the margins of the pleura mostly in the lower lung fields, are present. The roentgenographic pattern, although similar to that of hyaline membrane disease, differs from it because it does not usually show air bronchograms.

> Summary of clinical findings. This form of total anomalous pulmonary venous connection is very difficult to distinguish from neonatal pulmonary disease because of similar clinical and laboratory findings. In both, the patients present with respiratory distress and cyanosis in the neonatal period. No murmurs are present. The electrocardiogram may be normal for age; and the chest X-ray shows a normal-sized heart and a diffuse, hazy pattern. Echocardiography may be misleading, so cardiac catheterization and angiography may be necessary to distinguish pulmonary disease from this form of cardiac disease.

Echocardiogram. Because the intracardiac anatomy appears normal and visualization is often limited by pulmonary hyperinflation from aggressive mechanical ventilation used in these neonates, the echocardiographic detection of this lesion is challenging. An atrial septal defect with a right-to-left shunt exists, typical of total anomalous pulmonary venous return, but this finding may also be consistent with severe primary lung disease or persistent pulmonary hypertension. The atrial septal defect flow may be much lower than in the unobstructed form because pulmonary venous obstruction results in very low pulmonary blood flow. The ductus may be large and have bidirectional or predominantly pulmonary artery-to-aorta shunt because of elevated pulmonary arteriolar resistance from pulmonary venous obstruction. Doppler shows no pulmonary venous return to the left atrium; in the most common form, the pulmonary veins return to a common pulmonary vein that courses caudad to the abdomen, usually slightly to the left of the spine.

Cardiac catheterization. As in the unobstructed form, the oxygen saturations are identical in each cardiac chamber, but with this lesion oxygen saturations are extremely low. Pulmonary hypertension is present, and the pulmonary wedge pressure is elevated as well. Angiography shows the anomalous pulmonary venous connection, which is usually connected to an infradiaphragmatic site.

Operative considerations. Infants with total anomalous pulmonary venous connection to an infradiaphragmatic site often die in the neonatal period. As soon as the diagnosis is made, operation is indicated, using the technique described previously. In some infants, pulmonary hypertension persists in the postoperative period for a few days and requires management with mechanical ventilation, creation of an alkalotic state, and administration of nitric oxide and other pulmonary vasodilators.

Summary. Total anomalous pulmonary venous connection, although of several anatomic forms, presents with one of two clinical pictures. In one the pulmonary arterial pressures and right ventricular compliance are normal or slightly elevated. These patients' features resemble atrial septal defect but show mild cyanosis. In the second, pulmonary arterial pressure and pulmonary resistance are elevated because of pulmonary venous obstruction. Therefore, right ventricular compliance is reduced and pulmonary blood flow is limited. These patients show a radiographic pattern of pulmonary venous obstruction or severe cyanosis and major respiratory symptoms. The clinical and laboratory findings resemble neonatal respiratory distress or persistent pulmonary hypertension syndromes.

Truncus arteriosus

In persistent truncus arteriosus (Fig. 6.6), a single arterial blood vessel leaves the heart and feeds both the pulmonary and systemic circulations. This

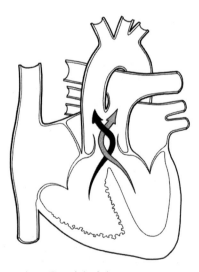

Figure 6.6 Truncus arteriosus. Central circulation.

malformation is always associated with a ventricular septal defect through which both ventricles empty into the truncus arteriosus. Because the defect is large and the truncus arteriosus essentially originates from both ventricles, the right ventricular systolic pressure is identical to that of the left ventricle.

The hemodynamics of persistent truncus arteriosus are similar to those of ventricular septal defect and patent ductus arteriosus because the respective volumes of systemic and pulmonary blood flow depend upon the relative resistances to flow into the systemic circulation and into the pulmonary circulation.

The resistance to flow through the lungs is governed by two factors: (1) the caliber of the pulmonary arterial branches arising from the truncus arteriosus and (2) the pulmonary vascular resistance. Although there are anatomic differences in the size of the pulmonary arterial branches as they originate from the truncus arteriosus, ordinarily their size does not offer significant resistance to pulmonary blood flow, so pulmonary arterial pressure equals that in the truncus arteriosus. Therefore, the pulmonary arteriolar resistance is the primary determinant of pulmonary blood flow. In the neonatal period, when pulmonary vascular resistance is elevated, the volume of blood flow through the lungs is similar to the systemic blood flow. As the pulmonary vasculature matures, the pulmonary blood flow becomes progressively larger.

Many of the clinical and laboratory findings of truncus arteriosus are dependent upon the volume of pulmonary blood flow. Increased pulmonary blood flow leads to three effects: (1) The degree of cyanosis and the volume of pulmonary blood flow are inversely related. The degree of cyanosis lessens as pulmonary blood flow increases because of the larger quantities of fully saturated pulmonary venous return mixing with the relatively fixed systemic venous return. (2) Congestive cardiac failure develops because of left ventricular volume overload. (3) The pulse pressure widens because the blood leaves the truncus arteriosus to enter the pulmonary arteries during diastole.

Although the truncal valve is usually tricuspid, it may become insufficient in some patients, allowing regurgitation into the ventricles. Therefore, an additional volume load that is proportional to the amount of regurgitation is incurred by the ventricles. Some truncal valves have four or more cusps; these are often stenotic as well as insufficient, adding pressure overload to the already volume-overloaded ventricles.

More than 75% of truncus patients show deletion of a portion of chromosome 22 and other laboratory findings of DiGeorge syndrome, such as hypocalcemia and reduced T lymphocytes.

History

The patient's symptoms vary with the volume of pulmonary blood flow. In the neonatal period, cyanosis is the major symptom because the elevated pulmonary vascular resistance limits the pulmonary blood flow. As pulmonary vascular resistance falls, cyanosis lessens, but congestive cardiac failure develops, usually after several weeks of age. Patients with truncus arteriosus and congestive cardiac failure mimic those with ventricular septal defect at this time because cyanosis is mild or absent. Dyspnea on exertion, easy fatigability, and frequent respiratory infections are common symptoms.

Patients whose pulmonary blood flow is limited, either by the development of pulmonary vascular disease or by the presence of small pulmonary arteries arising from the truncus, show predominant symptoms of cyanosis rather than congestive cardiac failure, unless significant regurgitation through the truncal valve coexists.

Physical examination
Cyanosis may or may not be clinically evident but is easily detected with pulse oximetry. Manifestations of a wide pulse pressure may appear if increased pulmonary blood flow or significant truncal valve insufficiency exist. Cardiomegaly and a precordial bulge are common. The auscultatory findings may initially resemble ventricular septal defect. The major auscultatory finding is a loud systolic murmur along the left sternal border. An apical mid-diastolic rumble that is present in most patients indicates large blood flow across the mitral valve due to increased pulmonary blood flow.

Truncus arteriosus shows three distinctive auscultatory findings: (1) The second heart sound is single since only a single semilunar valve is present. (2) A high-pitched early diastolic decrescendo murmur is present if truncal valve insufficiency coexists. (3) An apical systolic ejection click that is usually heard indicates the presence of a dilated great vessel, which in this case is the truncus arteriosus. The click, especially if heard early, suggests that the truncal valve is stenotic to some degree.

Electrocardiogram
The electrocardiogram usually reveals a normal QRS axis and biventricular enlargement/hypertrophy. The left ventricular enlargement is related to the volume overload of the left ventricle; the right ventricular hypertrophy is related to the elevated systolic pressure of the right ventricle. If pulmonary vascular disease develops and reduces pulmonary blood flow, the left ventricular enlargement may disappear. Truncal insufficiency and truncal stenosis modify these findings by augmenting the ventricular volume and by increasing ventricular pressures, respectively.

Chest X-ray
The pulmonary vasculature is increased. The prominent "ascending aorta" which is usually seen represents the truncus arteriosus. Because the branch pulmonary arteries arise from the truncus arteriosus, a main pulmonary artery silhouette is absent. Most patients show cardiomegaly proportionate to the

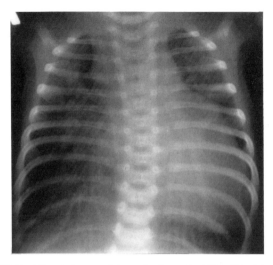

Figure 6.7 Chest X-ray in truncus arteriosus. Cardiomegaly, right aortic arch, and increased pulmonary vascularity.

volume of pulmonary blood flow and the amount of truncal insufficiency. Left atrial enlargement is found in patients with increased pulmonary blood flow.

A right aortic arch is found in one-fourth of patients; this finding, when combined with that of increased pulmonary vascular markings and the presence of cyanosis, is virtually diagnostic of truncus arteriosus (Fig. 6.7).

Summary of clinical findings. Persistent truncus arteriosus is suspected in a cyanotic patient who has a murmur suggesting ventricular septal defect and two characteristic features: a single second heart sound and a systolic ejection click. The volume of pulmonary blood flow is reflected by the degree of cyanosis and the amount of left atrial enlargement. The degree of cardiomegaly on chest X-ray or left ventricular hypertrophy on electrocardiogram is not the sole reflection of pulmonary blood flow, since coexistent truncal insufficiency can also cause these particular findings. DiGeorge syndrome is common.

Natural history
The course in truncus arteriosus resembles that in ventricular septal defect but is more severe; and development of pulmonary vascular disease, the ultimate

threat to longevity and operability, is greatly accelerated. Truncal insufficiency is usually progressive.

Echocardiogram

Cross-sectional echocardiography in views parallel to the long axis of the left ventricular outflow tract shows a large great vessel (the truncus) "overriding" a large ventricular septal defect, similar to images seen in tetralogy of Fallot. A pulmonary artery cannot be demonstrated arising from the heart; the pulmonary arteries arise from the truncus and their pattern of origin is seen by echocardiography. The ductus arteriosus is usually absent unless coexisting interruption of the aortic arch is present. The truncal valve may be trileaflet, with apparent movement similar to that of a normal aortic valve; or it may be deformed, usually as a quadricuspid or multicuspid, with both stenosis and insufficiency. Left atrial enlargement parallels the degree of pulmonary overcirculation.

Cardiac catheterization

Usually, a venous catheter is passed through the right ventricle into the truncus arteriosus and then into the pulmonary arteries. The systolic pressures are identical in both ventricles and in the truncus arteriosus, unless truncal valve stenosis is present. In that case ventricular systolic pressures exceed truncal systolic pressure. A wide pulse pressure is often found in the truncus arteriosus. An increase in oxygen saturation is found in the right ventricle with further increase in the truncus arteriosus. The blood in the truncus arteriosus is not fully saturated. Truncal root injection demonstrates the origin and course of the pulmonary arteries but requires a large volume of contrast that must be administered rapidly to overcome excessive dilution from high pulmonary blood flow.

Operative considerations

For infants manifesting severe cardiac failure who do not to respond to medical management, banding of the pulmonary artery is performed. Although the cardiac failure is improved and the infant grows, the band may complicate and increase the risk of repair. Banding surgery may also be difficult to perform, especially when the pulmonary artery branches arise from separate origins from the truncus.

Corrective operation by the age of 4 weeks is almost always preferable. In this procedure, the ventricular septal defect is closed so that left ventricular blood passes into the truncus arteriosus. The pulmonary arteries are detached from the truncal wall and connected to one end of a valved conduit; its other end is inserted into the right ventricle. If severe, truncal insufficiency can be corrected simultaneously by insertion of a prosthetic valve. The risk is considerably higher for patients with truncal insufficiency, stenosis, or any element of pulmonary vascular disease. Since the conduit from right ventricle to pulmonary arteries is a fixed diameter, reoperation is necessary as the child grows.

Summary. Persistent truncus arteriosus is an infrequently occurring cardiac anomaly whose clinical and laboratory features resemble ventricular septal defect and patent ductus arteriosus with similarities in hemodynamics and natural history. Early corrective operation is advised, but considerable operative risks remain, partially due to the frequent coexistence of DiGeorge syndrome.

CYANOSIS AND DIMINISHED PULMONARY BLOOD FLOW

Patients with cyanosis and roentgenographic evidence of diminished pulmonary blood flow have a cardiac malformation in which both obstruction to pulmonary blood flow and an intracardiac defect that permits a right-to-left shunt are found. The degree of cyanosis varies inversely with the volume of pulmonary blood flow. The amount that pulmonary blood flow is reduced equals the volume of blood shunted in a right-to-left direction.

The intracardiac right-to-left shunt can occur at either the ventricular or the atrial level. In patients with a ventricular shunt, the cardiac size is usually normal, as in tetralogy of Fallot, whereas those with atrial shunts show cardiomegaly, as in tricuspid atresia or Ebstein's malformation.

Tetralogy of Fallot

This is probably the most widely known cardiac condition resulting in cyanosis (Fig. 6.8).

Classically, tetralogy of Fallot has four components: ventricular septal defect; aorta overriding the ventricular septal defect; pulmonary stenosis, generally infundibular in location; and right ventricular hypertrophy. Because of the large ventricular septal defect, right ventricular systolic pressure is at systemic levels.

Hemodynamically, tetralogy of Fallot can be considered a combination of two lesions: a large ventricular septal defect, allowing equalization of ventricular systolic pressures, and severe pulmonary stenosis.

The magnitude of the shunt through the ventricular communication depends upon the relative resistances of the pulmonary stenosis and the systemic circulation. Because the pulmonary stenosis is frequently related to a narrowed infundibulum, it responds to catecholamines and other stimuli. Therefore, the amount of right-to-left shunt and the degree of cyanosis vary considerably with factors such as emotion and exercise. Many of the symptoms of tetralogy of Fallot are related to sudden changes in either of these resistance factors.

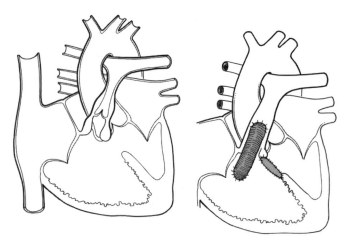

Figure 6.8 Tetralogy of Fallot. Central circulation and surgical repair.

Tetralogy of Fallot with pulmonary valve atresia (Fig. 6.9) has been called pseudotruncus arteriosus. In this anomaly, blood cannot flow directly from the right ventricle into the pulmonary artery, so the entire output from both ventricles is into the aorta. The pulmonary circulation of these patients is supplied either by bronchial arteries acting as collaterals or through a patent ductus arteriosus. Severe hypoxic symptoms may develop in the neonatal period if the patent ductus arteriosus closes or if the bronchial arteries are narrow.

History
The children often become cyanotic in the first year of life, some as early as the neonatal period. The time of appearance and the severity of cyanosis are directly related to the severity of pulmonary stenosis and the degree of reduction of pulmonary blood flow.

Patients with tetralogy of Fallot have three characteristic symptom complexes:

(1) The degree of cyanosis and symptoms are variable; any event that lowers systemic vascular resistance increases the right-to-left shunt and leads to symptoms associated with hypoxemia. Exercise, meals, and hot weather, for example, lower systemic vascular resistance; increase right-to-left shunt; and lead to increased cyanosis.

(2) Hypercyanotic or tetrad spells are uncommon in the current era of early operative correction or palliation with a shunt, but in unoperated patients they consist of episodes in which the child suddenly becomes quite dyspneic and

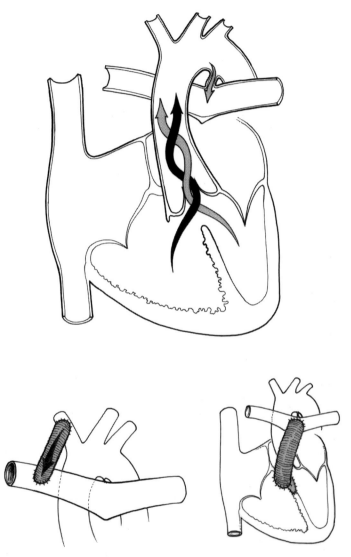

Figure 6.9 Tetralogy of Fallot with pulmonary atresia. Central circulation, showing a patent ductus. Palliative surgery and repair.

intensely cyanotic. Death caused by hypoxia may result unless the spell is properly treated. The mechanism for production of tetrad spells is probably multifactorial. Some believe they result from contraction of the right ventricular infundibulum, thus increasing the degree of pulmonary stenosis. This theory is supported by observations that beta-adrenergic blockers, such as propranolol, which decrease myocardial contractility, relieve the symptoms. Other evidence suggests that a fall in systemic vascular resistance plays an important role in the production of the spells; others attribute them to hyperpnea.

(3) Squatting is virtually diagnostic of tetralogy of Fallot but fortunately is rarely seen any more because of early diagnosis and surgery. During exercise or exertion, the unoperated child squats to rest. Squatting increases systemic vascular resistance, thereby reducing right-to-left shunt. It also briefly increases the systemic venous return; therefore, right ventricular stroke volume and pulmonary blood flow improve.

Congestive cardiac failure does not occur in patients with tetralogy of Fallot. The left ventricle handles a normal volume of blood. Although the right ventricle develops a systemic level of pressure, it tolerates the elevated systolic pressure well, since it has been developing this level of pressure since birth. Furthermore, no matter how severe the pulmonary stenosis, the right ventricular systolic pressure cannot rise above systemic levels because the right ventricle freely communicates with the left ventricle through the ventricular septal defect. Only when another abnormality, such as anemia or bacterial endocarditis, develops can congestive cardiac failure occur.

Children with unoperated tetralogy of Fallot fatigue easily; and as in all types of cyanotic heart disease, severe cyanosis can lead to stroke or brain abscess.

Physical examination

The examination reveals cyanosis and, in older children, clubbing. Cardiac size is normal. The most important auscultatory finding is a harsh systolic ejection murmur located along the middle and upper left sternal border. A thrill may be present. The murmur is caused by the pulmonary stenosis and not by the ventricular septal defect. Although the murmur is not diagnostic of tetralogy of Fallot, the loudness of the murmur is inversely related to the severity of the stenosis. The murmur is softer in patients who have more severe stenosis because the volume of flow through the stenotic area is reduced. This useful clinical fact allows assessment of the severity of the condition and verification that the murmur originates from the right ventricular outflow area and not from the ventricular septal defect.

During a "tetrad" spell, the murmur softens and may disappear.

Patients with tetralogy of Fallot with pulmonary valvar atresia have a continuous murmur representing either patent ductus arteriosus, bronchial collateral arteries, or an operative shunt; an ejection murmur is not heard.

Electrocardiogram
The electrocardiogram reveals right axis deviation, and in more severe cases, right atrial enlargement (Fig. 6.10). Right ventricular hypertrophy is always present and usually is associated with positive T waves in lead V_1.

Chest X-ray
The heart size is normal (Fig. 6.11). The cardiac contour is characteristic. The heart is boot-shaped (coeur en sabot-literally, "heart like a wooden shoe"). The apex is turned upward, and the pulmonary artery segment is concave because the pulmonary artery is small. Right ventricular hypertrophy and right atrial enlargement are evident. The ascending aorta is frequently enlarged, and in at least 25% of the cases, a right aortic arch is present.

> Summary of clinical findings. The history and roentgenographic findings are usually quite diagnostic of tetralogy of Fallot. Once this diagnosis has been made, the loudness of the murmur, character, severity, and frequency of symptoms, pulse oximetry, and level of hemoglobin and hematocrit provide the most reliable indications of the patient's course.

Natural history
Symptoms progress in patients with tetralogy of Fallot because of increasing infundibular stenosis. Increasing frequency or severity of symptoms, rising hemoglobin, and decreasing intensity of the murmur are signs of progression. However, the electrocardiogram and chest X-ray show no change.

Echocardiogram
Cross-sectional echocardiography in views parallel to the long axis of the left ventricular outflow tract shows a large aortic root "overriding" a large ventricular septal defect, similar to the images seen in truncus and double-outlet right ventricle. The pulmonary artery arises from the right ventricle; but the infundibulum, pulmonary valve annulus, and pulmonary arteries appear small.

Color Doppler shows accelerated, turbulent flow through the right ventricular outflow tract; a transition from laminar to disturbed color signals begins at the most proximal site of obstruction, usually the infundibulum.

Cross-sectional echocardiography can define the situs of the aortic arch and the anatomy and size of the proximal pulmonary artery branches. In neonates with tetralogy, the patent ductus often appears as a long, convoluted structure,

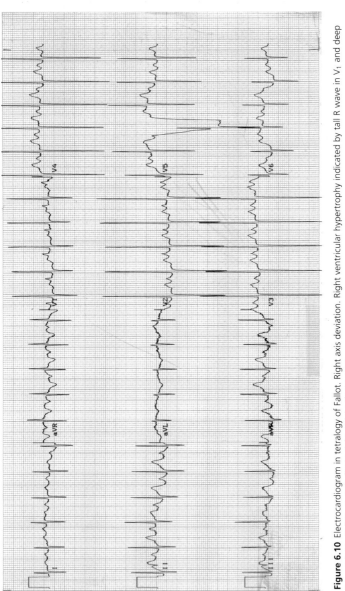

Figure 6.10 Electrocardiogram in tetralogy of Fallot. Right axis deviation. Right ventricular hypertrophy indicated by tall R wave in V_1 and deep S wave in V_6. Tall P waves indicate right atrial enlargement.

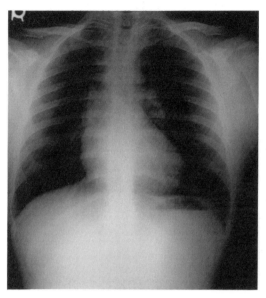

Figure 6.11 Chest X-ray in tetralogy of Fallot. Normal-sized heart and upturned apex. Decreased pulmonary vasculature and concave pulmonary artery segment.

in contrast to the normal neonate's ductal course, which is shorter and more direct.

Cardiac catheterization

The oxygen values through the right side of the heart show no evidence of a left-to-right shunt. Desaturation of aortic blood is found. A pressure drop is present across the outflow area of the right ventricle; the body of the right ventricle has the same pressure as the left ventricle, and the pulmonary arterial pressure is lower than normal; however, catheter placement across the right ventricular outflow tract is avoided to minimize the risk of infundibular spasm and hypercyanotic spells ("tetrad" spells).

Right ventricular angiography defines the anatomic details of the right ventricular outflow area. Such studies demonstrate the site of the stenosis in the right ventricle, outline the pulmonary arterial tree, and show opacification of the aorta through the ventricular septal defect. Aortic root injection may be indicated to define anomalies of coronary artery branching that occasionally occur and that may result in operative catastrophe if unrecognized.

Medical management

Most infants with tetralogy and favorable anatomy for repair require no medical therapy before corrective operation.

As in all patients with cyanotic cardiac malformations, the development of iron deficiency anemia must be prevented or promptly treated when it develops because increased symptoms occur in anemic patients.

> Remember that a cyanotic patient with a "normal" hemoglobin concentration (e.g., 12 g/dL) is functionally anemic: they may not have sufficient hemoglobin to counteract their level of hypoxemia.

Infants and children with tetrad spells (see Appendix C) should be treated by the administration of 100% oxygen (which increases systemic resistance while decreasing pulmonary resistance), by placing the child in a knee/chest position, and by having the parent console and quiet the child. Morphine or ultra-short-acting beta-blockers may be indicated. Systemic vascular resistance is increased with alpha-agonists like phenylephrine. Intravenous fluid by bolus injection may improve right ventricular performance; diuretics are contraindicated. Intractable tetrad spells may improve with intubation, paralysis, and ventilation to decrease oxygen consumption in preparation for performance of an emergency operation.

Operative considerations

Palliation. In very small infants, those with very small pulmonary arteries, or depending on the capabilities of the cardiac center, a palliative operation may be the initial surgical approach.

Several palliative procedures have been used since the first Blalock–Taussig shunt (anastomosing a subclavian artery to a branch pulmonary artery), performed in 1945. Because of early difficulties in anastomosing small subclavian arteries, the Waterston shunt (creating a communication between the right pulmonary artery and the ascending aorta) and the Potts procedure (creating a communication between the left pulmonary artery and the descending aorta) were developed. Neither the Potts nor the Waterston are currently used because of the tendency to create too large a communication, resulting in pulmonary vascular disease.

Modified Blalock–Taussig shunts, consisting of a synthetic tube (polytetrafluoroethylene or GoreTex), usually 4 mm in diameter, that connects a subclavian artery and a branch pulmonary artery, are commonly used to palliate infants with significant cyanosis. These procedures are also indicated for older children with tetralogy of Fallot whose pulmonary arteries are too small for corrective operation. Each of these operations allows an increased volume of pulmonary blood flow and improves arterial saturation.

Corrective repair. Tetralogy of Fallot can be corrected by closing the ventricular septal defect, by resecting the pulmonary stenosis, and often, by inserting a right ventricular outflow tract patch. Corrective operations are usually performed in infants in lieu of performing a palliative procedure. In the absence of complicating anatomy, such as small pulmonary arteries, the operative mortality in infants several months of age is less than 1%. Early operative results are good; very few patients have congestive cardiac failure as a consequence of the right ventriculotomy or require reoperation because of residual cardiac anomalies, such as persistent outflow obstruction or ventricular septal defect.

Patients with tetralogy with pulmonary atresia may require multiple operations to rehabilitate stenotic or disconnected pulmonary artery segments and may ultimately have conduits placed from right ventricle to pulmonary artery. Reoperation is frequently necessary as these patients outgrow and/or stenose the conduit.

Patients who have a normal pulmonary annulus diameter may have resection of the infundibular stenosis without right ventriculotomy and have good pulmonary valve function postoperatively. Long-term complications in patients repaired this way may be less than in those with classical repair with its accompanying transmural right ventricular scar and marked pulmonary valve regurgitation from removal of the valve and enlargement of the annulus using an outflow tract patch.

Despite highly successful corrective operations for tetralogy of Fallot that have been performed for a number of years, long-term risks still include right and left ventricular dysfunction, arrhythmias, and sudden death.

Summary. Tetralogy of Fallot is a frequent form of cyanotic congenital heart disease. The symptoms, physical examination, and laboratory features are characteristic. Several signs and symptoms permit evaluation of the natural progression of pulmonary stenosis. Several types of operations are available with a goal of complete correction. Long-term risks persist even for well-repaired patients.

Tricuspid atresia

In this malformation (Fig. 6.12), the tricuspid valve and the inflow portion of the right ventricle do not develop, so no direct communication exists between the right atrium and the right ventricle. Therefore, the circulation is severely altered. The systemic venous return entering the right atrium flows entirely in a right-to-left direction into the left atrium through either an atrial septal defect or a patent foramen ovale.

In the left atrium, the systemic venous return mixes with the pulmonary venous blood and is delivered to the left ventricle. The left ventricle ejects

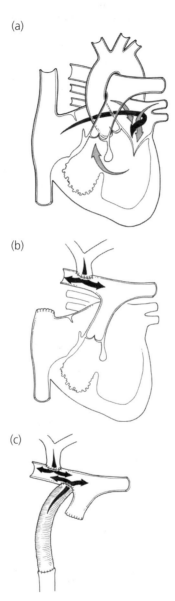

Figure 6.12 Tricuspid atresia and normally related great vessels. (a) Central circulation. Surgical options: (b) bidirectional Glenn; (c) Fontan.

blood into the aorta and, in most instances, through a ventricular septal defect, into a rudimentary right ventricle and then into the pulmonary artery. Usually, the ventricular septal defect is small. The right ventricle is hypoplastic, and frequently pulmonary stenosis coexists. Therefore, a high degree of resistance to blood flow into the lungs is present. In most patients with tricuspid atresia, the pulmonary blood flow is reduced.

In one-fourth of patients with tricuspid atresia, transposition of the great vessels coexists; therefore, the pulmonary artery arises from the left ventricle and the aorta arises from the hypoplastic right ventricle. In such patients, the pulmonary blood flow is greatly increased because of the relatively low pulmonary vascular resistance and the increased resistance to systemic blood flow caused by the systemic vascular resistance from a small ventricular septal defect and a hypoplastic right ventricle.

In all forms of tricuspid atresia, both the systemic and pulmonary venous returns mix in the left atrium; tricuspid atresia is an admixture lesion and the degree of cyanosis is inversely related to the volume of pulmonary blood flow. Therefore, the patient with tricuspid atresia and normally related great vessels is more cyanotic than the patient with tricuspid atresia and transposition of the great vessels. The degree of cyanosis is useful in following the course of the patient.

Two aspects of the circulation are important in influencing the course of patients and in directing the therapy. First, in many patients an ample-sized atrial septal defect is present, in contrast to patients who have only a patent foramen ovale, in which severe obstruction exists.

The second aspect relates to the volume of pulmonary blood flow. Usually, pulmonary blood flow is reduced, so the resultant hypoxia and related symptoms require palliation. But patients with markedly increased pulmonary blood flow, usually related to coexistent transposition of the great vessels, develop congestive cardiac failure because of volume overload on the left ventricle.

History
Children with tricuspid atresia are generally symptomatic in infancy and show cyanosis. Hypoxic spells may be present, but squatting is rare. In the patient with increased pulmonary blood flow, cyanosis may be slight; and the dominant clinical features relate to congestive cardiac failure. An unusual patient with the "proper" amount of pulmonary stenosis may be relatively asymptomatic for years.

Physical examination
The physical findings are not diagnostic of tricuspid atresia. Cyanosis is generally evident and is frequently intense. The liver is enlarged if congestive cardiac failure or an obstructing atrial communication are present. In a third of the patients, either no murmur or a very soft murmur is present, indicating marked

reduction in pulmonary blood flow. In patients with a large ventricular septal defect or with coexistent transposition of the great vessels, a grade 3/6–4/6 murmur is present along the left sternal border; in these patients an apical diastolic murmur may also be found. The second heart sound is single.

Electrocardiogram

Electrocardiogram is usually diagnostic of tricuspid atresia (Fig. 6.13). Left axis deviation is almost uniformly present and is typically between 0 and −60°. Tall, peaked P waves of right atrial enlargement and a short PR interval are common features. Because the right ventricle is rudimentary, it contributes little to the total electrical forces forming the QRS complex. Therefore, the precordial leads show a pattern of left ventricular hypertrophy with an rS complex in lead V_1 and a tall R wave in V_6. This precordial pattern is particularly striking in infancy because of the marked difference from the normal infantile pattern of tall R waves in the right precordium. In older patients, the T waves become inverted in the left precordial leads.

Chest X-ray

The pulmonary vasculature is decreased in most patients; but in those with transposition of the great vessels or large ventricular septal defect, it is of course increased. Cardiac size is almost universally increased, with a cardiac contour highly suggestive of tricuspid atresia because of the prominent right heart border (enlarged right atrium) and the prominent left heart border (enlarged left ventricle).

Summary of clinical findings. In patients with cyanosis, the electrocardiogram presents the most important diagnostic clue. The combination of left axis deviation and pattern of left ventricular enlargement/hypertrophy is highly suggestive of tricuspid atresia. The roentgenographic findings also help if the pulmonary vasculature is decreased. The auscultatory findings and history are not diagnostic but are useful for providing clues about the condition's severity.

Echocardiogram

The diagnosis is easily confirmed by demonstrating that the tricuspid valve is absent using the four-chamber cross-sectional view obtained from the apex. An atrial septal defect is seen, and an obligatory right-to-left atrial shunt is demonstrated by Doppler. If the great vessels are normally related, Doppler is used to define the degree of obstruction to pulmonary blood flow (at the ventricular septal defect, right ventricular infundibulum, and/or the pulmonary valve). If the great vessels are malposed, Doppler is used to estimate the degree

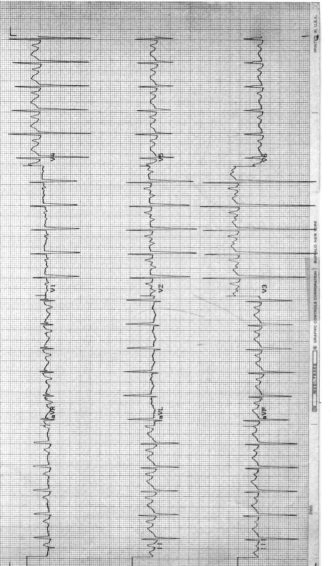

Figure 6.13 Electrocardiogram in tricuspid atresia. Left axis deviation (−45°). Right atrial enlargement.

of obstruction to aortic outflow. Doppler estimates of obstruction performed in neonates with tricuspid atresia may mislead the physician because the gradient is minimal in the presence of the large patent ductus and relatively high pulmonary vascular resistance at this stage of life and because narrowing of the muscular portions of the outflow pathway (ventricular septal defect and infundibulum) increases with age and hypertrophy.

Cardiac catheterization

Oximetry data reveal a right-to-left shunt at the atrial level. The oxygen values in the left ventricle, aorta, and pulmonary artery are similar; they are inversely related to pulmonary blood flow. In some cases the right atrial pressure is elevated, indicating a restricted interatrial communication. Patients who are surgical candidates for a cavopulmonary connection should have documented normal left ventricular end-diastolic pressure and normal pulmonary vascular resistance.

Left ventriculography shows simultaneous opacification of both great vessels and permits identification of the level of obstruction to pulmonary blood flow.

If cardiac catheterization is done in infancy, a balloon atrial septostomy may be performed at the same time to reduce obstruction to flow into the left atrium.

Operative considerations

Various palliative procedures are available for patients with tricuspid atresia.

Pulmonary artery banding. This is indicated in infants with increased pulmonary blood flow and is often performed by 1–3 months of age. It is an essential step in protecting the pulmonary vascular bed from high flow and pressure, in consideration for future palliative surgery.

Modified Blalock–Taussig (GoreTex interposition) shunt. This, or similar shunt, is performed in neonates with markedly reduced pulmonary blood flow.

After several weeks to months of age, when pulmonary resistance has fallen sufficiently, a cavopulmonary anastomosis (connecting systemic venous return directly into the pulmonary arteries without an intervening pump) is considered.

"Bidirectional" Glenn procedure or "Hemi-Fontan". This is an anastomosis of the end of the superior vena cava to the roof of the right pulmonary artery allowing systemic venous blood to pass into both pulmonary arteries. It is often done as the first part of a staged cavopulmonary anastomosis.

Complete cavopulmonary anastomosis (Fontan procedure). This is available for older patients with tricuspid atresia and normally related great vessels after a previous bidirectional Glenn procedure. With this operation, the inferior vena caval return is conducted to the pulmonary arteries, usually via a conduit coursing through or external to the right atrium. This effectively separates the pulmonary venous and systemic venous returns, like a normal heart; but unlike normal, no ventricle pumps blood between systemic veins and pulmonary arteries. Therefore, the Fontan procedure can be considered palliative but not corrective.

The long-term results of the Fontan procedure are variable. Some patients develop complications from chronically elevated systemic venous pressure, such as pleural, pericardial, and ascitic effusions; liver dysfunction; and protein-losing enteropathy. Stroke and arrhythmia are long-term risks. Many patients who appear well palliated for years after the Fontan procedure develop heart failure from left ventricular dysfunction of unknown cause, but it is probably independent of the type of palliation, since ventricular dysfunction develops in patients with Blalock–Taussig and other aorticopulmonary shunts. Some speculate that the myocardium is congenitally myopathic in many tricuspid atresia patients.

Summary. Children with tricuspid atresia present with cyanosis and cardiac failure. A murmur may or may not be present. The electrocardiogram reveals left axis deviation, right atrial enlargement, and left ventricular enlargement/hypertrophy. Chest X-rays show right atrial and left ventricular enlargement. Palliative, but not corrective, operations are available.

Pulmonary atresia with intact ventricular septum

In this malformation (Fig. 6.14), the pulmonary valve is atretic; no direct blood flow exists from the right ventricle to the pulmonary artery; and the right ventricle is usually hypoplastic. In a few neonates, significant tricuspid regurgitation is present; in these patients, the right ventricle is enlarged. An atrial communication, either foramen ovale or atrial septal defect that allows a right-to-left shunt, is present. Pulmonary blood flow depends entirely upon a patent ductus arteriosus. As the ductus arteriosus closes in the neonatal period, the infant becomes progressively more hypoxic.

History

Patients present in the neonatal period with progressive cyanosis and its complications. Features of congestive cardiac failure may appear if the atrial communication is small or if left ventricular dysfunction is present.

Physical examination

The infant presents with intense cyanosis and dyspnea. In many patients no murmur is present; however, in some a soft, continuous murmur of patent

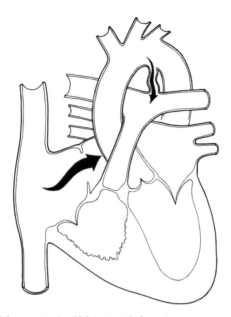

Figure 6.14 Pulmonary atresia with intact ventricular septum.

ductus arteriosus is found. In neonates with tricuspid regurgitation, a holosystolic murmur is heard along the lower left and right sternal border. The second heart sound is single. Hepatomegaly is present if the atrial septal defect is restrictive.

Electrocardiogram
The electrocardiogram usually shows a normal QRS axis. Peaked P waves of right atrial enlargement usually appear. Since the right ventricle is hypoplastic, the precordial leads show an rS complex in lead V_1 and an R wave in lead V_6. This pattern resembles left ventricular hypertrophy and contrasts strikingly with the normal pattern for a newborn. The T waves are usually normal. If tricuspid regurgitation and an enlarged right ventricle are present, a pattern of right ventricular hypertrophy is found.

Chest X-ray
The pulmonary vasculature is reduced. The cardiac contour resembles tricuspid atresia by showing prominent right atrial and left ventricular borders. The cardiac size is enlarged.

> Summary of clinical findings. In a cyanotic infant, the combination of roentgenographic findings of cardiomegaly and reduced pulmonary vascular markings and left ventricular enlargement/hypertrophy on electrocardiogram suggests the diagnosis of pulmonary atresia. This condition may be distinguished from tricuspid atresia by the difference in the QRS axis, but this distinction is not completely reliable.

Echocardiogram

Cross-sectional echocardiography shows a small hypertrophied, poorly contracting right ventricle and no motion at the location of the pulmonary valve, which appears platelike. The tricuspid valve motion may appear so limited by poor flow into the blindly ending right ventricle that, echocardiographically, the diagnosis may be confused with tricuspid atresia. In contrast to tricuspid atresia, Doppler usually demonstrates some tricuspid regurgitation. If marked tricuspid valve regurgitation is present, the right ventricle is enlarged. The right ventricular systolic pressure (which can be estimated from the tricuspid regurgitation velocity) is often suprasystemic (i.e., greater than that of the left ventricle).

As in tricuspid atresia and total anomalous pulmonary venous connection, an atrial septal defect with right-to-left atrial shunt is present.

The patent ductus, which shows a continuous aorta-to-pulmonary-artery shunt, appears long and convoluted, similar to that seen in tricuspid atresia and in tetralogy of Fallot with pulmonary atresia.

Left ventricular function may be subnormal, especially if abnormal right-ventricle-to-coronary-artery connections (sinusoids) are present. These connections are often demonstrated with color Doppler.

Cardiac catheterization

The oxygen saturation shows a right-to-left shunt at the atrial level and marked systemic arterial oxygen desaturation because of severe limitation of pulmonary blood flow. The right atrial pressure is often elevated because of a narrowed atrial communication. The hypoplastic right ventricle, entered with a catheter via the tricuspid valve, reveals high (often suprasystemic) pressure.

Right atrial angiography shows a right-to-left shunt at the atrial level and resembles tricuspid atresia. Left ventriculography usually distinguishes this defect from those conditions because the ventricular septal defect and right ventricular outflow areas are not visualized in pulmonary atresia; instead the aorta is opacified, and subsequently, the pulmonary artery opacifies by a patent ductus arteriosus. The right ventricle may be very cautiously injected by hand with a small volume. This allows determination of the distance between the right ventricle cavity and the main pulmonary artery (filled from the ductus with a separate injection). Abnormal connections, called sinusoids, between the right ventricular cavity and coronary arteries may be seen filling from the right ventricle. They represent a poor prognostic sign, since myocardial function may depend on retrograde perfusion, and limit operative efforts to return the right ventricular pressure to normal.

Operative considerations
Neonates require emergency palliation with prostaglandin to maintain ductal patency. A pulmonary valvotomy, usually surgical (or using various transcatheter methods to puncture and then balloon dilate the valve), is performed in the hope that the hypoplastic right ventricle will grow in size and compliance. Even if adequate pulmonary valvotomy is achieved, a large right-atrium-to-left-atrium shunt persists due to the small, poorly compliant right ventricle. A modified Blalock–Taussig shunt is then performed to take the place of the ductus. Pulmonary valvotomy may be contraindicated in infants with retrograde coronary artery flow via sinusoids, the so-called RV-dependent coronary circulation.

Summary. Pulmonary atresia resembles tricuspid atresia with normally related great vessels in hemodynamics, clinical and laboratory findings, and operative considerations. In both conditions the severity of symptoms is related to the adequacy of the communication between the atria and to the volume of pulmonary blood flow. The conditions are distinguished by the difference in the QRS axis.

Ebstein's malformation of the tricuspid valve
In Ebstein's malformation (Fig. 6.15), the leaflets of the tricuspid valve attach to the right ventricular wall rather than to the tricuspid valve annulus. The tricuspid valve is displaced into the right ventricle, so a part of the right ventricle between the tricuspid annulus and the displaced tricuspid valve (the "atrialized" portion) is functionally part of the right atrial chamber. An atrial septal defect is usually a component of the malformation.

The malformation has two hemodynamic consequences. First, the tricuspid valve frequently permits tricuspid regurgitation. Second, the portion of the right ventricle between the tricuspid and pulmonary valves is small and noncompliant. As a result, right ventricular inflow is impeded so that a right-to-left shunt exists at the atrial level and decreases pulmonary blood flow.

History
Patients frequently have a history of variable cyanosis being cyanotic in the first week of life, then acyanotic or minimally cyanotic for a variable period, only to become increasingly cyanotic later in life. As pulmonary vascular resistance

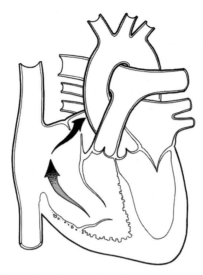

Figure 6.15 Ebstein's malformation. Central circulation.

decreases in the neonatal period, the symptomatic neonate improves from a decrease in resistance to pulmonary blood flow. In patients whose valve is more deformed and further displaced into the right ventricle, cyanosis is greater and survival less likely. Congestive cardiac failure may also be present in those with more severe forms but, transiently, in those neonates with less abnormal anatomy. Supraventricular tachycardia or atrial flutter, related to the right atrial dilation, and in some, to preexcitation (Wolf–Parkinson–White syndrome), may coexist.

Physical examination
Cyanosis is minimal or absent. A precordial bulge may be found. The auscultatory findings are characteristic. A quadruple rhythm is often present. Both the first and second heart sounds are split. A fourth heart sound may be present. Usually, a holosystolic murmur of variable intensity that indicates tricuspid insufficiency is found. In addition, a rough mid-diastolic murmur is often heard in the tricuspid area.

Electrocardiogram
The electrocardiographic features are characteristic (Fig. 6.16). Right atrial enlargement is evident and the P wave may be 8 or 9 mm in height. The QRS

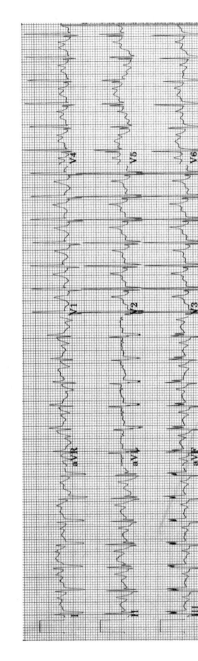

Figure 6.16 Electrocardiogram in Ebstein's malformation. Indeterminate frontal–plane QRS axis. Tall P waves indicate right atrial enlargement. Right bundle branch block with an rSR′ pattern in V$_1$.

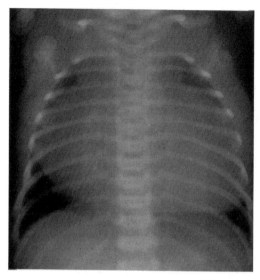

Figure 6.17 Chest X-ray in Ebstein's malformation. Massive cardiomegaly (so-called wall-to-wall heart) and decreased pulmonary vascularity.

duration is prolonged because of complete right bundle branch block or Wolff–Parkinson–White syndrome which is present in 20% of patients. The precordial leads show a pattern of ventricular hypertrophy and the R wave in lead V_1 rarely exceeds 10 mm in height.

Chest X-ray

The heart is enlarged, possibly having a boxlike configuration. The right atrium is enlarged. In neonates with severe right atrial enlargement, cardiomegaly may be massive (Fig. 6.17). The pulmonary vascular markings are diminished.

Echocardiogram

Cross-sectional four-chamber views demonstrate the apical displacement of the tricuspid valve within the right ventricle. The right atrium is markedly dilated. The cross-sectional area of the right atrium and the atrialized portion of right ventricle, when compared with the area of the remaining right ventricle, left atrium, and left ventricle, has been shown to correlate with survival. Patients with the most-displaced tricuspid valves and the largest right atria do less well. Doppler shows tricuspid regurgitation that varies in severity among patients. A right-to-left atrial shunt is generally present.

Cardiac catheterization

The oximetry data show a right-to-left shunt at the atrial level. Right ventricular pressure is normal, while right atrial pressure is elevated. Angiography may be diagnostic in showing the abnormal position of the tricuspid valve, reduced right ventricular size, enlarged right atrium, and right-to-left atrial shunt. Arrhythmias are common during catheterization, so the patient must be monitored carefully and treated promptly.

Operative considerations

The preferred approach is avoidance of operation. Shunt procedures should be avoided, since within the first few days of life, cyanosis may improve as pulmonary vascular resistance falls and right ventricular compliance improves somewhat. A shunt procedure is indicated for those patients with persistent and markedly reduced pulmonary blood flow. In some older patients, particularly those with congestive failure, an operation to reconstruct the tricuspid valve may be possible, otherwise, a prosthetic valve is placed in the tricuspid annulus; the huge right atrium is reduced in size by resection.

Summary. The diagnosis of Ebstein's malformation can usually be made clinically because of the history and auscultatory and electrocardiographic findings. Palliative procedures are available.

SUMMARY OF CYANOTIC LESIONS
Cardiac conditions with cyanosis generally present in the neonatal period or are recognized before birth by fetal echocardiography. While many are complex conditions, in most a corrective or palliative procedure can be performed. With prompt recognition of the neonate, correct diagnosis, medical management (usually including prostaglandin), operation can be performed with relatively low risk and good results considering the size and condition of the neonate.

Chapter 7
Other congenital cardiac anomalies

Congenitally corrected transposition of the great arteries (I-TGV)
Malposition of the heart
    Situs solitus
    Dextrocardia
    Levocardia
Splenic anomalies (heterotaxy syndromes; atrial isomerism)
    Asplenia syndrome (bilateral right-sidedness)
    Polysplenia syndrome (bilateral left-sidedness)
Vascular ring
    Right aortic arch
    Double aortic arch
    Aberrant subclavian artery
Vascular (pulmonary artery) sling

CONGENITALLY CORRECTED TRANSPOSITION OF THE GREAT ARTERIES (I-TGV)

As mentioned earlier, the term *transposition* means a reversal of anteroposterior anatomic relationships. Therefore, in transposition of the great arteries, the aorta arises anteriorly; and the pulmonary artery arises posteriorly. Normally, the anterior blood vessel arises from the infundibulum, which is the outflow portion of the morphologic right ventricle.

In congenitally corrected transposition of the great arteries, these abnormal anatomic relationships are present, but the circulation is physiologically correct (i.e., systemic venous return is delivered to the pulmonary arteries; pulmonary venous return is delivered to the aorta).

The anatomy of congenitally corrected transposition of the great arteries differs from complete transposition of the great arteries (d-TGV) because ventricular inversion coexists. The term *inversion* indicates an anatomic change in the left–right relationships. Therefore, inversion of the ventricles indicates that the morphologic right ventricle lies on the left side and that the morphologic

Pediatric Cardiology, by W Johnson, J Moller © 2008 Blackwell Publishing, ISBN: 978-1-4051-7818-1.

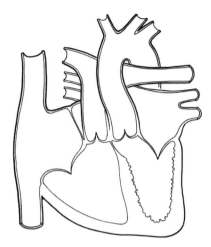

Figure 7.1 Congenitally corrected transposition of the great vessels (l-TGV). In addition to levo-transposed great vessels, ventricular inversion is found. The morphologic right ventricle (trabeculated) is left-sided and is connected to the left atrium (fully oxygenated blood) and the aorta. The morphologic left ventricle is right-sided and is connected to the right atrium (deoxygenated blood) and the pulmonary artery. Therefore, the circulation is physiologically correct.

left ventricle lies on the right side. The inversion of the ventricles in corrected transposition of the great arteries allows the circulation to flow in a normal pattern (Fig. 7.1).

The systemic venous return from the inferior and superior venae cavae passes into the normally positioned right atrium. This blood then flows into a ventricle that has these morphologic features of a left ventricle: it has a mitral valve; it is a finely trabeculated chamber; and it has a fibrous continuity between the atrioventricular and semilunar valves, which in this instance are mitral and pulmonary. This ventricle is located to the right of the other ventricle. This anatomic left ventricle ejects blood into a posteriorly and medially placed pulmonary artery (transposition).

The pulmonary venous blood returns into the normally placed left atrium. The flow then crosses a tricuspid valve into a ventricle having the morphologic features of a right ventricle: it is coarsely trabeculated; it has a tricuspid valve; and the atrioventricular and semilunar valves are separated by an infundibulum. The aorta arises from the infundibulum and lies anteriorly and leftward from the pulmonary artery.

The flow of blood, therefore, is normal and the anatomic relationship of the great vessels fulfills the definition of transposition of the great arteries. This type of transposition has also been termed levo-transposition because the aorta lies to the left of the pulmonary artery.

This condition alone would lead to no cardiovascular symptoms or murmurs (although there are concerns of the ability of the systemic ventricle to sustain the systemic circulation). However, virtually all patients with congenitally corrected transposition have other coexisting cardiac anomalies. Ventricular septal defect, pulmonary stenosis, and insufficiency of the left-sided atrioventricular valve are the most common cardiac anomalies in these patients.

These coexistent anomalies lead to clinical and laboratory findings similar to those found in patients with the same anomaly but with normal relationships among the ventricles and the great vessels.

Three clinical findings, however, allow detection of congenitally corrected transposition of the great arteries as the underlying cardiac malformation.

The second heart sound is loud and single and is best heard along the upper left sternal border (in the so-called pulmonary area). Because the aorta is located anteriorly and leftward, the aortic valve lies immediately beneath this area. The second sound appears single because the pulmonary valve is distant (posteriorly positioned), so its component is inaudible.

On chest X-ray, the left cardiac border is straight or shows only two rounded contours (the upper being the leftward positioned ascending aorta and the lower the inverted right ventricle). In contrast to that, patients with normally related great vessels have three contours—aortic knob, pulmonary trunk, and left ventricular border.

Electrocardiographic findings are distinctive, related to ventricular inversion. The bundles of His are also inverted, so the ventricular septum depolarizes from right to left, opposite of normal. This leads to a Q wave in lead V_1 and an initial positive deflection in lead V_6 (opposite the normal pattern of an initial R wave in lead V_1 and a Q wave in lead V_6). Such a pattern is present in almost all patients with congenitally corrected transposition of the great arteries. A word of caution: patients with severe right ventricular hypertrophy may also show such a pattern, so this electrocardiographic finding alone does not diagnose corrected transposition of the great arteries.

Patients with congenitally corrected transposition of the great arteries often spontaneously develop partial or complete heart block.

While the basic anatomic anomaly in congenitally corrected transposition of the great arteries does not require treatment, hemodynamically significant coexistent conditions do, generally by operation.

MALPOSITION OF THE HEART

The heart may assume an abnormal position in the thorax in either the left or the right side of the chest. Various classifications of cardiac malposition have been developed, but the authors favor the one presented here, although the terminology may differ from that of other authors.

Certain anatomic features are important in understanding cardiac malpositions. In normal patients and virtually all those with cardiac malposition, certain fundamental anatomic relations are constant.

The inferior vena cava (at the diaphragm), the anatomic right atrium, and the major lobe of the liver are located on one side of the body, whereas the aorta (at the diaphragm), the anatomic left atrium, and the stomach are located on the opposite side of the body.

The inferior vena cava is crucial in our considerations, as it is an important link between the abdominal and thoracic contents.

Situs solitus

Situs solitus (Fig. 7.2) describes the anatomic relationships in the normal individual wherein the liver, inferior vena cava, and right atrium are present on the right side of the body; meanwhile, the stomach, aorta, and left atrium are present on the left side.

Dextrocardia

This is a general term indicating that the cardiac apex is located in the right side of the chest.

Three anatomic variations associated with dextrocardia are presented here.

Situs inversus totalis (mirror image dextrocardia)

This condition is the opposite of the usual situs solitus (Fig. 7.2). The inferior vena cava, the major lobe of the liver, and the right atrium are located on the left side of the body. This has also been termed mirror image dextrocardia because the anatomic relationships are exactly the reverse of normal. Other anatomic findings include the presence of two lobes in the right lung, three lobes in the left lung, and of the appendix in the left lower quadrant.

Situs inversus is probably associated with an increased incidence of cardiac anomalies, but the type and distribution of the anomalies parallel those of patients with situs solitus.

About 40% of patients have ciliary dyskinesia, usually Kartagener syndrome, characterized by chronic sinusitis, bronchitis/bronchiectasis, and sterility.

Dextroversion with situs solitus

In this condition, the fundamental anatomic relationships of situs solitus are present; but the cardiac apex is directed toward the right (Fig. 7.2). The atria are anchored by the venae cavae, but the ventricles can rotate on the long axis of the heart and lie in the midline or right chest.

In dextroversion, the heart may show one of two anatomic forms.

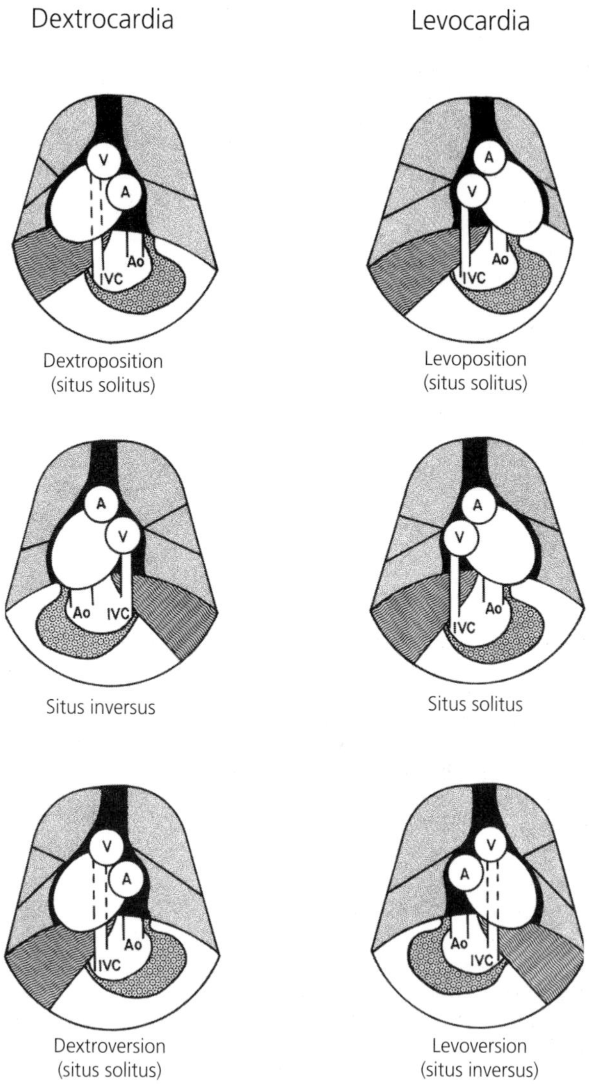

Figure 7.2 Diagrams of malposition of the heart. (Abbreviations: Ao, aorta; IVC, inferior vena cava; V, venous atrium; A, arterial atrium.)

In the first, the ventricles are normally related; and ventricular septal defect and pulmonary stenosis are common.

In the other form, corrected transposition of the great arteries and inversion of the ventricles are present. These patients show the type of cardiac anomalies commonly found with corrected transposition of the great arteries.

Dextroposition of the heart

This is another condition with the situs solitus relationship and the cardiac apex in the right side of the chest (Fig. 7.2). In this instance, cardiac displacement toward the right is caused by extrinsic factors, such as hypoplasia of the right lung. In many patients with dextroposition of the heart, cardiac anomalies coexist. The anomalies are often associated with a left-to-right shunt; the patients often develop pulmonary vascular disease. A common cause of dextroposition in the neonate with a structurally normal heart is left-sided congenital diaphragmatic hernia, in which distended gut in the left side of the chest forces the heart and mediastinal structures toward the right.

Levocardia

Levocardia is a general term indicating that the cardiac apex is located in the left side of the chest. Situs solitus is one form of levocardia; but, in other conditions, the cardiac apex may be located abnormally in the left side of the chest.

Levoversion of situs inversus

This anatomic relationship is the opposite of dextroversion of situs solitus (Fig. 7.2). The basic anatomic relationship is situs inversus, but the cardiac apex is located in the left side of the chest. As might be expected, many of these patients have corrected transposition of the great arteries.

Levoposition

In patients with situs solitus, the left lung may be hypoplastic, so the heart is displaced farther into the left hemithorax than normal. When this condition exists in a patient with a cardiac anomaly, a tendency to develop pulmonary vascular disease exists.

SPLENIC ANOMALIES (HETEROTAXY SYNDROMES; ATRIAL ISOMERISM)

In each of the conditions discussed earlier, the fundamental anatomic relationships are present among the inferior vena cava, liver, and right atrium and among the descending aorta, stomach, and left atrium. Unusual conditions are associated with cardiac malposition in which these anatomic relationships are not present and in which the spleen is usually abnormal. These conditions have been named after the type of splenic anomaly.

Asplenia syndrome (bilateral right-sidedness)

In this syndrome, the heart may be located in either the left or the right side of the chest, the spleen is absent, and numerous visceral and cardiac anomalies are found. The visceral anomalies reflect a tendency toward symmetrical organ development, with paired organs each having the form of the right-sided organ; left-sided structures are absent. Thus, each lung has three lobes (like a right lung); the spleen, a left-sided structure, is absent; and the liver is symmetrical. Malrotation of the bowel is often present.

Cardiac anomalies are complex, including atrial and ventricular septal defects, often in the form of endocardial cushion defect; severe pulmonary stenosis or atresia; transposition of the great arteries; and often total anomalous pulmonary venous connection. This combination of anomalies leads to clinical and roentgenographic features that resemble severe tetralogy of Fallot. Despite palliative procedures, the outlook for these patients is often bleak.

Because of the symmetry of the liver, malrotation of the bowel, and midline position of the inferior vena cava, the important anatomic relationships that allow definition of situs are disrupted, so classifying the type of cardiac malposition in patients with asplenia is difficult.

Polysplenia syndrome (bilateral left-sidedness)

In this syndrome, as in asplenia, the heart may be located in either the left or the right side of the chest. The spleen is present but is divided into multiple masses. A tendency to symmetrical organ development also exists, in this case bilateral left-sidedness, in which both lungs appear as the left lung, the gallbladder is absent, and there are multiple spleens. Malrotation of the bowel often occurs.

Cardiac anomalies include atrial and/or ventricular septal defect, partial anomalous pulmonary venous connection, and interrupted inferior vena cava with azygous continuation.

The clinical picture resembles that of left-to-right shunt. The prognosis is good and many patients undergo corrective operation.

As in asplenia, difficulty is encountered in determining situs because of the malrotation of the bowel and the fact that the inferior vena cava is interrupted at the level of the diaphragm.

VASCULAR RING

Normally, no vascular structure passes behind the esophagus, but in some anomalies the aortic arch or a major arch vessel lies behind the esophagus; this phenomenon is called vascular ring. Radiographic barium swallow and echocardiography are the most useful noninvasive means of confirming the diagnosis. CTA, MRI/MRA, or catheterization with aortography are often used to provide detailed anatomic information prior to surgical intervention.

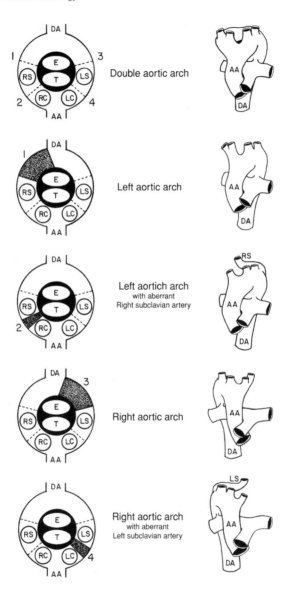

Double aortic arch

Left aortic arch

Left aortich arch
with aberrant
Right subclavian artery

Right aortic arch

Right aortic arch
with aberrant
Left subclavian artery

An understanding of the anatomic variations of vascular ring is gained by studying the development of the aortic arch (Fig. 7.3). Early in embryonic development, the ascending aorta gives rise to a right and a left aortic arch. These paired arches encircle the trachea and the esophagus and join to form the descending aorta. In addition, both a left and a right ductus arteriosus are found.

In the normal development, the right arch is interrupted beyond the right subclavian artery; and the right ductus arteriosus regresses. This leads to the normal left aortic arch. The proximal portion of the primitive right arch becomes the innominate artery, which in turn gives rise to the right carotid and right subclavian arteries. The other aortic arch vessels are the left carotid and left subclavian arteries; they arise from the left arch. The left ductus arteriosus persists, connecting the aortic arch beyond the left subclavian artery to the left pulmonary artery.

Right aortic arch

If the left aortic arch is interrupted beyond the left subclavian artery, the opposite aortic arch pattern occurs, a right aortic arch with mirror-image branching (Fig. 7.3). The ascending aorta arises; the first branch is an innominate artery representing the proximal portion of the left aortic arch. From this arise the left subclavian and left carotid arteries. The aortic arch passes toward the right and gives rise to the right carotid and right subclavian arteries. The ductus arteriosus may be on either the left or the right side.

Double aortic arch

On rare occasions, neither aortic arch is interrupted during embryonic life. The resultant anomaly is one form of vascular ring–double aortic arch. The ascending aorta divides into two aortic arches. One of the aortic arches passes anteriorly to the trachea and the other passes posteriorly to the esophagus. They join to form the descending aorta that then passes on either the left or the right side of the thorax. The trachea and esophagus are encircled by

←──

Figure 7.3 Diagram of development of aortic arch anomalies based on concept of primitive double aortic arch and the resultant aortic arch patterns. The primitive double aortic arch may be uninterrupted developmentally, and a double arch results. It may also be interrupted at any of four locations (1–4). These result, respectively, in a normal left aortic arch; left aortic arch with aberrant right subclavian artery; right aortic arch; and right aortic arch with aberrant left subclavian artery. (Abbreviations: AA, ascending aorta; DA, descending aorta; LC, left carotid artery; LS, left subclavian artery; RC, right carotid artery; RS, right subclavian artery; E, esophagus; T, trachea.)

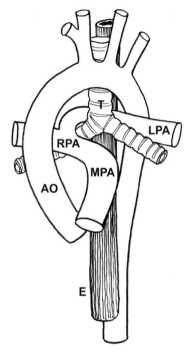

Figure 7.4 Pulmonary artery sling. The left pulmonary artery (LPA) arises anomalously from the right pulmonary artery (RPA) and courses between the trachea (T) and esophagus (E). (Abbreviations: MPA, main pulmonary artery; AO, aorta.) (Illustration courtesy of Dr David C. Mayer.)

vascular structures and can be compressed, leading to respiratory symptoms and difficulty in swallowing.

Aberrant subclavian artery

If the right aortic arch is interrupted between the right carotid and right subclavian arteries, the aortic arch is left-sided, but the right subclavian artery arises aberrantly. In this anomaly, no innominate artery is found; the first branch arising from the ascending aorta is the right carotid artery. The remaining arch vessels are, respectively, the left carotid artery, the left subclavian artery, and finally, the right subclavian artery. The right subclavian artery arises from the descending aorta and passes behind the esophagus to the right arm.

The opposite situation develops if the left aortic arch is interrupted between the left subclavian and left carotid arteries. This forms a right aortic arch and an aberrant left subclavian artery.

The vascular ring is often completed by a ductus arteriosus, either ligamentous or patent, that passes from the aberrant subclavian artery to the ipsilateral pulmonary artery.

Thus, vascular rings formed by aberrant subclavian arteries can also cause symptoms that are usually relieved by dividing the ductus arteriosus, which is usually ligamentous. However, most patients with this form of vascular ring require no treatment as they are asymptomatic.

In summary, a number of variations in aortic arch anatomy exist, depending upon the site(s) of interruption of the developmental aortic arches. If they are not interrupted, a double aortic arch is formed. If the aortic arches are interrupted at one site, a normal aortic arch, a right aortic arch, or an aortic arch with an aberrant subclavian artery can be formed. Rarely, the aortic arches are interrupted at two sites, yielding interruption of the aortic arch (see Chapter 8).

In many patients with vascular ring, symptoms such as wheeze or stridor suggest respiratory infection, bronchiolitis, or airway disease, and tracheobronchomalacia may indeed accompany vascular ring. After surgical relief of the ring, respiratory and/or airway symptoms may persist for weeks or months.

VASCULAR (PULMONARY ARTERY) SLING

This condition is not an anomaly of the aortic arch complex, but an anomalous origin of the left pulmonary artery from the right pulmonary artery (Fig 7.4). The left pulmonary artery then passes superior to the right mainstem bronchus and courses between the trachea and esophagus toward the left lung, creating tension on the tracheobronchial tree near the carina. Usually, one lung is over-inflated, and the other is underinflated, which results in respiratory symptoms.

It is the only vascular anomaly that creates an anterior indentation on the barium-filled esophagus. Sometimes, a plain lateral chest X-ray will suggest a mass (the left pulmonary artery) between the trachea and the esophagus, particularly if the position of the esophagus is outlined by a feeding tube.

Surgical reimplantation of the anomalous left pulmonary artery into the main pulmonary artery can relieve the sling effect, but tracheobronchomalacia and symptoms often persist.

Chapter 8
Cardiac conditions in the neonate

As indicated in Chapter 7, a variety of conditions may present in neonates, but they are not exclusively seen in that age period. In this chapter, we present conditions that are generally diagnosed exclusively in neonates.

NEONATAL PHYSIOLOGY

The distinctive and transitional features of the neonatal circulation may lead to cardiopulmonary abnormalities not only in newborn infants with cardiac malformations but also among those with pulmonary disease or other serious illnesses.

Understanding the anatomic and physiologic features of the transition from fetal to adult circulation aids the physician caring for critically ill neonates.

Normal fetal circulation

Normal fetal circulation differs from that of the postnatal state. In the fetus the pulmonary and systemic circulations are parallel, rather than occurring in series. In the fetal circulation, both ventricles eject blood into the aorta and receive systemic venous return. The right ventricle ejects a greater volume than

Pediatric Cardiology, by W Johnson, J Moller © 2008 Blackwell Publishing,
ISBN: 978-1-4051-7818-1.

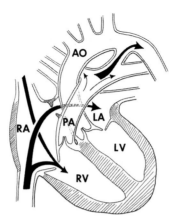

Figure 8.1 Central circulation in the fetus. Predominant flow from inferior vena cava is through the patent foramen ovale into the left atrium. Major portion of right ventricular flow is through the patent ductus arteriosus. (Abbreviations: Ao, aorta; LA, left atrium; LV, left ventricle; PA, pulmonary artery; RA, right atrium; RV, right ventricle.)

the left ventricle. Postnatally, the circulation is different in that the ventricles and the circulation are in series. The right ventricle receives the systemic venous return and the left ventricle alone ejects blood into the aorta. Left ventricular and right ventricular outputs are equal. The transition from a parallel to a series circulation normally occurs soon after birth; however, in distressed neonates the parallel circulation may persist, delaying the evolution to series circulation.

The fetal circulation also has three distinctive anatomic structures: the placenta, the patent ductus arteriosus, and the patent foramen ovale. The blood returning to the fetus from the placenta enters the right atrium and flows predominantly from the right to the left atrium through the patent foramen ovale (Fig. 8.1). This stream passes to the left ventricle and the ascending aorta, supplying the head with the proper level of oxygenated blood. The blood that leaves the head returns to the heart in the superior vena cava and flows principally into the right ventricle. Right ventricular output passes into the pulmonary artery, and the major portion (90%) flows through the ductus into the aorta, while a smaller amount (10%) flows into the lungs.

The major factor influencing the pattern and distribution of fetal blood flow is the relative vascular resistance of the pulmonary and systemic circuits. In contrast to the adult, the pulmonary vascular resistance in the fetus is very elevated, and the systemic vascular resistance is low. Prenatally, the lungs are airless, and the pulmonary arterioles possess thick media and a narrowed lumen. These anatomic features of the pulmonary arterioles are accentuated by the relative hypoxic environment of the fetus, as hypoxia is a potent stimulus for pulmonary vasoconstriction. The systemic vascular resistance is unusually low, primarily because of the large flow through the placenta, which has low resistance. In the fetus, the pulmonary vascular resistance is five times greater than the systemic vascular resistance, the reverse of the adult circulation.

Because the systolic pressures in both ventricles and great vessels are identical, the distribution of blood flow depends upon the relative vascular resistances. As a result, a relatively small volume of blood flows through the lungs and a large volume passes through the ductus from right to left into the aorta. A considerable portion (about 40%) of the combined ventricular output flows through the placenta.

The right-to-left shunt at the atrial level in the fetus depends in part upon the streaming effect caused by the position of the valve of the foramen ovale. This ridge tends to divert blood from the inferior vena cava into the left atrium through the defect. Since the atrial pressures are identical, the shunt also depends on the relative compliances of the ventricles. Approximately one-third of the total flow returning to the right atrium crosses the foramen ovale.

Transition to postnatal circulatory physiology

At birth the distinctive features of fetal circulation and the vascular resistances are suddenly changed. A major reversal of resistance occurs because of the separation of the placenta and the onset of respiration. The loss of the placenta, which has acted essentially as an arteriovenous fistula, is associated with a doubling of systemic vascular resistance. The expansion of the lungs is associated with a sevenfold drop in pulmonary vascular resistance, principally from vasodilation of pulmonary arterioles secondary to an increase in inspired air oxygen level to normal.

Coinciding with the fall in pulmonary vascular resistance, the volume of pulmonary blood flow increases; and thus the volume of blood returning to the left atrium increases. The left atrial pressure rises, exceeds the right atrial pressure, and closes the foramen ovale functionally. In most infants for up to several months, a small left-atrium-to-right-atrium shunt occurs via the incompetent flap of the foramen ovale. Anatomically, the atrial septum ultimately seals in 75% of children and remains "probe-patent" in 25%.

The ductus narrows by muscular contraction within 24 hours of birth, although anatomic closure may take several days. The closure of the ductus is associated with a lowering of pulmonary arterial pressure to normal levels. When the ductus and foramen ovale close, the pulmonary blood flow equals systemic blood flow, and the circulations are in series.

In the neonatal period, the changes that occur in the ductus, foramen ovale, and pulmonary arterioles are reversible. The pulmonary arterioles and the ductus arteriosus are responsive to oxygen levels and acidosis. Increase in the vascular resistance occurs in conditions associated with hypoxia. Although minor changes occur at pO_2 of 50 mm Hg, large increases in pulmonary vascular resistance occur at pO_2 less than 25 mm Hg. If acidosis coexists with hypoxia, the increase in pulmonary resistance is far greater than at comparable levels of pO_2 occurring at normal pH.

Persistent pulmonary hypertension of the newborn

Neonates with pulmonary parenchymal disease, such as respiratory distress syndrome, develop increased pulmonary vascular resistance and increased pulmonary arterial pressure because of hypoxia. If acidosis complicates the illness, the changes are even greater. This condition is often called persistent fetal circulation (PFC) or, by the more physiologically descriptive term, persistent pulmonary hypertension of the newborn (PPHN).

Because of elevation of right ventricular systolic pressure, right atrial pressure increases, causing a right-to-left shunt at the foramen ovale. In a similar way the ductus arteriosus of a neonate is also responsive to oxygen. With hypoxia, the ductus may open, and should the pulmonary resistance be simultaneously elevated, a right-to-left shunt could occur through the ductus arteriosus. Clinically, this is recognized by a lower PaO_2 (or pulse oximetry saturation) in the leg than the arm.

Thus, cyanosis in the neonate with pulmonary parenchymal disease can result from right-to-left shunting of blood, as well as from intrapulmonary shunting and diffusion defects. Administration of 100% oxygen improves both of these abnormalities, but often the improvement is not sufficient enough to exclude the diagnosis of cyanotic cardiac malformations. Oxygen administration to cyanotic patients with a cardiac anomaly generally also lessens the degree of cyanosis. With the development of echocardiography, the ability to distinguish these has been greatly enhanced.

CARDIAC DISEASE IN NEONATES

Cardiac malformations may lead to severe cardiac symptoms and death in the neonatal period. The types of cardiac malformations causing symptoms in this age group are generally different from those leading to symptoms later in infancy. Among the latter group, symptoms usually derive from a large volume of pulmonary blood flow, such as in ventricular septal defect (VSD), in which congestive failure develops at about 6 weeks of age. Other conditions, such as tetralogy of Fallot, await the development of sufficient stenosis before becoming symptomatic. In the neonate, congestive cardiac failure and hypoxia are the major cardiac symptom complexes.

Congestive cardiac failure

In the neonatal period, congestive cardiac failure results most commonly from (1) anomalies that cause severe outflow obstruction, particularly to the left side of the heart, and that are often associated with a hypoplastic left ventricle; (2) volume overload from an insufficient cardiac valve or systemic arteriovenous fistula; and (3) cardiomyopathy or myocarditis.

Cardiac conditions with a left-to-right shunt (e.g., VSD) almost never place large volume loads upon the ventricles and lead to symptoms in the neonatal period. Occasionally, in prematurely born infants, a patent ductus arteriosus may lead to signs of cardiac failure. Presumably, the pulmonary vasculature approaches normal levels more quickly than in full-term infants. The resultant large volume of pulmonary blood flow causes overload of the left ventricle.

Left heart obstruction
Hypoplastic left heart syndrome (HLHS). HLHS is the most frequent cause of cardiac failure in this age group (Fig. 8.2a). The term encompasses several cardiac malformations, each associated with a diminutive left ventricle and with similar clinical and physiologic features; included in these are aortic atresia, mitral atresia, and severe ("critical") aortic stenosis. In each, severe obstruction to both left ventricular inflow and outflow is present.

Whether from an atretic mitral valve or from a small left ventricle, filling of the left ventricle is impeded or made impossible. The foramen ovale is often small and restrictive, permitting only a small amount of blood to flow from the left to the right atrium. The volume of shunt is not sufficient to decompress the left atrium, so the pressure in this chamber rises leading to elevation of pulmonary capillary pressure and ultimately to pulmonary edema. Left ventricular outflow is either severely obstructed or rendered impossible.

Patent ductus arteriosus is a major component of all forms of hypoplastic left heart syndrome. The flow through the ductus occurs from right to left and represents the sole source of systemic arterial blood flow. The left ventricular output may be absent or is so small that the flow into the ascending aorta and to the coronary arteries is in a retrograde direction via the ductus arteriosus. Coarctation of the aorta may complicate the anatomic features.

History. These patients show severe congestive cardiac failure and/or low cardiac output, usually in the first week of life, with a clinical presentation similar to coarctation of the aorta.

Physical examination. The peripheral pulses are weak and the skin is mottled because of poor tissue perfusion. A soft, nonspecific murmur may be heard, but often no murmur is found. Systolic clicks may result from a dilated main pulmonary artery.

Electrocardiogram. The electrocardiogram may appear normal for age. The absence of a Q wave in V_6 is a common finding, but normal infants may lack this if the electrode for V_6 is not placed properly.

Chest X-ray. Chest X-rays show an enlarged heart and accentuated pulmonary arterial and venous markings.

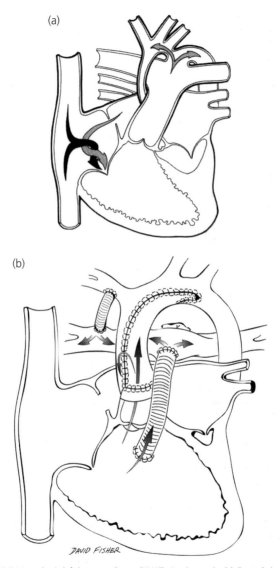

Figure 8.2 Hypoplastic left heart syndrome (HLHS). Aortic atresia. (a) Central circulation. (b) Norwood procedure (Stage 1). Both a modified Blalock-Taussig shunt and a Sano shunt are shown.

Natural history. Death usually occurs in the first week of life, although on rare occasions infants are not recognized with this condition for 2 or more weeks.

Echocardiogram. It demonstrates the hypoplastic ascending aorta and diminutive left ventricle, although in some patients no left ventricular cavity is seen. Doppler displays the typical pattern of pulmonary artery to aorta flow and retrograde blood flow in the aortic arch and ascending aorta.

Cardiac catheterization. Cardiac catheterization is usually unnecessary unless a restrictive atrial septum that requires blade atrial septectomy or balloon septostomy is found. Some infants awaiting cardiac transplantation require balloon dilation of the ductus or a ductal stent to maintain adequate ductal size.

Medical management. Prostaglandin should be administered to maintain ductal patency and thus systemic blood flow. Because the systemic and pulmonary circulations are connected at the great vessel level, systemic blood flow may suffer with any decrease in pulmonary vascular resistance; therefore, oxygen is avoided once the diagnosis is made because of its effect on lowering pulmonary vascular resistance.

Operative considerations. Corrective operations are not available for infants with hypoplastic left heart syndrome. Palliative operations include the Norwood procedure, which essentially converts the physiology from aortic atresia to pulmonary atresia by using the native pulmonary trunk as a neoaorta (Fig. 8.2b). Controlled pulmonary blood flow is supplied to the disconnected branch pulmonary arteries from a systemic artery via a prosthetic, usually Gore-tex, shunt. An alternative (Sano shunt) inserts a valveless prosthetic tube between the right ventricle and pulmonary artery to maintain pulmonary blood flow.

Infants palliated this way have a univentricular heart and later may be candidates for cavopulmonary anastomosis (Glenn and Fontan) operations.

Because results of these palliations are variable, many infants with HLHS may become candidates for cardiac transplantation. The long-term prognosis for children who have survived these two operative approaches is unknown. Some patients who are not considered for any intervention die in early infancy; controversy exists as to the most suitable management for HLHS.

Summary. Hypoplastic left heart syndrome is a common cause of shock and congestive heart failure in the neonate. Although palliative options, including Norwood operation and transplantation exist, mortality is higher than for most other cardiac malformations.

Coarctation of the aorta. Coarctation of the aorta (see Chapter 5), either isolated or coexisting with other cardiac malformations, is another common cause of congestive cardiac failure in the neonate.

Clinical diagnosis is difficult because the low cardiac output from congestive failure minimizes the blood pressure difference between the arms and legs. Following treatment with inotropes, a blood pressure differential may develop as the cardiac output increases. Prostaglandin also helps widen the juxtaductal area of the descending aorta. Cardiomegaly and an electrocardiographic pattern of right ventricular hypertrophy and inverted ST segment and T waves in the left precordium are found. Much less frequently, aortic and pulmonary stenosis may lead to congestive cardiac failure early in life.

Interrupted aortic arch. Interrupted aortic arch (Fig. 8.3), a complex anomaly resulting from the absence of a segment of aortic arch, is associated with various degrees of hypoplasia of the left ventricular outflow tract and aortic valve; a VSD is virtually always present. The aortic arch may be interrupted distal to the left subclavian artery origin (type A) or between the left carotid artery and the left subclavian artery (type B). Many patients, particularly those with type B, have DiGeorge syndrome. Blood flow to the descending aorta is only by way of the ductus arteriosus. As the ductus undergoes normal closure, flow to the lower body is markedly reduced.

History. All patients with interrupted aortic arch as neonates have a clinical presentation similar to coarctation of the aorta, characterized by signs and symptoms of low cardiac output and shock.

Physical examination. Neonates with interrupted aortic arch have a difference in oxygen saturation between the upper (normal saturation) and lower extremities (lower saturation) because the right ventricle supplies all the lower body cardiac output via the ductus.

As the ductus arteriosus narrows, decreased lower-extremity pulses become apparent, a finding similar to neonates with coarctation. In neonates with interruption occurring between the origin of the left carotid artery and the left subclavian artery (type B), only the right-upper-extremity pulses may be palpable, whereas in neonates with interruption distal to the left subclavian artery (type A), pulses in both upper extremities may feel equal.

Ventricular function becomes reduced and all pulses may be difficult to palpate. This stage is characterized by nonspecific signs of shock, including poor perfusion, cyanosis, listlessness, and marked tachypnea. A murmur and systolic click are not usually apparent.

Electrocardiogram. The electrocardiogram shows findings similar to those of coarctation, including right ventricular enlargement/hypertrophy.

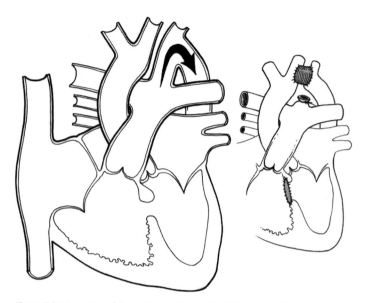

Figure 8.3 Interruption of the aortic arch. Central circulation and surgical repair.

Chest X-ray. The cardiac silhouette is enlarged and pulmonary vasculature is increased.

Natural history. Untreated, interrupted aortic arch is a uniformly fatal lesion in neonates. As with coarctation, temporary palliation is accomplished by maintaining ductal patency with prostaglandin.

Echocardiogram. All neonates with interrupted aortic arch have a large VSD, often one and one-half times larger than the diameter of the left ventricular outflow tract and the aortic valve annulus, both of which are typically smaller than normal. A spur of infundibular septum, which forms part of the rim of the VSD, may encroach upon the left ventricular outflow tract and cause obstruction. Because of this, the VSD is sometimes termed a malalignment VSD. The ascending aorta, which is small, courses cephalad and does not curve posteriorly to become the aortic arch, as in normal neonates.

 The ductus arteriosus, which is large, curves posteriorly to join the thoracic descending aorta so seamlessly that the ductus itself may be mistaken for the aortic arch; however, unlike a normal aortic arch, the brachiocephalic arteries cannot be seen arising from the ductus. As in coarctation, the ductal shunt is predominantly right-to-left (from pulmonary artery to descending aorta) because the right ventricle is the sole source of systemic artery blood flow to the lower body.

Cardiac catheterization. Oxygen data show a left-to-right shunt at ventricular level and a right-to-left shunt via the ductus arteriosus, with normal saturation in the ascending aorta and its branches and decreased saturation in the descending aorta, corresponding to the level of right ventricular saturation.

Left ventriculography demonstrates the location of the arch interruption, the origin and courses of the aortic branches, and the degree of left ventricular outflow tract hypoplasia; the latter is better demonstrated by echocardiography.

Operative considerations. Operation is designed to create an unobstructed connection from ascending to descending aorta and to close or to limit the flow through the VSD.

Two options exist: (1) primary repair of the arch and closure of the VSD, or (2) staged repair of the arch and pulmonary artery banding, with later debanding and VSD closure.

The latter approach may have less overall mortality risk, especially in neonates who have a hypoplastic left ventricular outflow tract that could grow in the interval between pulmonary artery banding and operative closure of the VSD. If the left ventricular outflow tract is of an inadequate size or is severely obstructed, a palliative operation, similar to a Norwood operation, can be done.

Summary. Interrupted aortic arch is a form of left heart obstruction that presents in neonates in a manner similar to coarctation of the aorta; it is highly associated with DiGeorge syndrome. The success of operative repair depends on the degree of left ventricular outflow tract hypoplasia and on whether associated noncardiac anomalies are present.

Volume overload

Volume overload placed on either ventricle may lead to neonatal cardiac failure.

Systemic arteriovenous fistula or malformation (AVM). AVM (e.g., in the great vein of Galen or in the liver) results in a high output failure; it is the most common noncardiac cause. The arteriovenous fistula is associated with low systemic arterial resistance and an increased volume of blood flow through the shunt. The increased flow through the right side of the heart leads to profound cardiac symptoms early in life.

Prior to birth, cardiac failure is absent because of the low systemic vascular resistance prenatally. With the loss of the placenta, systemic resistance increases and so does the volume shunted through the fistula. However, systemic resistance does not rise to normal postnatal levels because of the malformation, a circumstance that contributes to clinical findings of "persistent fetal circulation."

An arteriovenous fistula may be recognized by auscultation for a continuous murmur over the head, liver, or other peripheral sites and by increased pulse pressure, similar to that seen in large patent ductus arteriosus. Operative or transcatheter obliteration of the fistula, if possible, is curative.

Insufficiency of cardiac valves. Insufficiency of cardiac valves is an uncommon cause of neonatal cardiac failure. It is most likely associated with persistent atrioventricular canal defect or univentricular heart (in which the atrioventricular valves are insufficient); truncus arteriosus with marked truncal (semilunar) valve insufficiency; or rare aortic valve anomalies, including left ventricle–aortic tunnel.

Cardiomyopathy. Cardiomyopathy (including that from coronary artery anomalies) and myocarditis may cause neonatal heart failure. Rarely, tachy- or bradyarrhythmias present as neonatal cardiac failure.

Hypoxia

Severe cardiac symptoms also occur in the neonatal period because of hypoxia due to inadequate mixing, as is found in complete transposition of the great arteries with intact ventricular septum. Severe hypoxia can also occur in conditions with severe obstruction to pulmonary blood flow and an intracardiac shunt (see Chapter 6). In the neonate, tetralogy of Fallot, often with pulmonary atresia, pulmonary atresia with intact ventricular septum (hypoplastic right ventricle), and tricuspid atresia are the most common conditions leading to this state. Critical pulmonary stenosis is valvar pulmonary stenosis with a large right-to-left shunt via the foramen ovale and with various degrees of right ventricular hypoplasia and abnormal compliance; the physiology is similar to pulmonary atresia with intact ventricular septum.

Neonates with hypoxia show extreme cyanosis. Rapid, difficult respiration occurs from metabolic acidosis, which can develop quickly because of the hypoxia; cardiac failure is usually not a major problem. Administration of oxygen is usually of little benefit. Neonates with complete transposition of the great arteries require prostaglandins to keep the ductus patent and a Rashkind atrial septostomy to improve intracardiac mixing. Neonates with malformations causing inadequate pulmonary blood flow are improved with prostaglandin administration followed by an aorticopulmonary shunt to improve oxygenation or with corrective operation or catheter intervention.

Thus, a diverse group of cardiac conditions causes symptoms in the neonatal period. Because of the potential for correction or palliation, any neonate with severe cardiac symptoms should be stabilized, then studied by echocardiography and, in many cases, also by cardiac catheterization and angiocardiography to define the anatomic and physiologic details of the cardiac malformation. Although some risk (1% mortality) is involved in the performance of cardiac catheterization in neonates, it is outweighed by the benefits of the data obtained or the therapeutic interventions performed. Following definition of the malformation, appropriate decisions are made concerning surgical therapy; and in the case of certain malformations (e.g., critical aortic stenosis, critical pulmonary stenosis), balloon dilation of the obstruction is achieved.

An aggressive diagnostic and therapeutic approach is warranted in neonates. This approach begins with the prompt recognition of cardiac disease in the newborn nursery. Treatment, usually involving prostaglandin, should be initiated, and the infant should be immediately referred to a cardiac center for definitive diagnosis and therapy.

Chapter 9
Acquired cardiac conditions

Pediatric Cardiology, by W Johnson, J Moller © 2008 Blackwell Publishing,
ISBN: 978-1-4051-7818-1.

In pediatric cardiology, there has been much emphasis on congenital heart disease, arrhythmias, and murmurs. There is, however, an important wide spectrum of other conditions that affect the structure and/or function of cardiovascular system. These include genetic, infectious, and inflammatory diseases and in many instances the etiology is unknown. In some patients, a cardiac condition can be suspected because of a known association between the condition with a specific cardiac abnormality. In other instances, the family history may indicate the possibility of a genetic cardiac condition. Finally, the patient may present with cardiac symptoms or signs and the underlying cardiac condition recognized.

KAWASAKI DISEASE

Kawasaki disease (mucocutaneous lymph node syndrome) is a systemic vasculitis of unknown etiology. First described in Japan in 1967 by Dr Tomisaku Kawasaki, it is the most common cause of acquired cardiac disease among children in the United States, affecting at least 2500 children yearly. It is exclusively a childhood disease, with 80% of cases occurring by the age of 5 years. Occasionally, adolescents are diagnosed with this disease.

Coronary artery aneurysms are the most common and potentially dangerous sequelae of Kawasaki disease, occurring in one in four untreated patients. Mortality is 0.5%, usually from myocardial infarct, although severe myocarditis can occur. Other systemic arteries can be affected, and clinical overlap with a disseminated vasculitis, infantile polyarteritis nodosa, exists.

Diagnosis
Clinical features

The illness is characterized by the following features: (a) bilateral conjunctivitis without discharge; (b) erythematous mouth and dry, fissured lips; (c) a generalized erythematous rash; (d) nonpitting, painful induration of the

Table 9.1 Clinical Features of Kawasaki Disease.

Fever
Conjunctivitis, nonexudative, and bilateral
Erythematous and fissured oral changes
Erythematous rash
Painful hand and foot induration
Lymphadenopathy

hands and feet, often with marked erythema of the palms and soles; and (e) lymphadenopathy (Table 9.1). These occur with a high persistent fever without obvious origin, initially. It has been suggested that patients with 5 days or more of high fever and at least four of these five features have Kawasaki disease, analogous to the use of the Jones criteria for rheumatic fever diagnosis. Kawasaki disease is much more pleomorphic than rheumatic fever, and many cases of "atypical" Kawasaki disease occur. The diagnosis remains a clinical one, as no definitive laboratory test exists.

Natural history
Untreated, Kawasaki disease is self-limited, with a mean duration of 12 days for fever, although irritability and anorexia, both prominent during the febrile acute phase, often persist for 2–3 weeks after the fever ends. During the so-called subacute, or convalescent, phase, usually from day 10 to 20 after onset of fever, most patients have a highly specific pattern of desquamation of the hands and feet that begins periungual and proceeds proximally to involve the palms and soles. Occasionally, the perineal skin desquamates. The trunk and face do not peel, in contrast to scarlet fever.

Laboratory studies
Laboratory tests are only supportive but not diagnostic. The erythrocyte sedimentation rate (ESR), C-reactive protein (CRP), and other acute phase reactants are often very elevated. The platelet count is often normal throughout the acute phase (the first 10–14 days), so it cannot be used to exclude the diagnosis. An echocardiogram (or, if unavailable, a chest radiograph to screen for cardiomegaly) and 12-lead electrocardiogram are advisable at the time of diagnosis. Echocardiography during the acute phase usually does not show aneurysms; however, diffusely enlarged coronary arteries and other nonspecific signs of mild carditis may be present. Thus, echocardiography cannot be used to "rule out" Kawasaki disease. The echocardiogram should be repeated at about 1 month after onset of illness. Patients with carditis or aneurysms detected early require more frequent follow-up.

Treatment
Aspirin
Aspirin does not decrease the incidence of aneurysm formation, even in antiinflammatory doses (100 mg/kg/day), although it is indicated in low dose (3–5 mg/kg/day) for inhibition of platelet aggregation.

Intravenous gamma (immune) globulin (IVGG or IVIG)
IVIG is a preparation from human plasma containing mostly nonspecific polyclonal IgG from several thousand donors. Treatment with IVGG (2 g/kg as a single dose) within the first 10 days after onset of fever reduces the incidence of coronary artery aneurysm from 25 to ≤5%. Many patients show prompt and impressive resolution of fever and other acute-phase symptoms within hours after IVGG. Occasional patients require a second treatment because of failure to improve following a first dose.

The mechanism of action is unknown but probably involves attenuation of an autoimmune response that may be the prime pathophysiologic factor in Kawasaki arteritis.

Adverse effects of IVGG treatment are rare, but hepatitis C infection was associated with some preparations several years ago. Continuing concern over the possibility of as yet unknown transmissible agents and the high cost of IVGG have led to its overly conservative use in atypical Kawasaki disease, such that many patients are not treated in time and manifest aneurysms.

The authors recommend timely treatment with gamma globulin whenever a reasonable suspicion of Kawasaki disease exists, even if four of five classical criteria are not met.

Corticosteroids and other immune mediators
Steroids in high intravenous doses over several days have been used successfully in those patients (up to 10%) who fail to respond to IVGG. Oral steroids are not a substitute for IVGG, as data from the pre-IVGG era suggest the risk of aneurysms was unchanged or possibly higher than with aspirin alone.

Other agents, including monoclonal antibodies, infliximab and related drugs, often relieve signs of inflammation in children who appear to fail IVIG treatment, yet prevention of aneurysms is as yet unproven.

Follow-up care
Echocardiography
Because the peak time for detection by echocardiography or angiography of an aneurysm is approximately 30 days after onset of fever, well after most patients have had spontaneous resolution of fever, a normal echocardiogram during the febrile period does not exclude this vascular complication; and echocardiography should always be repeated 4–6 weeks after the onset of illness.

Laboratory

A striking finding during the convalescent phase, thrombocytosis (often $>1,000,000/mm^3$) does not peak until the second week after onset of fever; so a normal platelet count during the acute phase cannot be used as evidence against a diagnosis of Kawasaki disease. The ESR slowly falls to normal over several weeks.

Low-dose aspirin

Low-dose aspirin should be started for antiplatelet effect, although some have advocated high-dose aspirin for a variable period of time to aid in the resolution of inflammation before commencing low-dose aspirin.

Since occasional patients may manifest aneurysm several months later, an echocardiogram 4–6 months after onset of illness may be done; and if coronary arteries are normal, aspirin is discontinued.

Low-dose aspirin may confer a small risk during certain viral illnesses; it should be temporarily suspended during acute varicella or influenza and perhaps after varicella vaccination.

Recurrent disease

As in rheumatic fever, recurrent disease can develop, requiring retreatment with IVIG and aspirin and resetting of follow-up echocardiography. The risk is approximately 1:50, with most cases recurring within the first few months of the initial episode.

Coronary aneurysm

The natural history of patients who develop coronary artery aneurysms is variable. In 9 of 10 patients the aneurysms resolve on echocardiogram, although some of these have continued narrowing of the coronary artery lumen leading to stenotic lesions. Coronary artery stenoses may be impossible to image by echocardiography, and catheterization may be indicated.

In children with anginal symptoms or ECG abnormalities who have fully recovered from acute Kawasaki disease and who do not have echocardiographically apparent lesions, nuclear myocardial perfusion scans at rest and with exercise may be helpful in differentiating benign chest pain from true ischemia and/or infarct.

The effect of childhood Kawasaki disease (without aneurysms) on the risk of coronary atherosclerosis in later life is unknown.

RHEUMATIC FEVER

Rheumatic fever is a systemic disease affecting several organ systems, including the heart. It is a sequel of group A beta-hemolytic streptococcal infections, usually tonsillopharyngitis, developing in less than 1% of infected patients. Rheumatic fever usually develops 10 days to 2 weeks following a

Table 9.2 Modified Jones Criteria for the Diagnosis of Acute Rheumatic Fever.

Major Criteria
   Carditis*
   Arthritis
   Chorea*
   Erythema marginatum
   Subcutaneous nodules
Minor Criteria
   Arthralgia
   Prolongation of the PR interval
   Elevated acute phase reactants (e.g., ESR)
   Fever
Other
   Previous history of rheumatic fever*

---

*See exceptions noted.
Evidence of prior streptococcal infection is necessary before these criteria are considered.

streptococcal pharyngitis that almost always is associated with fever greater than 101°F (38.3°C), sore throat, and cervical adenitis. The pathogenesis of the systemic manifestations is unknown.

Despite a minor resurgence in the 1980s, the incidence of rheumatic fever in North America decreased markedly in the last half of the twentieth century. Worldwide, however, rheumatic fever remains the most common cause of acquired heart disease in the young.

Rheumatic fever is diagnosed by use of the modified Jones criteria (Table 9.2). These criteria comprise the various combinations of clinical and laboratory manifestations reflecting the multiple sites of disease involvement. There must be two major criteria or one major and two minor criteria, plus evidence of a preceding streptococcal infection, to diagnose acute rheumatic fever.

The proof of streptococcal infection can be established by either of two methods. The first is the recovery of beta-hemolytic streptococcus by throat culture. This finding must be interpreted with care because streptococcal carrier states exist and are not considered a streptococcal infection. The second method of proof is the finding of an increase in streptococcal antibodies. Following a streptococcal infection, antibodies to various streptococcal components, such as antistreptolysin-O (ASO) and antideoxyribonuclease B (DNase B), rise significantly. Titers for several antibodies should be measured because an individual may not form antibodies to each streptococcal product. Significant antibody rise indicates a recent streptococcal infection and is more meaningful than isolating beta-hemolytic streptococcus on a throat culture.

Diagnosis
Jones criteria
Five major and four minor criteria (Table 9.2) can be used to fulfill the Jones criteria.

Major criteria

Carditis. Carditis can involve any layer of the heart. Pericarditis can occur in this disease and can be suspected by the occurrence of chest pain that may be referred to the abdomen or shoulders. It is diagnosed by finding a pericardial friction rub, ST segment elevation/depression on the electrocardiogram, or thickened pericardium or effusion by echocardiogram.

Cardiac enlargement or cardiac failure without evidence of valvar anomalies is evidence of myocardial involvement. Rarely, cardiac failure occurs from myocardial involvement itself. Various degrees of heart block, gallop rhythm, and muffled heart sounds are other manifestations of myocarditis. Prolonged PR interval in itself is not a criterion for carditis.

Valvulitis is the most serious manifestation of carditis because it can lead to permanent cardiac sequelae. Both the aortic and mitral valves may be involved acutely. Three types of murmurs may be present that suggest acute rheumatic fever: (a) An apical holosystolic murmur of mitral insufficiency is the most frequently occurring murmur. (b) At times a mid-diastolic murmur may also be heard at the apex. The origin of this murmur is unknown, but it is perhaps related to turbulence either from the valvulitis or from the blood flow into a dilated left ventricle. (c) An early-diastolic murmur of aortic insufficiency may be found during the acute episode but is a more frequent late manifestation. Aortic stenosis does not occur during the acute episode of rheumatic fever.

These valvar abnormalities, particularly aortic and mitral insufficiency, may be demonstrated by echocardiography and color Doppler.

Arthritis. Arthritis is usually a migrating polyarthritis; several joints may be involved, often sequentially, but at a given time there may be involvement of only one joint. Usually the large joints are involved. Diagnosis of arthritis rests on finding warm and tender joints that are painful on movement. The changes are never permanent.

Chorea. Chorea is a late manifestation of rheumatic fever and often develops several months after the streptococcal infection. At that time, other manifestations of rheumatic fever may not be found. The presence of chorea alone is sufficient for the diagnosis of rheumatic fever, as there are virtually no other causes in childhood, although lupus must be excluded. Chorea is more common in females and prior to puberty.

Chorea is characterized by involuntary, nonrepetitive, purposeless motions, often associated with emotional instability. The parents may complain that their child is clumsy, is fidgety, cries easily, or has difficulty in writing or reading.

Classic physical findings of chorea exist. The milkmaid (or grip) sign describes the fibrillatory nature of a hand grasp. Other findings are related to exaggerated muscle movements, such as the hyperextension of the hands or apposition of the backs of the hands when the arms are extended above the head. Although lasting for months in some children, it is not usually permanent.

Erythema marginatum. Erythema marginatum is a fleeting, characteristic cutaneous finding. It is characterized by pink macules with distinct sharp margins; these change rapidly in contour. Warmth tends to bring out these lesions. With time the center fades, while the margin persists as a circular or serpentine border.

Subcutaneous nodules. Subcutaneous nodules are a rare manifestation of rheumatic fever, occurring late in the course of the disease. These are nontender, firm, pea-like nodules over the extensor surfaces, particularly over the knees, elbows, and spine. They have a strong association with chronic carditis.

Minor criteria

Arthralgia. The symptom of painful joints without subjective evidence of arthritis may be used as a minor criterion, if arthritis has not been used as a major one.

Prolongation of the PR Interval. This can be used as a minor criterion, if carditis has not been used as a major one.

Acute-phase reactants. Laboratory evidence of acute inflammation, such as elevated ESR or CRP, meets requirements for a minor criterion.

Fever. The temperature is usually in the range of 101–102°F (38.3–38.9°C).

Exceptions to the Jones criteria
A presumptive diagnosis of rheumatic fever may be made without strict adherence to the criteria in at least three circumstances:
(1) Chorea, which may be the only manifestation.
(2) Carditis and its sequelae in patients presenting long after an episode of acute rheumatic fever.

(3) Previous history of rheumatic fever and a recent streptococcal infection, but care must be taken that the diagnosis of the previous episode of rheumatic fever was carefully made according to the Jones criteria.

In any of these situations, other etiologies must be excluded by appropriate testing. As with all such diagnostic criteria, strict adherence to the Jones criteria may lead to under diagnosis of acute rheumatic fever. In the modern era, this is particularly pertinent when considering the increased identification of valvulitis by echocardiography, which is not evident by physical examination.

Treatment
Bedrest

This should be prescribed for the duration of the acute febrile period of the illness. Then gradual increases in activity should be allowed, provided that there is no recurrence of signs or symptoms. Serial determination of ESR is helpful in reaching decisions concerning activity levels. The return to full activity may be achieved by 6 weeks in patients with arthritis as the only major criterion; but in those with carditis, 3 months is advisable.

Salicylates

Salicylates are the preferred medication to reduce the inflammatory response, and they produce a prompt improvement in arthritis. However, evidence does not suggest that aspirin improves the natural history of carditis or valvulitis. Temperature associated with rheumatic fever returns to normal within a few days. Aspirin is administered in a dose sufficient to achieve a blood salicylate level of approximately 20 mg/dL (1.45 mmol/L); usually this dosage is about 75–100 mg/kg/day. Salicylates are continued until the ESR is normal, and then the dosage is tapered.

Corticosteroids

Steroids have been used in the treatment of acute rheumatic fever, but there is no evidence that they are superior to aspirin in preventing cardiac valvar damage. Steroids may, however, lead to a more prompt reduction in symptoms than does aspirin. Since steroids are more hazardous, their use should be reserved for patients with severe pancarditis.

The patient with acute rheumatic fever should be treated for streptococcal infection even if streptococcal cultures are negative, as described later under "Prevention of acute rheumatic fever."

Rheumatic fever prophylaxis ("secondary" prophylaxis)

Once patients have had an episode of rheumatic fever, they are at higher risk of developing a second episode, particularly within the first 5 years; however, some added risk continues throughout life. Since rheumatic fever develops following a streptococcal infection, preventive measures are directed at eliminating such infections in susceptible individuals.

The American Heart Association has recommended that all patients with a history of rheumatic fever be placed on long-term penicillin prophylaxis. The duration of prophylaxis is partly determined by the presence or absence of carditis, but for children it is a minimum of 5 years or until 21 years of age, whichever is longer; some authorities recommend lifelong prophylaxis in all patients.

Secondary rheumatic fever prophylaxis

Penicillin can be administered in two forms: (a) penicillin V, 250 mg orally twice a day; or (b) benzathine penicillin G, 1.2 million units, intramuscularly monthly. Some advocate a reduced dosage for children ≤60 pounds (27.3 kg) and ≤5 years of age (see Additional reading).
If the patient is allergic to penicillin, sulfonamides should be given. Although sulfa drugs are not bactericidal and should not be used for the treatment of a streptococcal infection, they are bacteriostatic for streptococcus and prevent colonization of the nasopharynx.
Patients allergic to penicillin and sulfonamides may receive erythromycin.

Prevention of acute rheumatic fever ("primary" prophylaxis)

The aim of physicians should be the prevention of the initial episode of rheumatic fever by recognition and proper treatment of group A beta-hemolytic streptococcal infections. Only by adequate treatment of such infections can rheumatic fever be prevented. The throat of any child with the symptoms and findings of tonsillopharyngitis should be tested, because the absolute clinical differentiation of streptococcal versus viral infection is not possible.

Two types of tests are available: culture and rapid screening tests. Rapid streptococcal tests that detect the group A carbohydrate antigen are highly specific, so positive results do not demand additional culture. But the rapid tests vary in sensitivity, so a negative result should be backed up with culture. If beta-hemolytic streptococcus is present, the throat culture becomes positive within 24 hours. The child with a positive culture may be treated then; to initiate treatment at the time of culturing the child is unnecessary, since antibiotic treatment does not alter the early course of acute streptococcal tonsillopharyngitis. The aim of treatment of this infection is the eradication of the streptococcus.

Primary rheumatic fever prophylaxis

This is done by administering either:

(a) Penicillin V, 250 mg (400,000 U) orally twice to three times daily for 10 days for children, and for adolescents and adults, 500 mg (800,000 U); or

(b) Benzathine Penicillin, 600,000 U for children weighing less than 60 pounds (27.3 kg) and for larger children and adults, 1.2 million U, intramuscularly in a single dose.

The intramuscular route is associated with a slightly better rate of eradication and is better for patients in whom compliance may be a factor. Mixtures containing procaine penicillin are often used to minimize the pain of injection.

Penicillin-allergic patients may receive erythromycin or other macrolides, but resistance is a problem in some parts of the world. First-generation cephalosporins may be used, but tetracyclines and sulfonamides are not advisable for acute streptococcal eradication.

Long-term care

After the acute episode of rheumatic fever, the patient should be seen periodically. The purposes of these visits are to (a) emphasize the continuing need of penicillin prophylaxis for rheumatic fever; (b) to emphasize the need for additional prophylaxis against bacterial endocarditis at the time of dental work or other procedures; and (c) to observe for the development of valvar rheumatic heart disease.

In half of the patients with evidence of valvar abnormality during the acute episode, the murmurs disappear; but over a period of years the other half may develop more severe cardiac manifestations, such as mitral stenosis, mitral insufficiency, or aortic insufficiency. These patients may ultimately require a cardiac operation or intervention.

MYOCARDIAL DISEASES

The term *myocardial disease* includes a variety of conditions affecting principally the myocardium and leading to similar clinical and physiologic states. It excludes obvious valvar heart disease, cardiac malformations, hypertension, and coronary arterial disease.

Despite the various etiologic factors of myocardial disease, the major signs and symptoms of myocardial diseases are similar. Because of the myocardial involvement, there is failure of the heart to (a) act as a pump, (b) initiate and maintain its rhythm, and (c) maintain its architecture. Each of these three effects of myocardial involvement has clinical and laboratory findings.

The inability of the myocardium to act efficiently as a pump is shown clinically by features of congestion and inadequate forward flow of blood. Signs of congestive cardiac failure are found: pulmonary edema, dyspnea, hepatomegaly, peripheral edema, and gallop rhythm. Symptoms of fatigue, angina, dizziness, and exercise intolerance indicate inadequate systemic output.

Cardiac arrhythmias are common in these patients. Two types of arrhythmias can be present. Slowing of conduction, particularly through the atrioventricular node, may occur, leading to first degree, or more advanced, heart block. Ectopic pacemaker sites may develop, leading to atrial or ventricular tachycardias. Low-voltage QRS complexes and abnormalities of repolarization are also common.

Finally, a group of signs and symptoms relates to the inability of the heart to maintain its normal muscular architecture. The most obvious finding on clinical examination is the displacement of the cardiac apex. Cardiomegaly is found on the chest X-ray and may be so extensive as to interfere with the left-sided bronchi, resulting in atelectasis of the left lower lobe. Mitral insufficiency may develop either from dilation of the mitral ring or from papillary muscle dysfunction. Prominent third and fourth heart sounds develop and are related to increased left ventricular filling pressure.

Typically, the patient presents with congestive cardiac failure, cardiomegaly (particularly involving the left side of the heart), absence of a cardiac murmur, and faint heart sounds.

The myocardial diseases may be divided into three broad categories: myocarditis, myocardial disease of obscure origin (idiopathic dilated, hypertrophic, and restrictive cardiomyopathies), and myocardial involvement with systemic disease.

Myocarditis

The myocardium may be involved in an inflammatory process related to infectious agents, autoimmune (collagen-vascular) disease, or unknown causes. Although many cases are considered to be of viral origin, this relationship has often been difficult to prove, even using molecular biologic techniques to evaluate for viral genome within diseased myocytes. Echo, Coxsackie, and rubella viruses have been associated with myocarditis in childhood. Myocarditis is generally a disease of the neonatal period or early infancy, but occurs sporadically thereafter. Onset may be abrupt, with sudden cardiovascular collapse and death within hours; or the development of congestive cardiac failure may be more gradual. The cardiac failure may respond well to treatment. The infant is mottled and has weak peripheral pulses. Evidence of cardiomegaly is found clinically, and the heart sounds are muffled. Sinus tachycardia is a regular feature, and episodic tachyarrhythmias are common.

The electrocardiogram shows normal or reduced QRS voltages. ST segment depression and T wave inversion are usually found in the left precordial leads. Cardiomegaly and pulmonary congestion are found on the chest X-ray. The echocardiogram shows a dilated left atrium and left ventricle with global decrease in contractility. Mitral regurgitation is almost always present, even in the absence of an audible murmur. Frequently, a mitral regurgitation murmur is noted only after treatment results in improved cardiac output.

The prognosis is variable. Corticosteroids and other immunosuppressants may be indicated when autoimmune disease is the etiology of myocardial dysfunction, but they have not been beneficial in apparent myocarditis. Intravenous gamma globulin has been suggested as a way to attenuate the inflammatory response in myocarditis. Some patients spontaneously improve to normal cardiac structure and function without treatment or with only symptomatic therapy. Treatment with anti-congestive heart failure drugs (see Chapter 11) usually improves the patient's status, although the course may be chronic with long-standing evidence of cardiomegaly. Many patients progress slowly over several months or years to irreversible severe myocardial dysfunction and death; cardiac transplant may be their only option for survival.

Dilated cardiomyopathy

This diffuse group of diseases, usually of unknown etiology, shows no evidence of myocardial inflammation. Most pediatric conditions in this category are clinically and pathologically indistinguishable with the following notable exceptions.

Anomalous origin of the left coronary artery

In the differential diagnosis of infants with manifestations of primary myocardial disease, anomalous origin of the left coronary artery from the pulmonary artery leads to similar findings but differs from the others in being a congenital anomaly and one that may be improved by operation.

In this condition, the left coronary artery arises from the pulmonary artery, whereas the right coronary artery arises normally from the aorta. As a result, the left ventricular myocardium is poorly perfused so that ischemia and infarction occur. Initially, the inadequate perfusion is related to the low perfusion pressure of the pulmonary artery. Subsequently, collaterals develop between the high-pressure right coronary arterial system and the low-pressure left coronary arterial system. In this situation, blood flows from the right coronary arterial system into the left coronary arterial system. The left ventricular myocardium is also poorly perfused because of the runoff of blood into the pulmonary artery.

History. Neonates are usually asymptomatic. Around the age of 6 weeks they typically develop episodes that have been described as angina, wherein the infant suddenly cries as if in pain, becomes pale, and perspires profusely. These episodes are short and are believed to represent transient myocardial ischemia. Other children may show no symptoms, but many of the patients have signs and symptoms of congestive cardiac failure. The lesion is sometimes recognized only at postmortem examination (e.g., in the adolescent patient who dies suddenly during sports).

Physical examination. The child usually appears normal. No abnormal auscultatory findings may exist, or a soft, apical holosystolic murmur of mitral insufficiency may be found.

Electrocardiogram. The electrocardiogram is usually diagnostic and shows a pattern of anterolateral myocardial infarction, manifested by deep Q waves and inverted T waves in leads I, aVL, V_5, and V_6). In a few cases it may show only left ventricular hypertrophy and strain or a pattern of complete left bundle branch block.

Chest X-ray. Chest X-ray reveals cardiomegaly and a left ventricular contour.

Echocardiography. Echocardiography shows nonspecific cardiac dilation and left ventricular dysfunction. Only the right coronary artery, which is enlarged, can be identified arising from the aorta. Using color Doppler, in some cases the origin of the anomalous coronary artery can be seen as a jet of flow from the left coronary artery into the pulmonary artery.

Management. Patients with cardiac failure should receive anticongestive therapy and should undergo cardiac catheterization. Surgical options include reimplantation of the left coronary artery to the aorta, or surgical creation of a tunnel within the pulmonary artery to establish continuity between the coronary artery and the aorta. Cardiac transplantation may be indicated in patients with severe irreversible left ventricular damage.

Anthracycline cardiotoxicity

Anthracycline chemotherapeutic agents such as doxorubicin (adriamycin) through unclear mechanisms possibly involving excessive oxygen radical formation can cause a cardiomyopathy. Most chemotherapeutic protocols limit the cumulative dose of these agents to 400 mg/m^2, because the incidence of cardiac dysfunction rises sharply with larger doses. A small number of patients, however, develop cardiac failure at levels below what is considered the threshold for toxicity, suggesting that the toxic effect is present at even low doses but only manifests clinically in certain patients. Patients may develop chronic congestive heart failure years after the conclusion of therapy.

Treatment is nonspecific, as with other dilated cardiomyopathies. Various drugs are being investigated that may prevent cardiac injury during chemotherapy.

Endocardial fibroelastosis

Endocardial fibroelastosis (EFE) is a disease of unknown origin that was a common cause of dilated cardiomyopathy in the 1950s and 1960s but that has virtually disappeared in recent decades. Some believe it results from a viral infection, possibly mumps. The endocardium, particularly of the left ventricle and left atrium, is thickened by a proliferation of fibrous and elastic tissue. The endocardium may be 2 mm thick, whereas in the normal individual it is only a few cells thick. The myocardium shows minimal change.

The disease usually presents in infancy as congestive cardiac failure. Electrocardiograms show left ventricular hypertrophy and inverted T waves in the left precordial leads. Gross cardiomegaly, particularly of the left atrium and left ventricle, is present on the chest X-ray.

The echocardiogram shows a strikingly echogenic endocardium, as well as chamber enlargement, decreased systolic function, and mitral regurgitation. (A similar echocardiographic picture, from subendocardial ischemia accompanying severe aortic stenosis, is often called "EFE.") With medical therapy, the prognosis for survival during childhood is good, although the authors have seen several children who died in adolescence after a long asymptomatic period.

Tachycardia-induced cardiomyopathy

Tachycardia-induced cardiomyopathy is a rare but curable type of dilated cardiomyopathy, caused by any incessant tachyarrhythmia of either ventricular or "supraventricular" types. Certain rare types of supraventricular tachyarrhythmias, automatic (ectopic) atrial tachycardia (AET or EAT), and the permanent form of junctional reciprocating tachycardia (PJRT) are particularly likely to cause myocardial dysfunction. Although PJRT has a distinctive electrocardiographic appearance—deep negative P waves in leads II, III, and AVF—other chronic tachyarrhythmias may be difficult to diagnose because they masquerade as sinus tachycardia, a common, nonspecific feature of dilated cardiomyopathy.

Elimination of the tachyarrhythmia usually results in recovery of normal cardiac function, although some degree of left ventricular dilation often persists.

Hypertrophic cardiomyopathy ("HCM"; idiopathic hypertrophic subaortic stenosis, "IHSS")

In this condition the myocardium is greatly thickened, but not in response to any pressure overload. This hypertrophy may be concentric, involving the ventricular walls diffusely, or asymmetric, affecting portions of the wall unevenly usually the ventricular septum.

In contrast to dilated cardiomyopathy, the left ventricular cavity has a normal or decreased size. During systole the hypertrophied myocardium bulges into the left ventricular outflow tract and may result in subaortic obstruction. Other names for this condition are hypertrophic obstructive cardiomyopathy and asymmetrical septal hypertrophy.

HCM has pleomorphic clinical features and course, with some patients progressing to obstruction, others to malignant arrhythmia, and still others to predominant diastolic dysfunction. The disease may be caused by one of many possible mutations of genes coding for various contractile proteins. This condition frequently occurs as an autosomal dominant or sex-linked condition (occurring in males). Multiple generations may be involved. The natural history and prognosis are variable; sudden death is not uncommon, even in patients who have no important obstruction or sentinel arrhythmia.

History
Syncope may be present, but congestive cardiac failure is rare unless an important diastolic dysfunction is found. Chest pain and palpitations, common benign symptoms in most children, may result from myocardial ischemia and/or obstruction and ventricular tachycardia associated with HCM. The family history may reveal other members with similar diagnosis or a history of sudden death.

Physical examination
The peripheral pulses are brisk, and palpation of the apex may reveal a double impulse. A long systolic ejection murmur is present along the left sternal border and faintly radiates to the base. The murmur varies in intensity with change in position; it is usually loudest with the patient standing, in contrast to functional flow murmurs. Third and fourth sounds may be present.

Electrocardiogram
The electrocardiogram shows a normal QRS axis, left ventricular hypertrophy, and occasionally left atrial enlargement. ST segment and T wave changes are common. Deep Q waves may be found in the left precordial leads. Conduction abnormalities of a nonspecific nature may alter the QRS complex.

Chest X-ray
The chest X-ray does not usually show cardiac enlargement related to the left ventricle and left atrium because hypertrophy alone may not alter the external silhouette. In contrast to other forms of aortic stenosis, the ascending aorta is usually of normal size.

Echocardiogram

The echocardiogram shows striking thickening of the left ventricular walls, particularly the interventricular septum, which may be 2–3 cm thick, compared with the normal ≤1 cm.

Systolic anterior motion (SAM) of the mitral valve anterior leaflet is a classic 2D echocardiographic finding. SAM results from the high velocity flow occurring in the left ventricular outflow tract. This creates low pressure which "pulls" the valve leaflet toward the interventricular septum during systole.

Color Doppler reveals disturbed flow within the left ventricular outflow tract, beginning proximal to the aortic valve, unlike other forms of aortic outflow obstruction. Spectral Doppler allows estimation of the systolic gradient by measurement of the maximal velocity; this may change as often as beat to beat because of the dynamic nature of the muscular obstruction.

Management

Because the following therapies increase the gradient, the use of digoxin or other inotropes is contraindicated in these patients. Beta-blockers, calcium channel blockers, and other "negative inotropes" have been advocated for these patients but do not necessarily prevent sudden death.

Implantable cardioverter/defibrillator (ICD) devices may abort potentially lethal arrhythmia in some patients.

Surgical excision of portions of the septal myocardium (myomectomy) has been helpful in some patients with obstruction. Alcohol injected via a coronary artery catheter can achieve a form of nonsurgical myomectomy by destroying myocardium. Ventricular pacing via a transvenous right ventricular electrode may reduce the gradient in some patients, presumably by altering the activation sequence of the left ventricular myocardium; but the response is variable, and few long-term studies of the procedure exist.

Restrictive cardiomyopathy

This is the rarest of the three general types of cardiomyopathy, characterized by poor ventricular compliance and limited filling. Some patients have a mutation of myocardial regulatory proteins, such as troponin, but most forms are idiopathic.

Symptoms are nonspecific and similar to those of congestive heart failure seen with dilated cardiomyopathy. In contrast to dilated cardiomyopathy, the left ventricle is of normal size and may have normal systolic function. Unlike HCM, the left ventricular walls are usually normal in thickness. This condition alters diastolic ventricular function, so the clinical manifestations are those of elevated left and right atrial pressures.

Examination reveals hepatic and splenic enlargement and jugular venous distension. Electrocardiographic abnormalities are usually limited to atrial enlargement. Chest X-ray shows pulmonary vascular congestion with a relatively normal cardiac silhouette.

The echocardiogram reveals striking dilation of the atria and great veins but normal or small ventricles. Physiologically, the condition is similar to restrictive pericarditis; differentiating the two can be difficult.

The prognosis is poor, as clinical decline is often rapid and mortality high. Cardiac transplantation is the only effective treatment.

MYOCARDIAL INVOLVEMENT WITH SYSTEMIC DISEASE

The myocardium of children with certain generalized diseases may be altered as a result of the particular disease process. Children may present clinically with features of dilated, hypertrophic, or restrictive pathophysiology. Inflammatory changes may occur in conditions such as lupus erythematosus. Abnormal substances may accumulate in the heart, as in glycogen storage disease type II or Hurler syndrome. Myocardial fibrosis may develop in neuromuscular disease such as Friedreich's ataxia or muscular dystrophy.

Glycogen storage disease, type II (Pompe disease)

A deficiency of acid maltase leads to the accumulation of glycogen in the myocardium, causing it to be thickened to more than twice normal dimensions.

The infants present within the first 3 months with congestive cardiac failure because of the cardiac involvement. Generalized muscular weakness is also prominent clinically because of the skeletal muscle involvement. The liver, which may contain increased glycogen content, may be enlarged out of proportion to the degree of cardiac failure.

Cardiac examination may be unrevealing except for evidence of cardiomegaly. The electrocardiogram is diagnostic and shows greatly increased QRS voltages and often, a shortened PR interval, and a delta wave consistent with Wolf–Parkinson–White (WPW) syndrome. Cardiomegaly, particularly left ventricular enlargement, is found.

The prognosis is poor; death occurs in the first year of life. Bone marrow transplantation or enzyme replacement therapy has been attempted in some infants but has had poor results.

Hurler syndrome, Hunter syndrome, and other mucopolysaccharidoses

These are storage diseases that affect the heart to a variable degree, but less severely than in Pompe disease. Valves may become thick and insufficient.

Neuromuscular disease

These include Friedreich's ataxia, a neurodegenerative disease, with an abnormal electrocardiogram (most commonly nonspecific ST–T changes) and variable expression of both hypertrophic and dilated cardiomyopathy. The cardiac findings may precede the onset of neurologic symptoms.

Duchenne muscular dystrophy and similar diseases frequently show electrocardiographic abnormalities (including ST–T changes, RBBB, and abnormalities of the QRS axis), some of which may relate to the chronic hypoventilation that accompanies the patient's progressive skeletal muscle weakness.

Both types of disorders may manifest dilated, hypertrophic, and/or restrictive type cardiomyopathy, and the severity of the cardiac dysfunction may be masked by the limitations imposed by the skeletal muscle disease. Although heart failure and arrhythmias can occur, these patients almost always succumb to progressive muscular weakness leading to respiratory failure.

Tuberous sclerosis

Tuberous sclerosis is a phacomatosis manifesting with seizures and skin findings, such as hypopigmented macules ("ash leaf spots") and a typical facial lesion, adenoma sebaceum.

The myocardium often contains benign tumors, rhabdomyomas, which can be extremely large, especially in neonates, but which tend to dwindle in size with age and may even disappear. Although rare patients may have obstruction or an arrhythmia from cardiac rhabdomyoma, myocardial performance is normal in most; the diagnosis is often made from incidental echocardiogram findings in a child being evaluated for other complaints, such as murmur.

Considerations in the differential diagnosis of cardiomyopathy
In infancy, the underlying cause of cardiomyopathy is often indicated by the electrocardiographic findings. Although most causes of cardiomyopathy are associated with ST segment and T wave changes, the QRS patterns may differ.

Myocarditis shows normal or reduced QRS voltages; glycogen storage disease, greatly increased voltages; EFE, left ventricular hypertrophy and strain; and anomalous left coronary artery, a pattern of anterolateral myocardial infarction. Infants with incessant tachycardia, especially with abnormal or frequently changing P wave axis, may have tachycardia-induced cardiomyopathy.

In the older child, other clinical signs and symptoms are related to the underlying disease, such as the characteristic facies and habitus of Hurler syndrome or the presence of the recurrent fever and antinuclear antibodies in a patient with myocardial involvement in lupus erythematosus. Often, however, no findings exist that allow an etiologic diagnosis because many cases are of unknown origin.

Therapy of myocardial disease

Therapy of myocardial disease is directed at the problems developing from the myocardial involvement. Specific treatment is rarely available for the underlying condition. The major therapeutic efforts address cardiac failure and diminished cardiac output. Mainstays of drug therapy include inotropes (e.g., digoxin) to strengthen myocardial contraction; diuretics, such as furosemide, to control pulmonary congestion; and afterload reduction (see Chapter 11).

Cardiomyopathies may lead to mitral insufficiency, probably not so much from dilation of the mitral annulus as from papillary muscle dysfunction. This condition may be related to infarction of the papillary muscle or subjacent ventricular wall or can result from ventricular dilation leading to an abnormal position of the papillary muscle. Regardless of the cause, if major mitral regurgitation results, the left ventricular volume load is further increased; and congestive cardiac failure may be worsened. In rare patients, annuloplasty (plication of the mitral ring) or replacement of the mitral valve may have a strikingly beneficial effect, but surgical mortality is high.

Cardiac arrhythmias, either heart block or tachyarrhythmias, may also occur in patients with cardiomyopathy and may require treatment. Heart block may not require treatment if the patient is asymptomatic. Should syncope occur or congestive cardiac failure worsen, pacemaker implantation may be indicated.

Tachyarrhythmias, such as premature contractions, are usually ventricular in origin and may be harbingers of ventricular tachycardia. Supraventricular tachyarrhythmias, such as atrial flutter or fibrillation, may develop secondary to atrial dilation and require treatment, as they often lead to worsening of the cardiac status. Except for treatment of incessant tachyarrhythmias as a cause for cardiomyopathy, treatment of secondary arrhythmias is controversial. Some studies suggest that aggressive drug therapy of secondary rhythm abnormalities increase mortality, perhaps because of the proarrhythmic effect of these drugs on the abnormal myocardium or by worsening of myocardial function, because most of these drugs are negative inotropes. Implantation of automatic defibrillators may slightly prolong survival in some patients but may not improve the quality of life.

The prognosis of primary myocardial disease as a group is unknown and variable, since a number of diseases cause this symptom complex. Without specific etiologic diagnosis, it is difficult to give a precise prognosis. Some conditions, such as idiopathic myocardial hypertrophy, are progressive and lead to death, whereas others, such as myocarditis, improve but may cause residual abnormalities.

Cardiac transplantation is reserved for patients who are severely ill and who have the worst prognosis for recovery based on worsening clinical course. Transplantation is often a difficult choice in a severely ill child who seems near death but who (rarely) might recover good cardiac function without transplantation. Recipients must have suitable pulmonary vascular resistance determined by pretransplantation catheterization; otherwise, the right ventricle of the donor heart fails acutely, and the patient dies. Since donor organs are in scarce supply, many children succumb to their disease before a suitable organ is available. Side effects of antirejection medication can be considerable and are a major factor in posttransplant mortality. Children who may have been bedridden for months or years with severe cardiac failure often become asymptomatic and return to normal activity within days of successful cardiac transplantation. Because rejection cannot be controlled completely, surveillance for its effects, particularly myocardial dysfunction and a unique form of coronary artery occlusive disease, is necessary over the long term.

INFECTIVE ENDOCARDITIS

Infective endocarditis involves infection of the endocardium or of the endothelium of the great vessels.

This condition usually occurs as a complication of congenital or rheumatic heart disease but occasionally develops without preexisting heart disease.

Infective endocarditis has been divided into subacute and acute forms—the latter is of shorter duration, is more commonly caused by a staphylococcus, and more frequently occurs without preexisting heart disease. This classification has limited use clinically because considerable overlap exists between acute and subacute types.

Streptococcus viridans is the most common causative agent; *Streptococcus faecalis* and *Staphylococcus aureus* occur less commonly. Rarely, other bacteria or fungi are involved. Fungal endocarditis occurs more commonly in immunocompromised patients and in those with indwelling lines or prosthetic valves.

Infective endocarditis usually occurs in cardiac conditions where a large pressure difference leads to a high-velocity jet creating an endocardial lesion susceptible to blood-borne bacteria. The cardiac malformations most often associated with endocarditis are ventricular septal defect, patent ductus arteriosus, aortic stenosis, and tetralogy of Fallot. Endocarditis can also occur in patients with aorticopulmonary shunts, such as a Blalock–Taussig shunt. It can involve the mitral or aortic valves in patients with rheumatic heart disease. Endocarditis is extremely rare in patients with atrial septal defect.

The cardiac lesions consist of vegetations of fibrin, leukocytes, platelets, and bacteria. Many clinical manifestations are related to destructive aspects of the infection or to embolization of portions of the vegetation. Endocarditis, particularly from staphylococcus, may cause valvar damage, such as perforation of the aortic cusps or ruptured chordae tendinae of the mitral valve. Embolization may occur into either the pulmonary or the systemic circulations and cause infarction, abscess, or inflammation of various tissues. Emboli to the lungs, kidneys, spleen, or brain are reported most frequently because in each location there are major clinical or laboratory findings of the phenomenon.

Major efforts should be made to prevent the development of bacterial endocarditis in children with cardiac anomalies (see Chapter 12).

History
Endocarditis occurs rarely before the age of 5 years. Fever, weight loss, anemia, and elevation of the ESR and CRP are common, but nonspecific, clinical findings in patients with bacterial endocarditis. The diagnosis should be suspected in any child with a significant cardiac murmur and a prolonged fever.

Physical examination
The appearance of a new murmur may indicate endocarditis, although a change in intensity of a murmur is not necessarily an indication of endocarditis, particularly as cardiac output, and murmur intensity, increases normally as a result of fever.

Congestive cardiac failure may develop, especially if aortic or mitral valve regurgitation is created by the infection. Signs and symptoms of embolic phenomenon should be sought. Signs of recurrent pneumonia or a pleuritic type of pain may indicate embolization of infected material to the lungs. Signs of systemic embolization, such as splenomegaly, hematuria, splinter hemorrhages, and central nervous system signs, should be sought in any febrile patient with a cardiac anomaly. Half of the patients with infective endocarditis show findings of embolization.

Laboratory findings
The diagnosis can be confirmed by obtaining the organisms from a blood culture. At least six blood cultures should be taken within the first 12 or 24 hours that endocarditis is suspected. It is not necessary to wait for a fever spike, since the chance of obtaining a positive culture is more dependent upon the volume of blood drawn.

Nonspecific acute-phase reactants like ESR, CRP, and rheumatoid factor are usually very elevated; the tests may also be useful in following the progress of therapy.

Echocardiography is not usually helpful in making a diagnosis, because the absence of valve changes or vegetations does not exclude endocarditis. Echocardiography can be helpful by confirming acute changes in valve function suspected clinically. When vegetations are seen, they may persist long after successful antibiotic treatment is concluded. Endocarditis is a clinical and a laboratory diagnosis, not an echocardiographic diagnosis.

Treatment
If the patient is very ill or if the clinical findings are typical, antibiotic treatment can be initiated immediately after the cultures are obtained and before the

results of cultures are available. If the diagnosis is questionable, initiation of therapy should await the results of the blood cultures.

Exact treatment depends upon the organism isolated and its antibiotic sensitivities. Usually, penicillin and nafcillin (until *S. aureus* is excluded) are the preferred antibiotics and are given in large dosages parenterally. Antibiotics may need to be changed if antibiotic sensitivities so indicate. For organisms sensitive to penicillin, low-dose gentamicin is sometimes added for its synergistic effect. Intravenous therapy is continued for 6 weeks. Following completion of therapy, blood cultures should be obtained to verify eradication of the infection.

Despite the availability of antimicrobials, endocarditis can lead to major complications, such as valvar damage or permanent sequelae resulting from embolization; occasionally, the disease is fatal.

MARFAN SYNDROME

Marfan syndrome is an autosomal dominant disease affecting connective tissue and leading to characteristic physical findings and cardiac lesions. A mutation of the gene coding for the structural protein fibrillin is usually the cause. These patients are tall and thin, showing a high incidence of kyphoscoliosis, pectus carinatum or excavatum, arachnodactyly, high-arched palate, and loose joints. Dislocation of the lens is common.

Cardiac anomalies occur in almost all patients and lead to premature death, although death rarely occurs in childhood. Aneurysmal dilation of the ascending aorta and aortic sinuses occurs and leads to aortic regurgitation. The degree of aortic insufficiency may become severe. Dissecting aneurysms can develop in the ascending aorta and lead to death. Mitral insufficiency and prolapse of the valve cusps are also common, resulting from elongated chordae tendinae.

Physical examination

Auscultation may be normal, or a systolic ejection click may result from aortic root dilation. If aortic insufficiency is present, an early diastolic murmur may or may not be audible. Mitral valve prolapse, if present, creates sounds as described in the next section (see Mitral Valve Prolapse).

Electrocardiogram

The electrocardiogram is usually normal, unless the heart is displaced by severe pectus excavatum or unless chamber enlargement from associated aortic or mitral insufficiency exists.

Chest X-ray

The chest X-ray may be normal or can show dilation of the ascending aorta. Pectus and other skeletal anomalies may be evident.

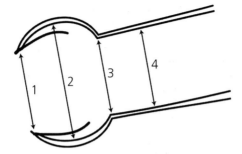

Figure 9.1 Two-dimensional echocardiographic assessment of the aortic root in Marfan syndrome. A parasternal long axis view of the aortic root in systole is used to measure diameter at four levels (1–4), named respectively as annulus (ANN), sinuses of Valsalva (SOV), supraaortic ridge (SAR), and ascending aorta (AAO). Ratios independent of body size and age, with normal upper 95% confidence limits: SOV/ANN =1.56, SAR/ANN =1.28, AAO/ANN =1.35. (Adapted from Sheil MLK, Jenkins O, Sholler GF. Echocardiographic assessment of aortic root dimensions in normal children based on measurement of a new ratio of aortic size independent of growth. Am J Cardiol 1995;75:711–715; Additional references for health professionals available at www.marfan.org.)

Echocardiogram

An echocardiogram is useful for screening and diagnosis of patients suspected of having Marfan syndrome (Fig. 9.1). For patients diagnosed with connective tissue disorder, periodic echocardiography is indicated to detect progressive aortic dilation and valve insufficiency.

Treatment

Many children with Marfan syndrome are asymptomatic, but treatment with beta-blockers (e.g., atenolol and propranolol) and other drugs (angiotensin receptor blockers) has been recommended to try to reduce or slow aortic dilation.

Aortic surgery is performed prophylactically to reduce the risk of sudden death by aortic dissection.

The timing of aortic surgery depends on family history and individual patient findings, such as the presence of aortic dissection, important valvar insufficiency, rapid enlargement of the aortic root, and absolute size of the aorta.

> Guidelines which have been proposed include:
>   In children, enlargement of the ascending aorta diameter by >1 cm/year
>   In adolescents and adults, enlargement of the ascending aorta
>   diameter by >0.5 cm/year or absolute aortic diameter by 4.5–5.0 cm.

Severe aortic or mitral regurgitation requires valve replacement. Replacement of the aortic valve is often combined with replacement of the ascending aorta with a prosthetic graft or homograft in order to prevent dissecting aneurysm. In some patients the aortic root is replaced with prosthetic material, leaving the native aortic valve in place. The long-term prognosis following these operations is good, but other segments of the aorta may remain at risk for aneurysm and dissection.

MITRAL VALVE PROLAPSE

Mitral valve prolapse has been described with increasing frequency in the last 35 years. Originally thought to occur predominantly in females, it may be as prevalent in males as in females. Usually first recognized in adolescence, it is rare in childhood; thus, it may represent an acquired condition or a congenital condition with late presentation, analogous to connective tissue disorder.

When a child is diagnosed with mitral valve prolapse, subtle congenital anomalies, such as mitral cleft or anomalous coronary artery, must be ruled out as well as acquired disorders such as hyperthyroidism or cardiac inflammatory diseases.

A positive family history may exist, but the etiology and pathology are largely unknown. Because of its seeming ubiquitous nature in young adults and the lack of consensus about what constitutes prolapse, controversy persists about the true incidence.

Various symptoms are often attributed to mitral valve prolapse, including chest pain, palpitations, near-syncope, syncope, and "panic attacks." Controlled studies have failed to show strong correlation between patients with these symptoms and those with mitral prolapse. The symptoms may represent a mild form of autonomic nervous system dysfunction, for which mitral prolapse is a weak marker.

Physical examination

The auscultatory findings are diagnostic. At the apex a mid- or late-systolic murmur exists that often begins with one or multiple mid-systolic to late-systolic clicks. The characteristics of the murmur are variable. Any maneuver that decreases left ventricular diastolic volume, such as a Valsalva maneuver, standing, or inhalation of amyl nitrate, causes the murmur to begin earlier and last longer. The increase in murmur intensity with the patient standing is similar to HCM, and is unlike innocent flow murmurs. The click occurs earlier with standing and later with squatting or in the supine position.

Laboratory findings

The electrocardiogram and chest X-ray are usually normal in the absence of significant regurgitation.

Echocardiography may show either one or both mitral valve leaflets prolapsing into the left atrium. The prolapse occurs maximally in mid-systole and may be associated with mitral regurgitation beginning in mid- or late-systole. Mitral regurgitation is easily demonstrated by color Doppler, yet current equipment is sufficiently sensitive that "physiologic" trace mitral regurgitation is commonly seen in normal individuals without prolapse.

Treatment

The prognosis is good for patients with mitral valve prolapse. There is virtually no risk of sudden death, provided that mitral regurgitation is not severe and that the mitral prolapse is not related to another condition, such as intrinsic cardiomyopathy, systemic disorder, or myocardial ischemic problem. Embolic stroke is so rare that the association with mitral prolapse remains controversial. Endocarditis is rare in individuals with mitral valve prolapse, and the indications for prophylactic antibiotics are controversial; the American Heart Association no longer recommends routine prophylaxis. Individuals with marked mitral insufficiency and/or myxomatous valve leaflets may be at greater risk and probably should receive prophylaxis.

PERICARDITIS

Pericarditis can result from a variety of diseases. The most common in our experience are (a) idiopathic, presumed viral; (b) purulent; (c) juvenile rheumatoid arthritis or systemic lupus erythematosus; (d) uremia; (e) neoplastic diseases; and (f) postoperative (postpericardiotomy syndrome).

In these conditions, both the pericardial sac and the visceral pericardium are involved. As a result of the inflammation, fluid may accumulate within the sac. The symptoms that result from pericardial fluid depend upon the status of the myocardium and the volume and the speed at which the fluid accumulates. A slow accumulation of a large volume is often better tolerated than the rapid accumulation of a small volume.

Cardiac tamponade can develop because of fluid accumulation within the pericardial sac. The pericardial fluid can compress the heart and/or interfere with ventricular filling. Three mechanisms compensate for the tamponade: (a) elevation of atrial and ventricular end-diastolic pressures; (b) tachycardia to compensate for lowered stroke volume; and (c) increased diastolic blood pressure from peripheral vasoconstriction to compensate for diminished cardiac output. These compensatory mechanisms must be considered in selecting medical treatment.

Clinical and laboratory findings are related to (a) the inflammation of the pericardium, (b) cardiac tamponade, and (c) etiologic factors.

Physical examination

Pericarditis is accompanied by pain in about half the patients. This pain may be dull, sharp, or stabbing. The pain may be located in the left thorax, neck, or shoulder and is improved when the patient is sitting.

A pericardial friction rub, a rough scratchy sound, may be present over the precordium. It is louder when the patient is sitting, or when the stethoscope is pressed firmly against the chest wall. The rub is evanescent, so repeated examinations may be needed to identify it. No direct relationship between the amount of pericardial fluid and the presence of a rub has been found, but with large effusions a rub is often not heard.

Cardiac tamponade is reflected by several physical findings. The patient may appear to be in distress and may be more comfortable when sitting. The neck veins are distended and, in contrast to normal, increase on inspiration. The heart sounds may be muffled. Hepatomegaly may be found. Tachycardia develops and is a valuable means of following the patient. As the stroke volume falls because of the tamponade, the heart rate increases to maintain cardiac output. The pulse pressure also narrows, and this can be measured accurately and serially to follow the patient's course. Peripheral pulses diminish as systemic vasoconstriction heightens and pulse pressure narrows. Central pulses diminish because of the narrow pulse pressure and decreased stroke volume.

Excess pulsus paradoxus, a decrease in pulse pressure of more than 20 mm Hg with inspiration (normal is less than 10 mm Hg), is also highly diagnostic of tamponade and can often be identified by palpation of the radial pulse. Excess pulsus paradoxus is not absolutely specific for tamponade; it often occurs in severe asthma, for example.

Historical and physical findings may suggest an etiology of the pericardial effusion, such as a history of neoplasm or uremia.

In many patients, no etiology is found for acute pericarditis. Certain viral agents, such as Coxsackie B, have been identified as causative agents for pericarditis. In these patients frequently a history of a preceding respiratory infection is found. Among patients with purulent pericarditis, *Hemophilus influenzae*, pneumococcus, and staphylococcus are the most common organisms. Purulent pericarditis usually occurs in infancy and may follow or be associated with infection at another site, such as pneumonia or osteomyelitis. The infants often show a high leukocyte count and appear to be very septic. An important clue in some infants and toddlers may be grunting respirations in the absence of auscultatory or radiographic evidence of pneumonia.

Pericarditis can develop secondary to juvenile rheumatoid arthritis and may occur before other manifestations of this disease. Usually, children show high fever, leukocytosis, and other systemic signs. Tamponade is rare.

Electrocardiogram

The electrocardiogram (Fig. 9.2) usually shows ST segment and T wave changes. Early in the course of the disease, the ST segment is elevated and the T wave is upright. Subsequently, the ST segments return to the isoelectric line, and the T waves become diffusely inverted. Reciprocal ST–T changes (elevation in one group of leads and depression in the opposite leads) are common early. Later, both ST segments and T waves return to normal. The QRS voltage may be reduced, particularly with a large fluid accumulation.

Chest X-ray

The chest X-ray may be normal, but the cardiac silhouette enlarges proportionately with accumulation of pericardial fluid.

Echocardiogram

Pericardial effusion can be recognized quite accurately by echocardiography, and this technique may be helpful in diagnosing suspicious cases. Often the fluid can be characterized as purulent versus serous because leukocytes are more echogenic (giving an echo-bright cloudy or smokey appearance) than fluid alone (which appears black by 2D echocardiography). Left ventricular diastolic diameter may be reduced because of inability of the ventricle to fill properly. The systolic function of the left ventricle is normal or even hyperdynamic. Tamponade is accompanied by dilation of the hepatic veins, vena cavae, and early diastolic "collapse" of the right atrium and right ventricle.

Treatment

Pericardiocentesis is indicated in many patients to confirm the diagnosis, to identify the etiology, or to treat pericardial tamponade. In patients with purulent pericarditis, pericardiocentesis is indicated, since reaching an etiologic diagnosis is imperative so that appropriate antibiotic therapy can be initiated. Other than in patients with neoplasm and purulent pericarditis, the analysis of the fluid rarely yields a diagnosis.

Pericardiocentesis is indicated often as an emergency procedure to treat the cardiac tamponade by removing fluid and thereby allowing adequate cardiac filling.

At times, particularly with recurrent tamponade, a thoracotomy with creation of a pericardial window is indicated to decompress the pericardial sac.

Pericardiectomy, removal of a large panel of the parietal pericardium, is sometimes performed, especially in purulent pericarditis, in the hopes of avoiding late restrictive pericarditis as the sac scars and contracts.

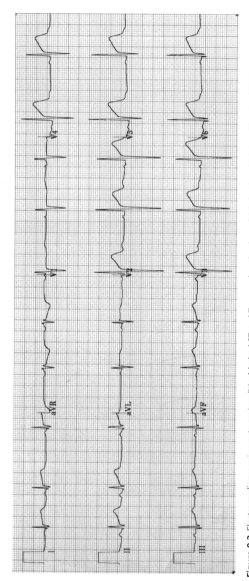

Figure 9.2 Electrocardiogram in acute pericarditis. Marked ST and T wave elevation in multiple leads, which is unlike the ST–T changes seen with acute myocardial ischemia or with coronary artery anomalies.

Other management may be indicated for pericarditis. Symptomatic relief of pain is indicated. Digoxin and diuretics are contraindicated because they slow the heart rate and reduce the filling pressure, contrary to the normal compensatory mechanisms for tamponade. High doses of antibiotics are indicated in purulent pericarditis, the type to be determined by antibiotic sensitivities, and open or closed drainage may be necessary. Appropriate cultures for mycobacteria and fungus should be performed, especially in immunocompromised patients. Skin tests for mycobacterial and fungus infection, with appropriate controls, may be helpful, especially if cultures prove negative.

ADDITIONAL READING

Baddour LM, Wilson WR, Bayer AS, et al., for Committee on Rheumatic Fever, Endocarditis, and Kawasaki Disease; Council on Cardiovascular Disease in the Young; Councils on Clinical Cardiology, Stroke, and Cardiovascular Surgery and Anesthesia; American Heart Association; Infectious Diseases Society of America. Infective endocarditis: Diagnosis, antimicrobial therapy, and management of complications: A statement for healthcare professionals from the Committee on Rheumatic Fever, Endocarditis, and Kawasaki Disease, Council on Cardiovascular Disease in the Young, and the Councils on Clinical Cardiology, Stroke, and Cardiovascular Surgery and Anesthesia, American Heart Association: endorsed by the Infectious Diseases Society of America. Circulation June 14, 2005;111(23):e394–e434.

Cilliers AM. Rheumatic fever and its management. BMJ 2006;333:1153–1156.

Ferrieri P, Gewitz MH, Gerber MA, et al. Unique features of infective endocarditis in childhood. Pediatrics May 2002;109(5):931–943, and Circulation April 30, 2002;105(17):2115–2126.

Newburger JW, Takahashi M, Gerber MA, et al., for Committee on Rheumatic Fever, Endocarditis and Kawasaki Disease; Council on Cardiovascular Disease in the Young; American Heart Association; American Academy of Pediatrics. Diagnosis, treatment, and long-term management of Kawasaki disease: A statement for health professionals from the Committee on Rheumatic Fever, Endocarditis and Kawasaki Disease, Council on Cardiovascular Disease in the Young, American Heart Association. Pediatrics December 2004;114(6):1708–1733, and Circulation October 26, 2004;110(17):2747–2771.

Pickering LK, Baker CJ, McMillan J, Long S. (eds.) Red Book: Report of the Committee on Infectious Diseases, 27th ed. Elk Grove Village, IL: American Academy of Pediatrics; 2006.

Roy CL, Minor MA, Brookhart MA, Choudhry NK. Does this patient with a pericardial effusion have cardiac tamponade? JAMA April 25, 2007;297(16):1810–1818.

World Health Organization. Rheumatic fever and rheumatic heart disease: Report of a WHO expert consultation. Geneva: WHO; October 29–November 1, 2001. WHO Technical Report Series 2004:923. Available from http://www.who.int/cardiovascular_diseases/resources/en/cvd_trs923.pdf. Accessed October 2007.

Chapter 10
Arrhythmias

Disturbance of cardiac rate and conduction occur in children with no history of preceding cardiac disease; as a manifestation of congenital or acquired cardiac disease; as a complication of drug therapy, particularly digoxin therapy; or as a manifestation of metabolic, particularly electrolyte, abnormalities.

Cardiac arrhythmias can be generally classified as (1) alterations in cardiac rate or (2) abnormalities of cardiac conduction.

ALTERATIONS IN CARDIAC RATE

Cardiac arrhythmias result from either of two mechanisms (a) automatic tachycardias—alterations in the rate of discharge of pacemakers at the atrial, junctional, or ventricular level, or (b) reentry mechanisms, occurring solely within the atria (primary atrial tachyarrhythmias), or ventricles (some types of ventricular tachycardia), or from reentry circuits involving atria, ventricles, junctional tissue, and abnormal atrial-to-ventricular connections (atrioventricular tachyarrhythmias).

Atrial and atrioventricular arrhythmias
Sinus arrhythmia
Sinus arrhythmia is a variation of normal sinus rhythm (SR; Fig. 10.1). It describes the normal increase in cardiac rate with inspiration and the slowing with expiration. Sometimes with expiration, nodal escape occurs.

Pediatric Cardiology, by W Johnson, J Moller © 2008 Blackwell Publishing,
ISBN: 978-1-4051-7818-1.

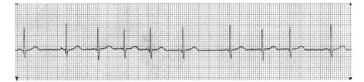

Figure 10.1 Electrocardiogram of sinus arrhythmia. Each QRS complex is preceded by a P wave, but the interval between each P wave is variable, usually changing with the respiratory cycle.

Premature atrial systole

Premature atrial systole (or contractions, PACs) (Fig. 10.2) occur commonly in the fetus and young infant less than 2 months of age but uncommonly in children past that age; they arise from ectopic (and automatic) atrial foci. On the electrocardiogram this condition is recognized by a P wave with an abnormal shape which is different in contour to the patient's usual P waves. They occur earlier than normal P waves do, so prematurely, in fact, that the atrioventricular node (AVN) is completely refractory, resulting in no QRS. PACs occurring during partial AVN refractoriness may be conducted aberrantly, mimicking multiform premature ventricular contractions (PVCs). PACs occurring after the AVN has ceased to be refractory are conducted normally with a narrow QRS. No treatment is required.

Sinus tachycardia

The normal sinoatrial node (SAN) can discharge at a rapid rate up to 210 beats per minute (bpm) in response to some stimulus such as fever, shock, atropine, or epinephrine. The increased heart rate does not require treatment, but the tachycardia should be considered a clinical finding that requires diagnosis and perhaps treatment of the root cause.

Paroxysmal supraventricular tachycardia

Paroxysmal supraventricular tachycardia (SVT, PSVT, PAT), often occurring with minimal or no symptoms, leads to death in rare cases if untreated. Typically, a

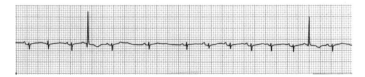

Figure 10.2 Electrocardiogram of premature atrial contractions.

previously healthy infant develops poor feeding, sweating, irritability, and rapid respiration. If the arrhythmia is unrecognized and untreated, congestive cardiac failure may progress to death in 24–48 hours. Recognition of arrhythmia is not difficult when examining the heart. The measured heart rate of 250–350 bpm (Fig. 10.3) is remarkably regular, showing no variation when the child breathes, cries, or becomes quiet.

The prognosis is excellent because many infants have no underlying cardiac malformation and recurrent episodes are rare or infrequent and are well tolerated, if of short duration. A few infants with Ebstein's malformation and/or Wolf–Parkinson–White (WPW) syndrome, however, may have repeated episodes of SVT.

The mechanism of this type of tachycardia is virtually always reentry via an accessory pathway between the atria and ventricles (Fig. 10.4). Normally, only one electrically conductive pathway—the penetrating bundle of His—exists between the atria and ventricles. In more than 95% of fetuses, infants, and young children with SVT, an abnormal accessory connection (AC) exists between the atria or ventricles, a possible vestige of the multiple connections that exist in the embryonic cardiac tube before separate chambers are formed.

This AC in participation with the AVN, the atria, and the ventricles may create a large reentrant circuit (Fig. 10.4). Impulses may conduct normally via the AVN (orthodromic conduction) but pass retrograde to the atria via the AC when the AVN is refractory. Then the impulse passes from atria through the AVN, to the ventricles, then to the atria via the AC, as the sequence is repeated. This creates orthodromic reciprocating tachycardia (ORT), the most common mechanism for childhood SVT. Because the tachycardia is not truly supraventricular (SV) but actually atrioventricular (AV) and is dependent on four components—atria, AVN, ventricles, and AC—any of these components can be altered slightly to terminate the tachycardia. In practical terms, the AVN is the component most amenable to intervention by vagal stimulation or medication such as adenosine.

The second most common tachycardia mechanism involves a small reentrant circuit within or near the AVN itself (Fig. 10.4). It can be thought of as an acquired form of SVT, since it has never been reported in children less than 4 years of age but does occur in half of adults with SVT. As in ORT, the tachycardia depends on atria, ventricles, and a fast and a slow pathway within the AVN; as an AV tachycardia, it is called atrioventricular nodal reentry tachycardia (AVNRT). The electrocardiogram shows a regular, narrow-QRS tachycardia similar in appearance to ORT. Conversion is best accomplished by altering AVN conduction via vagal stimulation or medication.

Atrial flutter

In atrial flutter, the atrial rate may be between 280 and 400 bpm with a 2–1, or greater, degree of AV block so that ventricular rate is slower than the atrial

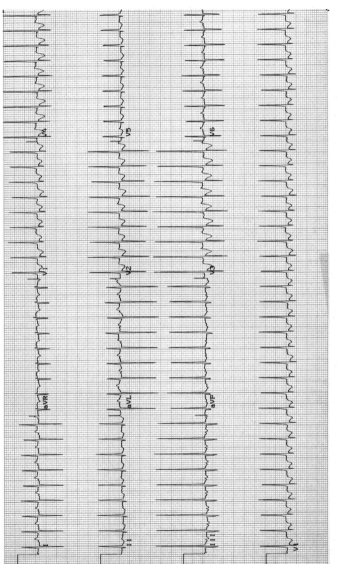

Figure 10.3 Electrocardiogram of supraventricular tachycardia. A regular narrow-QRS tachycardia without easily seen P waves.

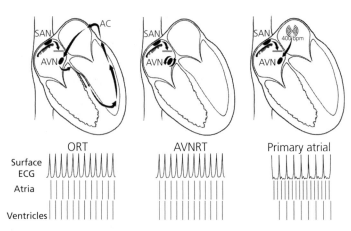

Figure 10.4 Mechanisms of supraventricular tachycardia. Orthodromic reciprocating tachycardia (ORT) is the most common in children. An abnormal accessory connection (AC) with the atrioventricular node (AVN) and the atria and ventricles constitutes a reentrant circuit. In atrioventricular node reentry tachycardia (AVNRT), the circuit includes two pathways within the AVN and also the atria and ventricles. Both types result in a regular narrow-QRS tachycardia without discernible P waves. Primary atrial tachycardia (e.g., atrial flutter) originates in the atria (true SVT) and conducts via the AVN to the ventricles—in this case, in a 2:1 ratio. P waves may or may not be seen. The lower panel allows simultaneous comparison of the surface ECG with electrograms recorded in the atria and ventricles. In each type, the sinoatrial node (SAN) is suppressed because of the more rapid SVT.

rate (Fig. 10.4). On the electrocardiogram, the atrial activity does not appear as distinct P waves; instead, it has a sawtooth appearance (Fig. 10.5).

This arrhythmia can occur in infants without an underlying condition or in children with conditions such as dilated cardiomyopathy, Ebstein's malformation, or rheumatic mitral disease that leads to a greatly enlarged atrium.

Digitalization usually slows the ventricular rate by slowing the AVN, but rarely does it result in conversion. Cardioversion (synchronized with the R wave to avoid induction of dangerous ventricular rhythms) with very low energy (usually 0.25 Joule/kg) converts the rhythm to a sinus mechanism.

Atrial fibrillation

Atrial fibrillation is associated with chaotic atrial activity at a rate of more than 400 bpm. Distinct P waves are not seen, but atrial activity is evident as small, irregular wave forms on the electrocardiogram (Fig. 10.6). The ventricular response is irregular. This arrhythmia results from conditions that chronically dilate

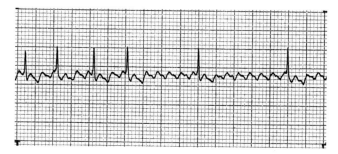

Figure 10.5 Electrocardiogram of atrial flutter. Regular P waves with less than 1-to-1 atrioventricular conduction.

the atria. Hyperthyroidism is a rare cause in childhood. Digoxin is indicated to slow the ventricular response. Cardioversion may require a high energy (1–2 Joules/kg) although biphasic shocks are often successful at lower energy compared to monophasic.

Reinitiation of atrial fibrillation is common, especially with underlying structural heart disease or cardiomyopathy. Antithrombotic therapy, usually with coumadin, is often used to minimize the risk of embolic stroke in patients with atrial fibrillation. In some patients, particularly those with complex postoperative disease, atrial fibrillation may be refractory to antiarrhythmic medication. Such patients may be candidates for a surgical or catheter (radiofrequency ablation) procedure to create multiple linear scars within the atria to prevent atrial fibrillation from becoming sustained (Maze procedure). In other patients, tolerance of chronic atrial fibrillation may be achieved by control of ventricular rate, using a variety of techniques, including medication, and AVN ablation and pacemaker implantation.

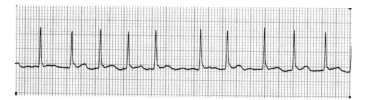

Figure 10.6 Electrocardiogram of atrial fibrillation. Wavy isoelectric line reflects the irregular and rapid atrial activity. Typically, the ventricular rate is "irregularly irregular."

Junctional arrhythmias

Ectopic (automatic) arrhythmias arise from the AVN; they are called nodal or junctional premature beats or tachycardia.

Premature junctional contractions

The QRS complex is normal because the impulses propagate along the normal conduction pathway. The P waves may appear with an abnormal form shortly before the QRS complex, may be buried within the QRS complex, or may follow the QRS complex.

Junctional ectopic tachycardia

This automatic tachycardia is sometimes seen in the early postoperative period after a cardiac operation where it can result in severe hemodynamic compromise. The rate of junctional ectopic tachycardia (JET), often around 200 bpm, may be difficult to control, requiring multiple interventions (including lowering of the core body temperature) and medications.

Permanent junctional reciprocating tachycardia

This rare form of incessant tachycardia is frequently associated with reversible myocardial dysfunction, although the heart rate is usually only 150–200 bpm. The P wave axis is always abnormal, with negative P waves in leads II, III, and AVF. Permanent junctional reciprocating tachycardia (PJRT) is actually an AV tachycardia caused by an accessory AV connection located near the os of the coronary sinus. Although rare, children may have spontaneous disappearance of the tachycardia, medication, or radiofrequency (RF), ablation is usually required.

Ventricular arrhythmias

Ventricular arrhythmias are characterized by widened QRS complexes and large abnormal T waves generally with opposite polarity to the QRS complex. They arise from ectopic foci in the His bundles, reentrant pathways within the ventricular myocardium, or from automatic foci in the myocardium.

Premature ventricular contractions

In children, PVCs are usually benign. They are recognized by bizarre QRS complexes falling irregularly in the normal cardiac rhythm (Fig. 10.7). This widened QRS has a different configuration from the normal QRS complex, does not follow a P wave, and is associated with a large T wave. Following the ectopic beat, a compensatory pause occurs. Generally, PVCs are unifocal, meaning that each of the aberrant QRS complexes has an identical configuration. PVCs occur more frequently at slow SR rates, happening as often as every other beat (bigeminy), and decrease in frequency or disappear at fast sinus rates, as with exercise. They do not usually occur in pairs (couplets).

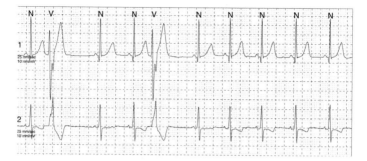

Figure 10.7 Electrocardiogram of premature ventricular contractions. These ectopic beats occur as wide-QRS premature complexes associated with abnormal T waves.

A useful office diagnostic technique to evaluate PVCs is to have the child perform mild exercise. Then, determine if the PVCs disappear with increased heart rate. Continue to listen or monitor with electrocardiogram following exercise, while the heart rate is returning to normal. The PVCs tend to return as the heart rate slows.

PVCs in children usually require no treatment, as the prognosis is excellent. Patients with a benign history (including family history) and normal physical examination should have an electrocardiogram to exclude the presence of multifocal PVCs (see later) and of abnormalities such as hypertrophic cardiomyopathy, WPW, or long QT syndrome. Patients with PVCs who otherwise have a normal evaluation are said to have benign PVCs of childhood.

In some patients, PVCs with QRS complexes of varying contours are present. These multifocal PVCs are often related to myocardial disease. They tend to increase with exercise and seek a cause by history, physical examination, electrolytes, and echocardiography, as indicated. PVCs may develop as a sign of a metabolic abnormality (e.g., hyperkalemia) or drug toxicity (especially digoxin) and require treatment of the metabolic abnormality or discontinuance of the medication, followed by careful monitoring. Occasionally, multifocal PVCs result from a right atrial central venous catheter tip intermittently entering the right ventricle in diastole.

Ventricular tachycardia

Ventricular tachycardia (VT) arises as a rapidly discharging ventricular focus at a rate of 150–250 bpm. These arrhythmias are usually serious and associated with symptoms of chest pain, palpitations, or syncope. This rhythm may occur in normal children as a manifestation of digoxin or other drug toxicity,

(a)

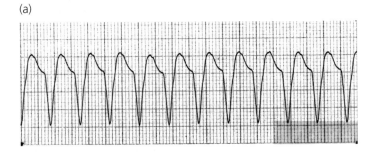

(b)

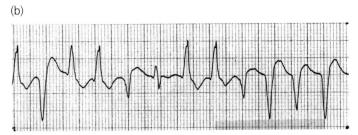

Figure 10.8 Electrocardiogram of ventricular tachycardia. Wide-QRS complexes occurring at regular intervals without evidence of atrial activity. (a) Monomorphic ventricular tachycardia, the most commonly seen. (b) Torsades de pointes (literally, "twisting of the points").

in myocarditis, or as a terminal event after a catastrophic injury or metabolic derangement.

The electrocardiogram shows regular wide-QRS complexes (Fig. 10.8a) and often P waves that occur at a slower rate (AV dissociation). Patients with antiarrhythmic drug toxicity (particularly procainamide) and those with the long QT syndrome may have a distinctive type of VT called torsades de pointes (literally, "twisting of the points" or axis) (Fig. 10.8b).

Rare patients, usually infants, have a self-limited, apparently benign, monomorphic VT that usually requires no treatment. In almost all other patients, VT requires cardioversion, either by external direct current shock, intracardiac pacing in the catheterization laboratory, or drug therapy; the immediacy and type of cardioversion depend on whether or not the child is hemodynamically stable and, if stable, upon the degree of symptoms.

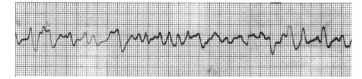

Figure 10.9 Electrocardiogram of ventricular fibrillation. Irregular disorganized ventricular activity.

Ventricular fibrillation

The electrocardiographic finding of ventricular fibrillation often represents a terminal event and appears as wide, bizarre, irregularly occurring wave forms of various amplitudes (Fig. 10.9). Cardiac output is markedly decreased. VT may degenerate into ventricular fibrillation. It is treated by the methods used for management of cardiopulmonary arrest and by external nonsynchronized direct current shock.

CONDUCTION DISTURBANCES

Most major conduction disturbances occur between the atrium and the ventricles at the level of the AVN.

Shortened atrioventricular conduction (preexcitation syndromes)

In preexcitation syndromes, conduction through or around the AVN is accelerated; such patients tend to develop episodes of paroxysmal supraventricular tachycardia.

One of these conditions, the WPW syndrome, has three electrocardiographic features: (1) a shortened PR interval; (2) a widened QRS complex; and (3) a delta wave, a slurred broadened initial portion of the QRS complex (Fig. 10.10).

WPW syndrome results from a microscopic accessory AV connection (Fig. 10.11), consisting of working myocardium (i.e., lacking the electrical properties of the AV nodal tissue that allow for normal delay in atrial to ventricular impulse transmission). Such a delay, called the PR interval, is necessary for efficient movement of blood from atria to ventricles before ventricular systole.

In WPW, the AC conducts antegrade from atria to ventricles, much faster than the AVN, allowing a portion of the ventricle to depolarize early, thus creating the slurred delta wave and short PR interval.

When impulses conduct retrograde, from ventricles to atria via the AC, SVT may occur by the identical mechanism as in those patients whose concealed AC only conducts one way.

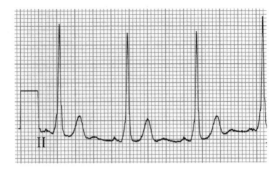

Figure 10.10 Electrocardiogram in Wolff–Parkinson–White (WPW) syndrome. Short PR interval and wide-QRS complex with a delta wave, indicated by slurred initial portion of QRS complex.

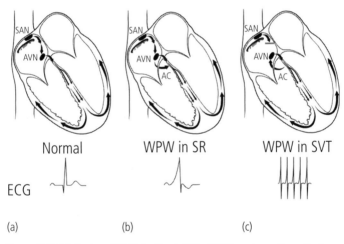

Figure 10.11 Mechanism of Wolff–Parkinson–White (WPW) syndrome. Normal is shown for comparison (a). During sinus rhythm (SR), WPW patients have early activation (preexcitation) of a portion of the ventricular myocardium via an abnormal accessory connection (AC) that conducts more rapidly from atrium to ventricle than the atrioventricular node (AVN) (b). If a WPW patient has "supraventricular tachycardia" (SVT), the AC conducts from ventricle to atrium; therefore, a delta wave is not present, and the QRS is narrow, similar to other patients with this type of SVT (orthodromic reciprocating tachycardia) (c). (Abbreviation: SAN, sinoatrial node.)

WPW patients have a manifest AC only evident electrocardiographically during SR; SVT appears the same for WPW patients as for those with concealed connections.

In rare patients with WPW, conduction via the AC is so rapid—much faster than that which occurs via the AVN—that rapid atrial arrhythmias like atrial flutter may result in very rapid atrial-to-ventricular conduction, ventricular fibrillation, and sudden death.

Patients with concealed ACs do not risk sudden death during primary atrial tachyarrhythmias because the only atrial-to-ventricular conduction is via the normal AVN, limiting the ventricular rate to 210 bpm or less.

Many cardiologists discourage the use of verapamil or digoxin in WPW patients, since these drugs may speed conduction through the AC in rare WPW patients and thus increase the risk of life-threatening arrhythmia.

WPW syndrome may be present in patients without other cardiac anomalies and in patients with Ebstein's malformation or other structural malformations.

In the other preexcitation syndromes, the PR interval is short, but the QRS is of normal duration.

Prolonged atrioventricular conduction

Several forms of prolonged AV conduction have been described.

First-degree heart block

First-degree heart block (Fig. 10.12) is represented by prolongation of the PR interval beyond the normal range; each P wave is also followed by a QRS complex. Digoxin, acute rheumatic fever, and acute infections can cause first-degree heart block. Certain neuromuscular diseases may also cause it, but it is also seen in a small number of otherwise normal individuals. It does not require treatment.

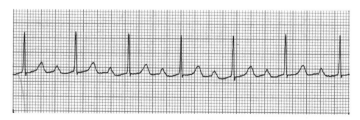

Figure 10.12 Electrocardiogram in first-degree heart block. Prolonged PR interval and 1:1 atrioventricular conduction.

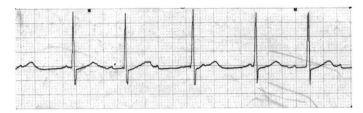

Figure 10.13 Electrocardiogram in second-degree heart block, type I (Wenckebach). The PR interval lengthens each beat until conduction fails and a "beat is dropped." The QRS is typically "regularly irregular."

Second-degree heart block

In this form of heart block, each P wave is not followed by a QRS complex. A 2:1, 3:1, or greater block may exist between the atria and the ventricles.

Two types occur, often named Mobitz types.

Type I. Type I (Wenckebach; Fig. 10.13) is characterized by a progressively lengthening PR interval until a P wave fails to conduct to the ventricles and a ventricular beat is "dropped" (absent). Type I second-degree block is usually benign and is often seen during drug therapy (especially digoxin) or minor metabolic derangements. It may occur in asymptomatic individuals with a structurally normal heart. Treatment is not indicated in asymptomatic patients.

Type II. Type II (Fig. 10.14) is characterized by sudden failure of AVN conduction without any sentinel abnormalities of the preceding beats. Type II second-degree AV block is often associated with serious AVN disease, and the

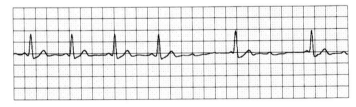

Figure 10.14 Electrocardiogram in second-degree heart block, type II. The PR interval is normal and constant, until sudden failure of conduction from atria to ventricle occurs.

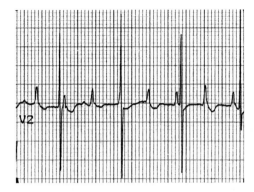

Figure 10.15 Electrocardiogram in complete heart block. P waves and QRS complexes are occurring independently, and the ventricular rate is slow.

propensity for progression to complete AV block is high. Patients often have syncopal episodes. A pacemaker is usually indicated.

Third-degree heart block

This condition is complete AV block with dissociation between the atria and the ventricles, and the atrial impulse does not influence the ventricles (Fig. 10.15). Since the ventricular rate is slow, ventricular stroke volume is increased, leading to a soft systolic ejection and a mid-diastolic murmur and cardiomegaly.

Third-degree heart block can occur congenitally, often associated with maternal autoimmune disease (see Chapter 2). It has a good prognosis except in those cases with a family history of heart block from neuromuscular disease or myopathy or in neonates with major cardiac structural anomalies. It may also develop from digoxin toxicity or may follow a cardiac operation. The prognosis for recovery from postoperative block is poor. Complete heart block may be associated with syncopal episodes (Stokes–Adams attacks) but is usually not tied to congestive cardiac failure, unless additional cardiac abnormalities exist, particularly those placing volume loads on the ventricles.

If the heart rate is persistently low (less than 40 bpm) or if syncopal episodes occur, a permanently implanted pacemaker is indicated. A pacemaker is usually indicated in children with postoperative heart block because of the high incidence of sudden death. Waiting for 2 weeks after operation, with careful monitoring, before implanting a permanent pacemaker is wise, as within that time SR may return.

GENERAL PRINCIPLES OF TACHYARRHYTHMIA DIAGNOSIS AND MANAGEMENT

Initial clinical assessment

Patients with tachycardia should be immediately assessed for hemodynamic stability. Stable infants and children may have no symptoms or minimal complaints, such as palpitations in a child old enough to articulate them. In a preverbal child the parents may observe rapid forceful precordial activity.

Children showing hemodynamic compromise from their tachycardia have increased respiratory rate, resulting from pulmonary congestion and/or compensation of the metabolic acidosis that follows from inadequate cardiac output.

Inadequate cardiac output is reflected by poorly palpable pulses, decreased skin perfusion, agitation, listlessness, or unconsciousness.

A normal oxygen saturation by pulse oximeter is the rule and therefore is an unreliable means of assessing the hemodynamic effect of tachycardia, except in patients with a cyanotic cardiac malformation, such as unrepaired tetralogy of Fallot, or following a "fenestrated" Fontan or partial Fontan operation. In these cyanotic patients, oxygen saturation (as well as cardiac output in the patients with a cavopulmonary anastomosis) falls dramatically during tachycardia.

Patients with significant reduction of cardiac output during tachyarrhythmia are obviously unstable; they die without immediate cardioversion (usually best accomplished by external direct current shock) and other resuscitative and support measures.

Stable patients in tachycardia should be assessed using the 12-lead electrocardiogram (Table 10.1) to obtain valuable diagnostic and therapeutic information that cannot be gathered by a single-lead rhythm strip or by counting the heart rate during physical examination.

Differential diagnosis and management in stable patients

Most tachyarrhythmias in children are regular (each R–R interval varying by less than 10 ms). Stable regular tachycardia with wide QRS is either SR with preexisting bundle branch block, a variety of SVT with bundle branch block,

Table 10.1 Electrocardiographic Differential Diagnosis of the Most Common Narrow-QRS (Supraventricular) Tachycardias in Neonates, Children, and Adolescents.

Rhythm	P Waves	Ventricular Rate	Minute-to-Minute Rate Variation	Ventricular Rhythm	Response to Adequate Adenosine Dose or Vagal Stimulation
Sinus tachycardia	Distinct	≤230 bpm neonates ≤210 infants and children ≤180–200 adolescents	Yes	Regular	*Gradual* slowing of atrial and ventricular rate ± transient 2° AVB
AV re-entrant tachycardia					
ORT (any age)	Indistinct	240–280 bpm	No	Regular	*Sudden* conversion to sinus
AVNRT (≥4 years)	Indistinct	160–240 bpm	No	Regular	*Sudden* conversion to sinus
Primary atrial tachycardia					
Atrial flutter	Regular uniform flutter waves	120–280 bpm	No	Regular	Transient 2° AVB, no change in atrial rate, atrial rate usually a multiple of ventricular rate
Atrial fibrillation	Irregular low voltage	120–280 bpm	±	Irregular	Transient ventricular slowing, no change in atrial rhythm
Automatic or "Chaotic"	Irregular multiform	160–280 bpm	±	Irregular	Transient ventricular slowing, no change in atrial rhythm

2° AVB, second-degree atrioventricular nodal block; AVNRT, atrioventricular nodal reentry tachycardia; bpm, beats per minute; ORT, orthodromic reciprocating tachycardia.

or VT. The last should be suspected first, even in asymptomatic patients. The presence of AV dissociation (atria and ventricles contracting at different rates) during wide-QRS tachycardia is virtually pathognomonic of VT.

A regular narrow-QRS tachycardia is either SR (but not at rates greater than about 210 bpm), a primary atrial tachyarrhythmia (e.g., atrial flutter), or most commonly, one of the AV reentrant tachyarrhythmias.

Sinus tachycardia varies in rate from minute to minute, whereas the latter two tachyarrhythmias tend to have no rate variation, despite changes in the infant's activity level.

A 12-lead electrocardiogram allows better definition of P waves than a single-lead recording. P waves are usually easily seen in sinus tachycardia, can appear, obvious or not, as a "sawtooth" pattern in atrial flutter, and are generally not well seen in AV tachycardias.

Adenosine or vagal maneuvers that slow AVN conduction can be used to differentiate these three main types of narrow-QRS tachycardia and can convert an AV tachycardia (see Table 10.1). Adenosine is an endogenous purine that must be rapidly injected intravenously; its qualities include an ultrashort (seconds) duration of action, low risk, and effectiveness in patients when vagal stimulation fails.

An electrocardiogram, preferably using at least three leads, must be recorded during adenosine or the vagal maneuver; otherwise valuable information is lost.

(a) In sinus tachycardia, adenosine or a vagal maneuver transiently slows the sinus rate because of direct effects on the SAN, and transient second-degree AV block may be seen, yet the P wave morphology remains unchanged.

(b) In atrial flutter or other primary atrial tachycardia, the AVN fails to conduct some atrial depolarizations (second-degree AV block), making the diagnosis obvious but not producing conversion. As soon as the adenosine or vagal effect subsides, the rapid ventricular rate resumes.

(c) In AV tachycardias, adenosine or vagal stimulation may produce a lasting conversion to SR, or a transient conversion to SR, followed by rapid reinitiation of tachycardia.

Failure to record an adequate electrocardiogram during these interventions may lead to the erroneous conclusion that the maneuvers had no effect, as the brief decrease in ventricular rate may not be apparent by examination alone.

Long-term management

Following conversion to SR, many infants and children do not have recurrent SVT.

The need for prophylactic antiarrhythmic medication is based on the hemodynamic severity of the tachycardia (or degree of symptoms in older children), the frequency of SVT episodes, the difficulty and/or risk of tachycardia conversion, and the possibility of whether or not the tachycardia poses other risks for the patient (e.g., the adolescent who has tachycardia-induced near-syncope and who wishes to drive a car).

Many patients require no prophylactic therapy as they can be easily converted with simple vagal maneuvers during infrequent mild episodes.

Patients with troublesome or potentially risky SVT, who fail drug therapy, or who have unacceptable side effects can essentially be cured using RF ablation at the time of electrophysiologic study in the catheterization laboratory.

By probing using a catheter-mounted electrode, the location of an AC is mapped by determining the site of earliest electrical activation during tachycardia. A burst of RF energy is delivered through the catheter to heat the AC and destroy it.

Unlikely complications include destruction of the AVN (complete AV block). Some patients with automatic foci can be cured by RF ablation.

In children with malignant forms of VT that do not respond well to antiarrhythmic drugs, implantation of an implantable cardioverter-defibrillator can be life-saving, however, these devices have important risks and limitations.

ADDITIONAL READING

Deal BJ, Johnsrude CL, Buck SH. Pediatric ECG Interpretation: An Illustrative Guide. Oxford: Blackwell-Futura; 2004.

Tipple M. Paediatric ECG of the week. 2007. Available from www.paedcard.com.

Walsh EP. Interventional electrophysiology in patients with congenital heart disease. Circulation 2007;115;3224–3234.

Walsh EP, Saul JP, Triedman JK. (eds.) Cardiac Arrhythmias in Children and Young Adults with Congenital Heart Disease. Philadelphia: Lippincott, Williams, and Wilkins; 2001.

Wren C, Campbell RWF. (eds.) Paediatric Cardiac Arrhythmias. Oxford: Oxford University Press; 1996.

Chapter 11
Congestive cardiac failure

Congestive cardiac failure is a frequent emergency problem occurring in children with cardiac disease and demands a similar level of care and attention as for infants and children with an arrhythmia.

> Among children who develop cardiac failure, 80% do so in the first year of life, most commonly from congenital cardiac anomalies; of the 20% who develop cardiac failure after 1 year of age, in half it is related to congenital anomalies, and in the other half, to acquired conditions.

PATHOPHYSIOLOGY

Mechanisms
Two basic mechanisms are involved. In each type, certain physiologic principles, such as the Laplace and Starling relationships (see Chapter 4), describe the derangements that occur with ventricular dilation.

Increased cardiac work
Many infants experience heart failure from increased cardiac work (e.g., left-to-right shunts and valve insufficiency) despite normal or increased myocardial

Pediatric Cardiology, by W Johnson, J Moller © 2008 Blackwell Publishing,
ISBN: 978-1-4051-7818-1.

contractility. This type of heart failure is sometimes referred to as "high-output failure."

Reduced myocardial contraction

This includes dilated cardiomyopathy. Most adults and some children have failure because of this type. Myocardial failure may result from myocarditis, chemotherapy, or familial cardiomyopathies.

In the neonate and young infant, severe failure may result from obstructive lesions including aortic stenosis and coarctation, or from severe systemic hypertension. Myocardial function often improves in these infants following gradient relief of obstruction or treatment of hypertension.

Patients with a morphologic right ventricle acting as the systemic pump (e.g., Norwood palliation of hypoplastic left heart syndrome, and the atrial switch repair of d-Transposition) frequently experience systolic heart failure. Longstanding pulmonary insufficiency in postoperative tetralogy of Fallot patients may also lead to right ventricular failure, but since these patients have a two-ventricle heart, the clinical manifestations are generally less acute.

Unfortunately, the basic cellular abnormalities responsible for weak myocyte contractility are poorly understood; and usually, no specific therapy is available to repair the cellular problem.

Most therapy, either nonspecific or supportive, is designed to counteract elevation of systemic and pulmonary vascular resistance that accompany neurohumoral abnormalities (including increased sympathetic tone and activation of the renin–angiotensin system) common to the two types of failure.

Clinical features

> The clinical diagnosis of congestive cardiac failure rests upon the identification of the four cardinal signs: tachycardia, tachypnea, cardiomegaly, and hepatomegaly.

In addition, the patient often has a history of poor weight gain, fatigue upon eating (dyspnea on exercise), and excessive perspiration. Table 11.1 presents the most common classifications, which are often referred to in deciding management and studying outcomes of patients.

MEDICAL MANAGEMENT

Once the diagnosis of cardiac failure has been made, treatment should be initiated with up to four types of medication: an inotrope; a diuretic; an agent to reduce afterload; and in those with chronic heart failure, a beta-blocker.

Table 11.1 Clinical Classifications of Heart Failure.

	NYHA (Functional Capacity)*	Ross†
Class	Adults and older children	Infants and children
I	No imitation of physical activity; no symptoms with ordinary activity	No limitations or symptoms
II	Slight limitation of physical activity; comfortable at rest; symptoms with ordinary activity	Mild tachypnea and/or diaphoresis with feedings, dyspnea on exertion in older children; no growth failure
III	Marked limitation of physical activity; comfortable at rest; symptoms with less-than-ordinary activity	Marked tachypnea and/or diaphoresis with feedings or exertion; prolonged feeding times with growth failure
IV	Inability to carry on any physical activity without discomfort; symptoms may be present at rest; symptoms increase with any activity	Symptomatic at rest with tachypnea, retractions, grunting, or diaphoresis

*New York Heart Association (NYHA) Functional Class. Adapted from American Heart Association Medical/Scientific Statement. 1994 Revisions to classification of functional capacity and objective assessment of patients with diseases of the heart. Circulation 1994;90:644–645. The Criteria Committee of the New York Heart Association. Nomenclature and Criteria for Diagnosis of Diseases of the Heart and Great Vessels, 9th ed. Boston: Little, Brown; 1994:253–256.
†"Ross Classification" data from Ross RD, Daniels SR, Schwartz DC, et al. Plasma norepinephrine levels in infants and children with congestive heart failure. Am J Cardiol 1987;59:911–914.

Inotropes

Inotropes include beta-receptor agonists like dopamine and dobutamine; inhibitors of myocardial phosphodiesterases, such as milrinone and amrinone; and digoxin preparations, which inhibit cell wall sodium–potassium pumps.

The common end-effect of all these inotropes is the increase in intracellular calcium ions available to the myocardial contractile proteins.

Inotropes, however, have severe limitations. The child with cardiac failure usually has maximal activation of compensatory mechanisms, including elevated catecholamines, and in chronic heart failure, beta-receptors and contractile elements show a blunted response to adrenergic stimulation. Administration of therapeutic inotropes in such children may have little added benefit.

Patients with certain types of heart failure, including ischemic cardiomyopathy, may actually fare worse with inotropes and may have a better long-term prognosis with beta-receptor blockers than with beta-stimulants.

Other adverse effects of inotropes include increased heart rate and metabolic work with little increase in myocardial performance. High doses of some inotropic drugs, particularly digoxin or dopamine, may result in adverse increases in systemic vascular resistance.

Intravenous inotropes

These include dopamine (1–15 μg/kg/min) and dobutamine (5–20 μg/kg/min). Neither has superior inotropic effect, yet dopamine may increase renal blood flow more than dobutamine. Dopamine doses in excess of 15 μg/kg/min stimulate alpha-receptors and may lead to adverse increases in systemic vascular resistance. Milrinone and amrinone, inotropic by inhibition of the breakdown of phosphorylated "messenger" compounds within the cell, may exert their greatest beneficial effect by vasodilation (see section "Afterload Reduction").

Oral therapy

Digoxin is the preferred oral drug for pediatric use. Other than the digitalis glycosides, no other useful oral inotropes exist, although oral phosphodiesterase inhibitors are in development.

Digoxin may exert its greatest beneficial effect through vagal stimulation and slowing of conduction and heart rate. Although it may be given orally, intramuscularly, or intravenously, digoxin is safest given orally. Digoxin can be initiated at the maintenance dose without a loading dose. This is a safer method of starting outpatient therapy but requires several days to reach full digitalization.

Digoxin loading dose

Great care must be exercised in the calculation of dosage and ordering the medication; dose errors have a potentially greater adverse effect than with many other drugs.

Except in premature infants, the dosage is greater on a weight basis for infants than for older children.

Recommended oral *total digitalizing doses* (TDD) per kilogram of body weight of digoxin:

premature infants, 20 *micro*grams (μg)

term neonates, 30–40 *micro*grams (μg)

children up to 2 years of age, 40–60 *micro*grams (μg)

children more than 2 years of age, 30–40 *micro*grams (μg)

If given parenterally, these doses are reduced by 25%.

Usually, half of the total digitalizing dose is given initially;

one-fourth at 6–8 hours after the first dose; and the final one-fourth at 6–8 hours following the second dose.

If necessary, in emergency cases, three-fourths of the digitalizing dosage may be given initially.

Maintenance digoxin dose. Twenty-four hours after the initial dose of digoxin, maintenance therapy is started. The recommended maintenance dose is 25% of the total digitalizing dose, in divided doses, with one-half the maintenance dose given in the morning and one-half in the evening.

These recommendations are merely guidelines, and the dose may have to be altered according to the patient's response to therapy or the presence of digitalis toxicity.

Digoxin maintenance dosing
Except for premature infants and those with renal impairment, generally 10 μg/kg/day are given in two divided doses.

In children taking the elixir (50 μg/mL), a convenient dose is 0.1 mL × body weight in kilograms, twice daily. The authors round off the dose to the nearest (usually the lowermost) 0.1 mL. For example, a 4.4-kg infant may be given 0.4 mL bid. A 2.8-kg infant can safely receive 0.3 mL bid.

Toxicity. During digitalization, monitoring the patient clinically is important. If indicated, an electrocardiographic rhythm strip is used before the administration of each portion of the digitalizing dose to detect digitalis toxicity.

Slowing of the sinus rate and alterations in the ST segments are indications of digitalis effect but not of toxicity.

Digitalis toxicity is indicated by a prolonged PR interval or higher degrees of AV block and by cardiac arrhythmia, such as nodal or ventricular premature beats. Clinical signs of digitalis toxicity are nausea, vomiting, anorexia, and lethargy.

Digoxin should not be used in the presence of hypokalemia. Toxic effects, especially ventricular arrhythmias, are much more likely during hypokalemia, even with therapeutic digoxin levels.

Because digoxin is almost completely eliminated by the kidney, it should be used with caution and with appropriate dose modification in patients with renal impairment.

Diuretics

Diuretics are also indicated in many patients with congestive cardiac failure. Although peripheral edema is uncommon in infants and children with cardiac failure, perhaps because they are supine much of the time, they do retain sodium and fluid. The major manifestations of tissue edema are tachypnea and dyspnea.

Furosemide (Frusemide; Lasix), the diuretic most commonly used in the acute treatment of cardiac failure, is usually given parenterally, 1 mg/kg/dose. The oral dosage is 2–4 mg/kg/day. Furosemide effect begins promptly.

For infants who also commonly receive digoxin, parental stress is minimized by giving the same volume of furosemide suspension (10 mg/mL) as of digoxin at each dose, twice daily. For example, an infant weighing 3 kg can be given digoxin 0.3 mL and furosemide 0.3 mL orally twice a day.

With repeated use, serum sodium, chloride, and potassium levels become abnormal; and a contraction metabolic alkalosis may develop. Patients receiving chronic diuretic therapy may develop hypokalemia, and the low potassium enhances digitalis toxicity, even with normal digoxin blood levels.

Potassium supplementation should be given to such patients. Older children should be encouraged to eat potassium-rich foods, such as oranges, bananas, and raisins, as part of their regular diet.

The central fluid volume in some children may actually be low, leading to higher renin (and angiotensin) levels than occur from heart failure alone. These adverse effects of chronic high-dose diuretics may contribute to increased systemic vascular resistance and paradoxically, worsen cardiac failure (see later).

A variety of other diuretics, including hydrochlorothiazide or spironolactone, are used for chronic long-term management of congestive cardiac failure. Although they produce less electrolyte disturbance, their beneficial effect relative to that of furosemide has been questioned.

Furosemide and a potassium-sparing diuretic are often used in combination. Potassium-sparing diuretics must be used with caution if other aldosterone antagonists (ACE inhibitors) are used (see the next section, "Afterload Reduction").

Afterload reduction

Natural mechanisms that produce vasoconstriction and redistribution of organ blood flows occur in patients with hypotension. Although such events may be beneficial during acute hemorrhage, for example, vasoconstriction may be disadvantageous in chronic heart failure.

Vasoconstriction increases the impedance to forward arterial flow that myocytes must overcome to propel blood from the heart. The mechanical load on the myocytes is known as afterload, which is increased in heart failure.

Reducing the afterload on failing myocardial cells may improve their performance, lessen ongoing myocyte injury, and allow for recovery of injured myocytes, depending on the mechanism of the heart failure.

Afterload reduction is achieved by the administration of vasodilator drugs, which produce relaxation of smooth muscle in the systemic arterioles, leading to a decrease in the systemic vascular resistance.

These drugs may also partially redistribute blood flow toward more normal patterns. Increasing renal blood flow may lessen the overproduction of renin, a factor in elevated afterload.

Afterload reduction is titrated to prevent lowered blood pressure; as systemic resistance (R_S) falls, myocyte performance is enhanced, cardiac output (Q_S) increases, and blood pressure (P) remains constant or rises, according to the equation, $P = Q_S \times R_S$.

In infants with a large left-to-right shunt via a ventricular septal defect, reduction of the systemic vascular resistance (as long as the pulmonary vascular resistance does not also fall by a similar degree) decreases the volume of blood shunted and relieves cardiac failure by lessening the left ventricular volume overload.

Angiotensin-converting enzyme (ACE) inhibitors block the conversion of renin to its vasoconstrictor form, angiotensin, thereby producing afterload reduction. The prognosis for patients with chronic heart failure treated with ACE inhibitors appears better than that for those treated with direct vasodilator agents, such as nitrates. Presumably, ACE inhibitors prevent maladaptive changes within the myocardium that occur as nonspecific responses to failure from widely differing causes.

The authors use a solution of captopril for infants, but care must be observed in its preparation and storage, since captopril degrades rapidly in solution.

A similar solution can be compounded for enalapril. Oral enalapril can be used once daily in children able to take tablets. An intravenous form, enalaprilat, is available.

Disadvantages of ACE inhibitors include an increase in bradykinins (also metabolized by ACE), which may worsen pulmonary symptoms, and renal injury. These drugs have an antialdosterone effect on the kidney, so they must be used with caution in patients receiving other potassium-sparing diuretics or potassium supplements.

Beta-receptor antagonists

Beta-receptor antagonists (beta-blockers) benefit some children with chronic heart failure of moderate degree (class II–III; see Table 11.1), usually patients with cardiomyopathy. Beta-blockers may reverse some of the neurohumoral derangements that occur in chronic heart failure, especially the detrimental effect of high levels of endogenous catecholamines on the heart. Some drugs (e.g., carvedilol) have both alpha-antagonist (promoting vasodilation and afterload reduction) and beta-antagonist properties.

Beta-blockers are for long-term use. Short-term treatment of heart failure may require an inotrope, including a beta-agonist (e.g., dopamine); the simultaneous use of beta-agonists and antagonists is irrational. Identifying patients who can benefit from beta-blockers (i.e., those who are not dependent on high levels of catecholamines) can be clinically challenging.

These drugs are not useful for and may have adverse effects in most children with high-output-type heart failure (such as left-to-right shunts). These children usually can be managed definitively with surgery.

Supportive measures
Other therapeutic measures may be useful in the treatment of children with congestive cardiac failure.

Oxygen. Oxygen should be administered initially. Long-term use of oxygen may be counterproductive, perhaps because of its effect as a systemic vasoconstrictor (thereby increasing afterload). Oxygen is administered using a rigid plastic hood in neonates and nasal cannulae in older children. The least aggravating method of delivery should be sought since increased patient agitation in the face of limited cardiac output will be counterproductive.

Mechanical ventilation. In the acute management of severe cardiac failure, endotracheal intubation and mechanical ventilation may be indicated. Children may present in extremis with respiratory failure due to fatigue of overworked ventilatory muscles. After intubation and mechanical ventilation, paralysis and deep sedation can reduce these patients' requirements for cardiac output, allowing time for more definitive management of their heart failure.

Morphine. Morphine (0.1 mg/kg) and other sedatives may be useful in treating the tachypneic, dyspneic, and dusky infant who has severe respiratory distress associated with congestive cardiac failure and pulmonary edema.

On the other hand, sedation may result in apnea in children who have impending respiratory failure from fatigue and in those with underlying pulmonary disease.

> Close monitoring and preparations for emergency intubation are warranted if sedatives are used.

Management of pulmonary consolidation. Conditions associated with increased pulmonary blood flow have an increased incidence of pneumonia. Atelectasis occurs more commonly in children because of bronchial compression from enlarged pulmonary arteries or cardiac chambers. Pneumonia, atelectasis, or other febrile illnesses are events that can precipitate a decompensation of previously stable congestive cardiac failure. Pulmonary consolidation should be sought in children with cardiac failure and treated appropriately if present.

Fever. Fever should be treated aggressively in children with heart failure if it has been demonstrated to result in decompensatory episodes. Fever increases cardiac output approximately 10–15% per degree centigrade.

Anemia management. Anemia occurs often in children with chronic cardiac failure. It is usually a mild normochromic anemia, not related to iron or nutrient deficiency, and may be similar to the "anemia of chronic disease." It may improve with heart failure treatment.

In patients with severe uncompensated heart failure, severe anemia imposes a cardiac volume overload proportional to the degree of anemia; the effects of compensatory changes in hemoglobin affinity for oxygen are negligible compared with the hemoglobin concentration.

> For example, if a child's hemoglobin concentration is 10 g/dL rather than 15 g/dL, cardiac output will be approximately one-third greater to deliver the same amount of oxygen to the tissues in the same amount of time.
>   A dysfunctional left ventricle may lack the contractile reserve to compensate for anemia by increased cardiac output.

Transfusion is usually well tolerated if given slowly. Unfortunately, the small number of leukocytes that contaminate packed erythrocyte transfusions expose the patient to foreign antigens and may make tissue matching for subsequent cardiac transplantation problematic. Steps should be taken to filter the transfused erythrocytes.

DEFINITIVE DIAGNOSIS AND MANAGEMENT

Congestive cardiac failure is not a disease but a symptom complex caused by an underlying cardiac condition. After treatment of congestive cardiac failure, consideration must be given to the type of cardiac disease that produced the failure.

Operable lesions, such as coarctation of the aorta or patent ductus arteriosus, may cause the cardiac failure. Therefore, following the treatment of congestive failure in any infant, appropriate studies should be performed to establish the diagnosis.

Once a diagnosis is made, either a palliative or a corrective procedure should be completed. For lesions with a favorable natural history (e.g., the infant with a moderate-sized ventricular septal defect that might close spontaneously, thereby avoiding operation) and if he or she gains weight and does well, a conservative approach may be appropriate.

Since in older children congestive cardiac failure often results from acquired cardiac conditions, cardiac catheterization may not be required because the etiology is frequently evident from history, physical examination, or laboratory findings. Catheterization may be indicated to determine pulmonary resistance in consideration for cardiac or cardiopulmonary transplantation.

If appropriate, specific treatment should be undertaken for the condition (e.g., fever from infection) triggering the failure.

ADDITIONAL READING

Rosenthal D, Chrisant MR, Edens E, Mahony L, Canter C, Colan S, Dubin A, Lamour J, Ross R, Shaddy R, Addonizio L, Beerman L, Berger S, Bernstein D, Blume E, Boucek M, Checchia P, Dipchand A, Drummond-Webb J, Fricker J, Friedman R, Hallowell S, Jaquiss R, Mital S, Pahl E, Pearce B, Rhodes L, Rotondo K, Rusconi P, Scheel J, Pal Singh T, Towbin J.. International society for heart and lung transplantation: Practice guidelines for management of heart failure in children. J Heart Lung Transplant 2004;23:1313–1333.

Chapter 12
Preventive cardiology and health promotion

In this chapter we discuss prevention of cardiac disease, both for patients with cardiac malformations and cardiac disease acquired during childhood, as well as for children and adolescents with normal hearts who may be at risk for the development of atherosclerotic heart disease in adulthood. In this chapter, we discuss the environmental and genetic factors that influence cardiac disease in these two groups of patients.

Pediatric Cardiology, by W Johnson, J Moller © 2008 Blackwell Publishing,
ISBN: 978-1-4051-7818-1.

PREVENTION FOR CHILDREN WITH NORMAL HEARTS

Risk factors for adult-manifest cardiovascular disease

Many risk factors have been identified for the development of atherosclerotic disease of coronary and other systemic arteries. Some of these factors are of greater importance and/or prevalence in childhood than others, and their impact in adulthood begins with exposure in childhood and adolescence. We discuss factors that are generally regarded to have the greatest preventive benefit if effective modification can be achieved early in life. Many factors are strongly interrelated (e.g., obesity and abnormal lipid and glucose metabolism).

Tobacco

Tobacco use is the single most important independent risk factor for development of atherosclerotic cardiovascular disease that is purely environmental, and thereby potentially modifiable. Adults who smoke have a two- to fourfold increased risk of myocardial infarction (MI).

Smoking and tobacco use

The mechanism of adverse cardiovascular effect is related to multiple factors:

(1) Endothelial cell dysfunction and injury from various toxins and oxygen free radicals.

(2) Hypercoagulable effects and platelet activation.

(3) Induced hyperlipidemia.

(4) Increased myocardial work, caused by nicotine.

(5) Decreased oxygen delivery, caused by carbon monoxide.

Because of the poor rate of recovery from addiction, prevention of first-use of smoking and other tobacco products among children and adolescents is the single most important means of avoiding adverse health effects in adulthood.

The reported long-term abstinence rate among adults without physician-based intervention is less than 5% and yet with intervention is only about 40%.

Passive smoking is risky for children, so family members and household contacts should be counseled not to smoke. The cardiovascular risk is related to both dose and duration, but a safe lower limit of passive exposure has not been determined.

Factors in tobacco addiction

Nicotine is highly addictive and shares features common to other addictive substances:

(1) Psychoactive properties—substance use causes pleasurable central nervous system response.

(2) Tolerance—(Tachyphylaxis) occurs by multiple physiologic mechanisms including receptor down-regulation, and is overcome by increased dose.

(3) Physiologic dependency—results in physiological reaction and adverse withdrawal symptoms upon cessation of use.

Other factors have been observed regarding tobacco addiction:

(1) Genotype. Certain individuals may be biologically predisposed to addiction; a familial tendency has been demonstrated.

(2) Age of introduction. Patients who begin smoking as children or adolescents are more likely to continue smoking as adults. Prevention of addiction must begin in childhood.

(3) Chemical dependency. Chemical dependency on other substances is associated with increased rates of tobacco addiction.

(4) Depression, other mental illness, and high emotional stress are associated with increased rates of tobacco addiction.

(5) Other smokers in the household.

(6) Lack of access to smoking-cessation resources.

Cessation management

The risk of cardiovascular disease declines after cessation and, after a number of years, may approach the risk level of those who have never smoked.

The reported long-term abstinence rate of counseling, psychotherapy, and/or nicotine replacement (chewing gum, transdermal patches, nasal spray, etc.) is 20% or less (for adolescents, it is less than 5%).

The addition of antidepressants, such as bupropion (a dopamine reuptake inhibitor), increases success rates to just over 20%.

The use of drugs (e.g., varenicline) which act on the nicotine receptor increases success rates to more than 40%. Such drugs are partial nicotine receptor agonists (which serve to blunt withdrawal and craving) and receptor blockers (which prevent nicotine binding, eliminating the positive reinforcement from tobacco use).

Hypercholesterolemia

Coronary atherosclerosis is a highly prevalent problem in developed societies and relatively less common in other cultures, suggesting that diet, lifestyle, and other environmental factors are important; however, a strong genetic component also influences the metabolism of lipids, which in turn has an important effect on individual risk of disease.

Mechanism of cardiovascular effect. Atheroma, the basic lesion of coronary and other arteriosclerosis, is an erosion of the arterial endothelium that is capped by a lipid-laden plaque. These plaques may slowly narrow the coronary arterial lumen, leading to intermittent insufficiency of arterial blood flow (creating myocardial ischemia and symptoms of angina), or they can rupture, leading to acute thrombosis and occlusion of the artery, resulting in MI and/or sudden cardiac death. The exact role of lipids in the initial endothelial injury is unclear. Atheromas are known to begin in childhood; therefore prevention of adult cardiovascular disease should begin in childhood.

Heart-diet theory
Coronary atherosclerosis is strongly associated with high blood levels of certain lipids. Dietary fats influence the concentration of circulating lipids, which are transported by lipoproteins:
(1) Low-density lipoprotein cholesterol (LDL-C), the "bad cholesterol," promotes atheroma formation, transports cholesterol to tissues like the endothelium, binds to the LDL receptor on cells, and thereby allows the cholesterol to enter the cell.
LDL receptors on liver cells can be modified by drugs (statins) to reduce circulating LDL-C.
LDL-C can be measured but is often estimated using the Friedewald formula: LDL-C = TC − (HDL-C + triglycerides/5), where TC represents total cholesterol and HDL-C, high-density lipoprotein cholesterol. This formula is invalid if the patient is nonfasting, if abnormal lipoprotein is present (type III, see later), and when triglycerides exceed 400 mg/dL.
(2) High-density lipoprotein cholesterol (HDL-C), the "good cholesterol," may inhibit atheroma formation by transporting cholesterol away from tissues like the endothelium and into the liver for excretion as bile acids. It can be measured in nonfasting children. HDL-C levels may be congenitally low, but more commonly they fall with smoking, obesity, or lack of exercise, and conversely, rise with intervention for these factors.
(3) Other lipids, including triglycerides, transported by very-low-density lipoproteins (VLDL), and chylomicrons, are less strongly associated with cardiovascular risk, and blood levels are more subject to dramatic postprandial shifts. Screening of these lipids in otherwise healthy children is not uniformly recommended; interventions targeting LDL-C, HDL-C, and total cholesterol generally improve levels of these lipids also.
(4) Total cholesterol (TC) is a collective measure of LDL-C, HDL-C, and VLDL.
Measurement of LDL-C, HDL-C, VLDL, and triglycerides must be done after a 12-hour fast (nothing to eat or drink except water).

> But, because TC is less affected by postprandial change, it can be drawn in fasting and nonfasting patients. Therefore, total cholesterol is the test most often used for screening.

> Adults with MI, 25% have LDL-C $\leq$ 130 mg/dL (corresponding to TC $\leq$ 200 mg/dL).
> MI is rare in adults with LDL-C $\leq$ 100 mg/dL (TC $\leq$ 150 mg/dL).

Screening and intervention. The goals of screening include identification of children with familial dyslipidemia (1–2% of patients) or secondary causes of hyperlipidemia (1%) and of those at highest risk for adult-manifest cardiovascular disease (10–25% of all children).

Screening of blood lipid levels in children has been controversial because of lack of consensus about which children to screen and at what ages, as well as the lipid level limits (cutpoints) at which to consider a patient for further testing or intervention.

A recent approach has been to risk-stratify children according to their BMI, BP, family history, and the presence of conditions associated with increased risk of coronary artery disease such as diabetes, familial hypercholesterolemia, renal disease, Kawasaki disease, chronic inflammatory disease such as lupus, cancer-treatment survivors, and heart transplant recipients. Depending on the individual child's level of risk, differing cutpoints for lipids, blood pressure, and so on, are then targeted for intervention.

Controversy also exists as to the most appropriate intervention when hyperlipidemic children are identified. This discussion includes concerns about the safety and efficacy of dietary restriction of essential fatty acids on the child's growth and central nervous system development and about the advisability and safety of drug therapy. Recommendations continue to evolve as more data become available.

> The National Cholesterol Education Program (NCEP) is but one approach. It has two components:
> A population approach (with the goal of lower lipid levels in all persons through population-wide education and changes in diet and lifestyle) and an individual approach (identification and treatment of children at the highest risk for adult-manifest heart disease) using these steps:
> (1) Assess child's risk, by family history.
> (2) Measure TC (nonfasting; for children whose parents have TC $\geq$ 240 mg/dL) or lipoproteins [fasting] for those with parents or

grandparents with coronary artery disease that manifests at 55 years of age or less and for children with TC > 200 mg/dL).

(3) Repeat TC if "elevated" (>200 mg/dL) or "borderline" (170–199 mg/dL) and measure lipoproteins (fasting) if repeat TC $\geq$ 170 mg/dL.

(4) Repeat lipoprotein measurement (fasting) and average the LDL-C values.

(5) LDL-C < 110 mg/dL "acceptable"

Retest in 5 years.

LDL-C 110–129 mg/dL "borderline"

Such a level suggests dietary intervention.

Retest in 1 year.

LDL-C $\geq$ 130 mg/dL "high"

Rule out secondary causes (see below), screen other family members, and evaluate for familial disorder. Begin intervention and intensify if necessary.

(6) NCEP guidelines for adults advise that nonfasting HDL-C levels be measured and interventions targeted to achieve HDL-C of 35 mg/dL or more (approximately the 5th to 10th percentiles for adults).

The NCEP guidelines have been criticized for fixed lipid cutoff values, which, depending on the age of the child at screening, identify not just the top quartile, but up to 75% of children as being at risk. Concerns about the number of blood samples required and about the potential for a large number of children to experience "medicalization" of a preventive health issue that will not be manifest for decades have been expressed.

Adults in the upper quartile for lipid concentration are at the highest risk for cardiovascular disease. Most of these adults and their children do not have a specific lipid metabolism disorder. Children of these adults tend to be those with lipid levels in the highest quartile and usually "track" along similar percentiles into their adult years. Screening and preventive measures are designed to identify and improve risk for these 25% of all children.

Fredrickson classification (Types I through V)

This system describes five major phenotypes of hyperlipidemia, but more than one genotype (or acquired condition, such as diabetes) can be associated with a particular phenotype. Cardiovascular risk tends to correlate better with genotype.

Strictly applied, all patients in the top quartile for TC and LDL-C can be classified as Type II, but traditionally, the Fredrickson classification is used only for those with lipid levels more than the 98th percentile. It is not useful for most children screened in a general practice but may be helpful

in the management and referral of the uncommon patient with a recognized primary lipid disorder. It requires a fasting blood sample.
Type I (high chylomicrons),
Type III (high abnormal VLDL), and
Type V (high VLDL and chylomicrons), are rare (less than one in 1 million children).
Type II (high TC, high LDL-C, ± high triglycerides) and
Type IV (normal TC, high triglycerides) are more common
(1:200–1:100), but only Type II patients have significantly increased risk of cardiovascular disease.

Familial hypercholesterolemia (FH)
Type II patients may have FH involving an LDL receptor defect; they may be heterozygotes (TC 250–500 mg/dL) or more rarely, homozygotes (TC 500–1200 mg/dL).
Children can present with xanthomas (nodular deposits of lipid in skin or tendons), arcus juvenilis (and other ocular deposits of lipids), and diffuse atherosclerosis.
These children (including heterozygotes) need referral to a specialist experienced in the management of dyslipidemias, as diet and first-line drugs (bile sequestrants) often prove inadequate. Higher risk of additional therapy requires careful monitoring and consideration of whether the potential long-term benefit outweighs the risk.

Primary versus secondary hyperlipidemia
Secondary causes of hyperlipidemia that must be ruled out include the following:
(1) Nonfasting sample.
(2) Metabolic—renal failure, nephrotic syndrome, anorexia nervosa, inborn errors of metabolism.
(3) Hepatic disorders—biliary atresia, hepatitis.
(4) Drug—corticosteroids, hormone contraceptives, retinoic acid, anticonvulsants.
(5) Endocrine disorders—diabetes mellitus, thyroid disease, pregnancy.

Blood lipid levels vary by age, gender, and to some extent ethnicity. However, ethnicity may involve environmental factors (diet and lifestyle may vary between cultures) as well as genetic factors.

In general, lipid levels in the late teenage years best predict adult levels, but for younger children, the lipid percentile level correlates better with adult

Table 12.1 Blood Lipid Levels in a Sample of US Children.

	Age (Years)	Males (Percentiles)					Females (Percentiles)				
		5	25	50	75	95	5	25	50	75	95
TC	0–4	114	137	151	171	203	112	139	156	172	200
	5–9	121	143	159	175	203	126	146	163	179	205
	10–14	119	140	155	173	202	124	144	158	174	201
	15–19	113	132	146	165	197	120	139	154	171	200
	20–24	124	146	165	186	218	122	143	160	182	216
LDL-C	0–4										
	5–9	63	80	90	103	129	68	88	98	115	140
	10–14	64	81	94	109	132	68	81	94	110	136
	15–19	62	80	93	109	130	60	78	93	110	135
	20–24	66	85	101	118	147	—	80	98	113	—
HDL-C	0–4										
	5–9	38	49	54	63	74	36	47	52	61	73
	10–14	37	46	55	61	74	37	45	52	58	70
	15–19	30	39	46	52	63	35	43	51	61	73
	20–24	30	38	45	51	63	—	43	50	60	—
TG	0–4	29	40	51	67	99	34	45	59	77	112
	5–9	30	40	51	65	101	32	44	55	71	105
	10–14	32	45	59	78	125	37	54	70	90	131
	15–19	37	54	69	91	148	39	52	66	84	124
	20–24	44	63	86	119	201	36	51	64	84	131

TC, total cholesterol; LDL-C, low-density lipoprotein cholesterol; HDL-C, high-density lipoprotein cholesterol; TG, triglycerides.

Plasma lipid values are expressed as mg/dL and are based on a sample of White males and females (not taking hormone contraceptives). Values for Black males and females (not shown) were based on a smaller sample size, but tended to be up to 5% higher for TC in the 0–9 age group.

From Lipid Research Clinics Population Studies Data Book, Vol. I, NIH Publication 80-1527, 1980.

For TC, LDL-C, and HDL-C, to convert from mg/dL to mmol/L, multiply mg/dL by 0.0259.

For TG, to convert from mg/dL to mmol/L, multiply mg/dL by 0.0113.

percentile rank. Values by age and gender are presented in Table 12.1. However, lipid levels alone are not perfect predictors of future coronary artery disease.

For the child identified with a lipid abnormality, three levels of care may be advisable: primary care, referral, and/or comanagement with a lipid specialist.

In general, healthy children with a family history of coronary artery disease and/or LDL-C values in the top quartile should be counseled and followed by their primary care provider.

Children with secondary causes of hyperlipidemia (e.g., diabetes, nephrotic syndrome) may be followed jointly by other subspecialists (e.g., pediatric

Table 12.2 Nutritional Guidelines for Children >5 Years and Adults.

Nutrient	Recommended Intake	
Fat, total	≤30%	
Saturated	<10%	
Polyunsaturated	≤10%	Of total calories
Monounsaturated	≤15%	
Carbohydrates	≥55%	
Cholesterol	≤300 mg/day	
Calories, total	Adults—to achieve and maintain desirable weight	
	Growing children—should not be placed on calorie restriction	
Salt	<6 g/day (adults)	

Adapted from Deckelbaum J, Fisher EA, Winston M, et al. Summary of a scientific conference on preventive nutrition: Pediatrics to geriatrics. Circulation 1999;100: 450–456.
This is essentially the "Step 1 diet" advocated in the management of hyperlipidemia. The effect of these restrictions on fat and cholesterol for children <5 years is not known to compromise growth and development but remains under evaluation.

endocrinologist, nephrologist) and usually do not require further evaluation by a specialist in dyslipidemia.

Those children with heterozygous FH can be managed jointly, but the rare child with homozygous FH or another rare lipid disorder requires intensive therapy by a lipid specialist who works with dietitians specializing in the treatment of primary hyperlipidemia. The mainstays of therapy are diet, and for selected children, drug therapy.

Diet, although simple in concept, remains difficult to execute, requires a high level of compliance and cooperation from the family and child, and usually represents a considerable commitment in counseling. A professional dietitian is helpful but is a resource not usually available to the primary care provider.

The American Heart Association Step 1 and 2 diets are advocated as interventions for children with primary hyperlipidemia:

Step 1 diet is the same as that recommended for the population approach (Table 12.2) and should be used for children whose LDL-C is borderline or high for more than 3 months. The goal is reducing LDL-C to the acceptable range.

Step 2 diet is advocated for patients who have been compliant with a Step 1 diet but who have persistently high LDL-C levels. Nutrient guidelines are similar to the Step 1 diet, except that the level of saturated fat is 7% or less and of polyunsaturated fat is 10% or less of total calories, with cholesterol intake of 200 mg/day or less. A detailed assessment by a trained specialist, such as a dietitian, is required; the diet must be carefully monitored to ensure adequate nutrient intake.

Drug therapy is inappropriate for most children with hyperlipidemia, as most respond to diet. When drugs are indicated, they are most effective in combination with diet therapy.

(1) Bile-binding agents like cholestyramine prevent enterohepatic recycling of bile acids, thus leading to increased conversion of blood and hepatic cholesterol to bile acids.

   Though relatively safe with few side effects, they are usually not necessary if dietary compliance can be achieved. They are useful in FH children and in management of some secondary hyperlipidemias. Side effects include gastrointestinal symptoms.

(2) Nicotinic acid (niacin) lowers lipid levels by an unknown mechanism. It has unpleasant side effects, including vasodilation, hepatic toxicity, and hyperuricemia, and is usually reserved for children with homozygous FH.

(3) 3-Hydroxy-3-methylglutaryl coenzyme A (HMG-CoA) reductase inhibitors ("statins") result in lower hepatocyte cholesterol levels. This decrease causes an increase in the LDL receptors on the liver cell and leads to increased uptake of LDL-C by the liver. Blood levels of TC, LDL-C, and triglycerides decrease; HDL-C increases.

Although statins have become first-line drugs for adults, they are not recommended for use in children, except in those children with FH, in consultation with a lipid specialist. Side effects include skeletal muscle, hepatic, and gastrointestinal toxicity.

Other drugs commonly used in adults have had limited use in children, usually in those with severe forms of hyperlipidemia. These drugs include Fibrates, which lower TG (by accelerating enzymatic clearance of triglyceride-rich particles) and raise HDL, and Ezetimibe, a molecular inhibitor of cholesterol absorption in the small bowel.

Nonpharmacologic treatments have included stem cell (bone marrow) transplantation for children with rare metabolic errors, such as homozygous FH.

Obesity
Mechanism of cardiovascular effect and definitions of obesity. Obesity, strongly associated with cardiovascular disease, may act through multiple interrelated mechanisms, including hyperlipidemia, hypertension, increased left ventricular mass, diabetes and insulin resistance, and obstructive sleep apnea (OSA) which may cause increased pulmonary resistance and right heart abnormalities.

Obesity is the presence of excess body fat, usually expressed as a proportion of total body mass. Like hyperlipidemia, the definition of obesity is somewhat arbitrary and dependent on population "normals." Although controversial, a commonly used definition of the term *overweight* in children is a proportion of body fat greater than the 85th percentile; the term *obesity* is reserved for those above the 95th percentile.

Comparing children in the 1990s with children studied in the 1960s, the number of "obese" children doubled.

Obesity is multifactorial: 30% of factors are estimated to be genetic, but 70% are environmental factors that respond to intervention.

Techniques for assessing obesity include indices of weight or mass compared with some reference, such as height, and also various measures of the portion of body mass that is consisted of fat. The indices, though rapid and simple to perform, do not reliably express adiposity, especially in children with lean body mass who are at the highest percentiles for age. More difficult to perform, body fat proportion measurements require special equipment and/or training and have limited reproducibility. Clinical observation of body fat and habitus is important in interpreting measures of obesity.

Body mass index (BMI or Quetelet index) is most often used in adults. Normal values are published for children.

$$BMI = \frac{\text{weight in kg}}{(\text{height in m})^2}$$

or

$$BMI = \frac{[(\text{weight in pounds}) \; 705/\text{height in inches}]}{\text{height in inches}}$$

For adults, overweight is defined as BMI $\geq$ 25 kg/m^2 and obesity is BMI $\geq$ 30 kg/m^2.
Note that in this index, the denominator *does not* represent body surface area.

Ideal weight for height can be calculated from a standard growth chart showing both height and weight for age.

Ignore the child's true age, plot the child's true height along the 50th percentile line, then find the "ideal weight" along the 50th percentile for the age corresponding to the plotted height (draw a perpendicular line from the height to the weight curve to find the "ideal weight").

Overweight is defined as weight $\geq$ ideal body weight $\times$ 1.2 (which corresponds to approximately the 85th percentile for BMI).

Obesity is weight $\geq$ ideal body weight $\times$ 1.3.

Body fat proportion requires estimation of the percentage of body mass that is fat. Varying with age and gender, it may be as much as 25% in normal infants. Triceps skin-fold thickness and bioelectric impedance are commonly used methods, but they require special equipment and training.

Management. Management of the obese child has become an important preventive medicine priority given the rising prevalence of obesity in developed societies, yet effective intervention remains challenging, in part because of the difficulty in changing the strong societal factors that influence obesity in individual patients.

Although the definition of overweight and obese is to some degree arbitrary, avoid classifying as obese any large-for-age child with high lean body mass who appears nonobese.

Rule out rare hormonal and genetic causes (i.e., Klinefelter syndrome, hypothyroidism, etc.); this can be done clinically, as most such affected children will be short (height ≤5th percentile) with other physical clues to the diagnosis.

Increased physical activity rather than direct dietary intervention is the primary therapy for simple obesity. This treatment is most effective when the patient has time prescribed for unstructured outdoor play, away from television and other sedentary pursuits. It may work by (1) increasing energy expenditure; (2) decreasing total caloric intake (presumably because the child is spending less time near food); and (3) altering the type of food ingested (e.g., lower percentage of fat calories) by an unknown mechanism.

Morbidly obese children or those who prove refractory to simple management techniques benefit from an intensive team approach and require referral to a specialist in pediatric obesity.

Nutrition
Nutrition is an independent risk factor for cardiovascular disease through multiple mechanisms, most of which are interrelated to the other known risk factors, such as hyperlipidemia and obesity.

In general, the risk increases with a diet high in total calories, total fat, saturated fat, and salt and low in fiber, complex carbohydrates, antioxidants, and certain vitamins.

Commonsense guidelines for improving diet include eating a wide variety of foods; increasing the proportion of whole grains, fruits, and vegetables; and reducing overall fat intake, saturated fat, simple sugars, and salt (Table 12.2).

Some specific nutrients have been associated with increased risk of cardiovascular disease, notably increased dietary consumption of trans-fatty acids. These fatty acids are chemically different than cis-fatty acids, leading to straighter and stiffer molecules when they are incorporated into cellular structures such as membranes.

Exercise
Even moderate-intensity exercise, if regularly performed, exerts a beneficial protective effect against adult-manifest cardiovascular disease, mediated through

lower blood pressure, less risk of obesity and diabetes, and more favorable lipid profile (particularly increased HDL-C). Exercise may confer a direct benefit to the endothelium, a tissue responsive to mechanical changes, such as increased blood flow and pressure. Children who pursue regular physical activity are more likely to remain active as adults.

Light and moderately intense exercise has low risk. The risks of more intense physical activity, particularly competitive sports participation, have been studied in relation to sudden death in young athletes, which is estimated to occur at a rate of 1:300,000–1:100,000 each year. Most of these children had conditions such as asthma or unrecognized heart disease.

Sports preparticipation evaluation

This examination is designed to identify young athletes who may be at risk for death with intense exercise. Various screening guidelines have been proposed. Heart disorders causing sudden death include hypertrophic cardiomyopathy and coronary artery anomalies which together account for more than 50% of cases. Other rare causes (e.g., myocarditis and arrhythmogenic right ventricular dysplasia) are difficult to diagnose. Unfortunately, not all patients at risk can be identified by screening tests. AHA recommendations include the following screening elements (Table 12.3).

Laboratory studies have not been accepted as universal screening tools, but the 12-lead electrocardiogram (ECG) has been proposed, as 95% of hypertrophic cardiomyopathy patients will have an abnormal ECG. The ECG is often abnormal in coronary artery anomalies, and it is the most effective means of screening for LQTS and Wolf–Parkinson–White syndrome. Because ECG is not very specific and requires age-appropriate interpretation, many normal children could face unnecessary referral for "borderline" ECGs.

Other risk factors for acquired atherosclerotic disease

Family history and gender. Genetics determines an individual child's future risk for adult-manifest cardiovascular disease in an important but variable fashion. Even when familial risk factors (such as hyperlipidemia) cannot be identified, family history remains an independent risk factor that cannot be modified. With greater understanding of lipid metabolism and endothelial function, many of these patients may become candidates for therapy to lessen their risk. Premenopausal women are relatively protected from atherosclerotic disease when all other risk factors are equal.

Diabetes. Juvenile and adult-onset diabetes are major independent risk factors for cardiovascular disease in adults, as they damage endothelium by

Table 12.3 The 12-Element AHA Recommendations for Preparticipation Cardiovascular Screening of Competitive Athletes.

Medical history*
Personal history
1. Exertional chest pain/discomfort
2. Unexplained syncope/near-syncope[†]
3. Excessive exertional and unexplained dyspnea/fatigue, associated with exercise
4. Prior recognition of a heart murmur
5. Elevated systemic blood pressure
Family history
6. Premature death (sudden and unexpected, or otherwise) before age 50 years due to heart disease, in one relative
7. Disability from heart disease in a close relative 50 years of age
8. Specific knowledge of certain cardiac conditions in family members: hypertrophic or dilated cardiomyopathy, long-QT syndrome or other ion channelopathies, Marfan syndrome, or clinically important arrhythmias
Physical examination
9. Heart murmur[‡]
10. Femoral pulses to exclude aortic coarctation
11. Physical stigmata of Marfan syndrome
12. Brachial artery blood pressure (sitting position)[§]

* Parental verification is recommended for high school and middle school athletes.
[†] Judged not to be neurocardiogenic (vasovagal); of particular concern when related to exertion.
[‡] Auscultation should be performed in both supine and standing positions (or with Valsalva maneuver), specifically to identify murmurs of dynamic left ventricular outflow tract obstruction.
[§] Preferably taken in both arms.
Reprinted with permission from Maron BJ, Thompson PD, Ackerman MJ, et al. Recommendations and considerations related to preparticipation screening for cardiovascular abnormalities in competitive athletes: 2007 update: A scientific statement from the American Heart Association Council on Nutrition, Physical Activity, and Metabolism: Endorsed by the American College of Cardiology Foundation. Circulation March 27, 2007;115(12):1643–1655.

hyperglycemia and glycosylation and less directly, via hyperlipidemia, hypertension, and autonomic neuropathy, which may worsen microvascular dysfunction.

Insulin resistance is a spectrum of metabolic derangements (type 2 diabetes is at one end), including hyperinsulinemia, that are related to obesity, inactivity, and advancing age and are associated with a greater risk of coronary artery atherosclerosis.

Rarely, young adults and adolescents may have angina and other symptoms of coronary arterial insufficiency but without narrowed proximal coronary arteries—the so-called syndrome X. This condition may represent an abnormality of the coronary microvascular bed and has been associated with insulin resistance.

Systemic hypertension. This is a risk factor for adult-manifest cardiovascular disease, and children with a strong family history of essential hypertension tend to "track" into adulthood with the highest blood pressures relative to their same-age peers. Some other risk factors, such as obesity and dyslipidemia, usually associate with essential hypertension, leading to speculation that a group of abnormal genes is responsible.

Renal disease. Chronic and end-stage kidney disease is associated with early onset coronary artery disease, likely due to multiple mechanisms including systemic hypertension, abnormal lipid and calcium metabolism, elevated homocysteine, and the effects of inflammation and uremia on endothelial function. Calcification of soft tissues, including coronary arteries, can develop in children with chronic renal disease, especially those on dialysis.

Homocysteine and hypercoagulable states. High blood levels of this amino acid are associated with atherosclerosis and a hypercoagulable state. The observation was first made in homocystinuric children, rare individuals with an inborn metabolic error. For most individuals, adequate dietary intake of folate and other vitamins can decrease homocysteine levels.

Heart transplantation. A diffuse form of coronary artery narrowing occurs in most children and adults following transplantation and may be due primarily to low-grade chronic rejection. In at least a third of children it is a major factor for death or need for retransplantation. Although the pathology of transplant vasculopathy differs from that of atheroma, modifying traditional risk factors such as systemic hypertension and lipids has been proposed as a means to improve the outcome for these patients.

Substance abuse. In addition to tobacco, excessive alcohol consumption may adversely affect other risk factors, such as lipids, but it also has a direct toxic effect on the myocardium, which can result in a dilated cardiomyopathy. Cocaine and similar illicit drugs are associated with acute myocardial ischemia and sudden death. Anabolic steroids may result in systemic hypertension and dyslipidemia.

Dental disease and bacterial infection. Dental disease and bacterial infection are speculative factors in the genesis of atheromas, presumably by direct (infection) or indirect (toxin or inflammatory) injury to the endothelium.

ISSUES FOR CHILDREN AND YOUNG ADULTS WITH HEART DISEASE

General considerations
Almost all the preventive health issues discussed earlier apply to children and young adults with congenital or acquired heart disease, and in some, such

as children with coronary artery abnormalities from Kawasaki disease, these preventive issues become even more important.

Optimum care of the child with congenital cardiac disease entails attention to the effect of the disease upon the behavioral, psychological, and intellectual growth of the child and on the family. Other considerations include the proper definition of the disease and medical and surgical management.

In this age of sophisticated diagnostic and surgical procedures, the common psychological factors of chronic disease are frequently overlooked.

Some patients undergo expensive and extensive operative procedures to correct their cardiac malformations but suffer from the "crippling" effect of the severe emotional problems common to many children with chronic disease. Because of a murmur or cardiac disease, many potential problems can develop in the family. The physician must make the recognition of these problems of utmost importance.

On the initial visit, following the review of the clinical and laboratory findings with the parents, the parents should be given ample opportunity to express their feelings and to ask questions. Listening to them and reassuring them is wise. A feeling of guilt, although seldom expressed, is often present. Many parents are helped by the practitioner who, when explaining cardiac anomalies, points out that, except for rare cases, the medical community knows little of the etiology of the condition. Parents should be told that their child's malformation was not the result of something they did wrong or that they did not do right.

Many parents, because of feelings of guilt or sympathy, assume an overprotective and solicitous attitude toward the child with cardiac abnormalities; in part, this can be fostered by the physician's attitudes. Unless there are contraindications, the child should be treated the same way as his siblings or peers in chores, responsibilities, and discipline. He should partake as fully as possible in family activities. Family life should not center on the cardiac patient. Stressing the emotional needs of other children in the family is also important. Whenever possible, the affected child should attend regular school. Grandparents in particular must be cautioned of the dangers of an overly sympathetic or solicitous approach.

In summary, the child must be treated like other children to the fullest possible extent.

Family counseling

This involves consideration of the type and severity of maternal heart disease, the risk to the mother and fetus, and the recurrence risk in offspring.

Both maternal and fetal risk largely depend on the type of cardiac disorder. In general, for women with well-repaired congenital malformations with normal or near-normal hemodynamics, the risk of pregnancy is similar to that of unaffected women.

Disorders conferring the highest risk of maternal and fetal death include Marfan syndrome, severe dilated cardiomyopathy, pulmonary vascular obstructive disease (PVOD) or primary pulmonary hypertension, and severe unrepaired malformations (e.g., severe left ventricular outflow tract obstruction), especially those with severe cyanosis and polycythemia.

Maternal cardiovascular medications (e.g., certain antiarrhythmics and antithrombotic therapy) may confer high risk to the fetus.

Recurrence risk varies with lesion and even with which parent is affected. In general, maternal congenital heart disease is more likely than paternal to recur in offspring. Some lesions, such as ventricular septal defect (VSD) and atrial septal defect (ASD), have a relatively low recurrence risk, except in families where multiple members are affected despite the absence of a recognizable syndrome. Left heart obstructive lesions, such as aortic stenosis, have a relatively high recurrence risk (estimated at 10–15%). A parent affected by DiGeorge or Noonan syndrome has a 50% risk of recurrence.

Following the discovery of congenital cardiac disease in one of their children, parents become concerned with the risks of having a second child that would be similarly affected. If, in the proband, the cardiac malformation is not part of a recognized syndrome (including microdeletions of chromosome 22 or translocation-type trisomies) and no previous family history of cardiac anomalies exists, the risk of a second affected child is probably twice that of the first. The incidence of congenital heart disease in the population is 0.7%, reflecting an incidence of 1:135. If a second child in a family is affected, the form of cardiac anomaly will be concordant in half. Some families have several members of one generation who show the same form of cardiac malformation. Interestingly, one exception seems to be complete transposition of the great vessels, where the occurrence of multiple, or even two, instances in a family is rare. If a second child does have a cardiac anomaly, the risk of a subsequent child also having cardiac anomaly is even higher.

If the child shows one of the recognizable syndromes associated with cardiac malformations, specific genetic counseling should be given. The physician's responsibility is not to instruct parents about whether they should or should not attempt to have more children, but they should be advised of the available information so that they can reach an appropriate decision.

Exercise limitations
These have been based on limited evidence and much speculation. Wide differences exist in the advice given to parents regarding exercise.

General exercise. Most children with a cardiac anomaly can be allowed a normal range of physical activity; however, they should realize that the anomaly may limit their ability to exercise. The child may be permitted to participate in physical education in school, but teachers must understand that the child may have to stop and rest sooner than the other children. The child should not be pushed to extremes of physical activity or to perform in unfavorable situations, such as extreme heat or cold; and dehydration should be avoided. More severe exercise restrictions are indicated for children with disorders, such as severe aortic stenosis, hypertrophic cardiomyopathy, and Marfan syndrome, as exertion can be fatal in these children.

Sports. Some pediatric cardiologists advise avoidance of any competitive sports activity for all unrepaired and some repaired patients (such as those with tetralogy of Fallot); these patients may participate in fun physical activities as long as they are in charge of when they cease activity, but presumably they are at greater risk if they are "pushed" to more intense exertion, as during a competitive sports situation. The 26th Bethesda Conference in 1994, and revised as the 36th Conference in 2005, sought to determine eligibility for athletic competition based on the type and severity of the cardiac abnormality and the type and intensity of the sport (Tables 12.4 and 12.5).

Inappropriate restriction. Children with cardiac abnormalities may be inappropriately restricted by school authorities, even when the school has been informed that no need for exercise restriction exists. This reflects an unrealistic fear that teachers sometimes have about children with cardiac disease, which arises from ignorance of cardiac anomalies and from the association of all cardiac disease with heart attacks and sudden death. In any correspondence regarding a child with cardiac abnormality, whether to a referring physician or to a school, the recommended level of exercise should be clearly defined.

Postoperative. Following pediatric cardiac operations, the level of exercise can be gradually increased to full participation 4–6 weeks postoperatively, if no major complication (e.g., congestive cardiac failure or pericardial effusion) is present. After recovery from operation, the child should be permitted normal activity as tolerated and dictated by the postoperative hemodynamics.

Modified bedrest. This has very limited indications. In the presence of an active inflammatory disease involving the myocardium, such as acute rheumatic carditis or myocarditis, it may be advisable. Complete bedrest is difficult to achieve because of a child's natural activeness; it may even have adverse consequences compared with modified bedrest. As an alternative, children can spend most of their time sitting or lying on the couch and can be allowed up to the bathroom and dinner table.

Nutrition
Diet. Most children with cardiac anomalies do not require a special diet, except for those with cardiac failure, in whom a high-caloric-density diet and

Table 12.4 Classification of Sports—36th Bethesda Conference.

	A. Low (<40% Max O$_2$)	B. Moderate (40–70% Max O$_2$)	C. High (>70% Max O$_2$)
III. High (>50% MVC)	Bobsledding/Luge*†, Field events (throwing), Gymnastics*†, Martial arts*, Sailing, Sport climbing, Water skiing*†, Weight lifting*†, Windsurfing*† (1)	Body building*†, Downhill skiing*†, Skateboarding*†, Snowboarding*†, Wrestling* (2)	Boxing*, Canoeing/Kayaking, Cycling*†, Decathlon, Rowing, Speed-skating*†, Triathlon*† (3)
II. Moderate (20–50% MVC)	Archery, Auto racing*†, Diving*†, Equestrian*†, Motorcycling*† (4)	American football*, Field events (jumping), Figure skating*, Rodeoing*†, Rugby*, Running (sprint), Surfing*†, Synchronized swimming† (5)	Basketball*, Ice hockey*, Cross-country skiing (skating technique), Lacrosse*, Running (middle distance), Swimming, Team handball (6)
I. Low (<20% MVC)	Billiards, Bowling, Cricket, Curling, Golf, Riflery (7)	Baseball/Softball*, Fencing, Table tennis, Volleyball (8)	Badminton, Cross-country skiing (classic technique), Field hockey*, Orienteering, Race walking, Racquetball/Squash, Running (long distance), Soccer*, Tennis (9)

Increasing Static Component ↑

Increasing Dynamic Component ⟶

This classification is based on peak static and dynamic components achieved during competition. It should be noted, however, that higher values may be reached during training. The increasing dynamic component is defined in terms of the estimated percent of maximal oxygen uptake (Max O$_2$) achieved and results in an increasing cardiac output. The increasing static component is related to the estimated percent of maximal voluntary contraction (MVC) reached and results in an increasing blood pressure load. The lowest total cardiovascular demands (cardiac output and blood pressure) are shown in Cell 7 and the highest in Cell 3. Cells 4 and 8 show low moderate; Cells 1, 5, and 9 show moderate; and Cells 2 and 6 show high moderate total cardiovascular demands.

* Danger of bodily collision.
† Increased risk if syncope occurs.

perhaps a low-sodium diet may be indicated. In older children, salt restriction varies from recommendations of no added salt and avoidance of foods with high salt content, such as potato chips and pizza, to a modified diet limiting sodium. Sodium restriction has less impact on symptoms and prognosis than once thought; it is less important (and more difficult to achieve) than avoiding excess sodium intake.

Infants with congestive heart failure (CHF). Nutrition is most critical for infants with CHF because of large left-to-right shunts, such as VSD. These

Table 12.5 Sports Recommendations for Athletes with Cardiovascular Abnormalities.

Condition	Sport
ASD, untreated	
Small defects, nl RV volume, no PA htn	All
Large ASD, nl PA pressure	All
ASD, mild PA htn	IA
ASD, PVOD, cyanosis, R-to-L shunt	None
ASD, symptomatic arrhythmia or MR	Individualize
ASD, closed at operation or catheterization	
After 3–6 months, if no PA htn, arrhythmia, AVB, or myocardial dysfxn	All
Or, if residual abnormalities	Individualize
VSD, untreated	
VSD, nl PA pressure	All
VSD, large, with R_P allowing repair	Repair first
VSD, closed at operation or catheterization	
After 3–6 months, if no sxs, no or small residual defect, no PA htn, no arrhythmia, and no myocardial dysfxn	All
Symptomatic arrhythmias, AVB, PA htn, myocardial dysfxn	Individualize
PDA, untreated	
Small PDA, nl LV size	All
Moderate or large PDA with LV enlargement	Repair first
Moderate or large PDA, severe PA htn, cyanosis	See Elev Rp
PDA, closed at operation or catheterization	
After 3 months, if no sxs, with nl exam, no PA htn or LV enlargement	All
With residual PA htn	See Elev Rp
PS, untreated	
≤40 mm Hg peak systolic gradient, nl RV fxn, no sxs; reeval annually	All
>40 mm Hg peak systolic gradient	IA, IB; prior to gradient relief
PS, treated by operation or balloon valvuloplasty	
No or mild (≤40 mm Hg gradient) residual PS, no sxs, nl RV fxn	All (2–4 weeks after BD; 3 months after surgery)
>40 mm Hg peak systolic gradient and/or severe PI with RV enlargement	IA, IB
AS, untreated (reevaluate annually)	
Mild (≤30 mm Hg peak-to-peak gradient), no sxs, nl ECG, no exercise intolerance, no arrhythmia	All
Moderate (30–50 mm Hg gradient), no sxs, mild or no LVE by echo, nl ECG, nl exercise test	IA, IB, IIA
Moderate, with arrhythmia at rest or exercise	IA, IB
Severe (>50 mm Hg gradient)	None

(*continued*)

Table 12.5 (*cont.*)

Condition	Sport
AS, treated by operation or balloon valvuloplasty (reeval annually)	
Mild, moderate, or severe residual AS	See untreated AS
Moderate to severe AI	See AI
AI	
Mild AI, no sxs, nl LV size	All
AI, moderate LVE (adult LVEDD 60–65 mm), no arrhythmia or sxs on GXT to at least exertion level of competition	IA-C, IIA-C
AI, with asymptomatic nonsustained ventricular arrhythmia at rest or exercise	IA
Mild to moderate AI, with symptoms	None
Severe AI, and LVE (adult LVEDD >65 mm)	None
Bicuspid aortic valve	
No aortic root dilation (>40 mm, or z-score > +2), no significant AS or AI	All
Dilated aortic root 40–45 mm (adult)	IA, IB, IIA, IIB (+ no collision)
Dilated aortic root >45 mm (adult)	IA
Coarctation, untreated	
Mild, no large collaterals, aortic root diameter z-score ≤ +3.0, resting gradient ≤20 mm Hg, nl exercise test and max exercise peak systolic BP ≤230 mm Hg	All
Resting gradient ≥20 mm Hg, or exercise-induced htn ≥230 mm Hg	IA, until treated
Coarctation, treated by surgery or balloon angioplasty	
At least 3 months to 1 year after treatment, no sxs, resting gradient ≤ 20 mm Hg, nl resting and exercise systolic BP	Avoid III A, B, C and collision
Significant aortic dilation, wall thinning, or aneurysm	IA, IB
Elevated pulmonary resistance with congenital heart disease*	
PA systolic ≤30 mm Hg	All
PA systolic ≥30 mm Hg	Perform full evaluation and individualize
Ventricular dysfunction after cardiac surgery (reeval periodically)	
Normal or near-normal function (EF ≥50%)	All
Mild depression of function (EF 40–50%)	IA, IB, IC
Moderate to severe depression of function (EF <40%)	None
Cyanotic congenital heart disease	
Unoperated	None or IA
Palliated, if sat >80%, no sxs, no LV dysfunction, no arrhythmia	IA

Table 12.5 (cont.)

Tetralogy of Fallot	
Normal or near-normal right heart pressure, no or mild RV volume overload, no significant shunt, no arrhythmia on ambulatory ECG or exercise test	All*
Marked PI with RV volume overload, and/or RVp ≥ 50% systemic, and/or arrhythmia	IA
d-TGV, repaired*	
Venous switch, if nl heart size, no arrhythmia, no syncope, nl exercise test (nl duration, workload, etc. for age/gender)	IA, IIA
Venous switch, if any of above abn	Individualize
Arterial switch, if nl ventricular fxn, no arrhythmia, nl exercise test	All
Arterial switch, with > mild hemodynamic abn, ventricular dysfxn, but nl exercise test	IA, IB, IC, IIA
l-TGV ("Corrected" transposition) (reeval periodically)	
No sxs, no systemic ventricle enlargement, no arrhythmia, and nl exercise test (including nl VO$_2$ max)	IA, IIA
Post operative Fontan	IA (IB if nl sat and ventricular fxn)
Ebstein's	
Mild; no cyanosis, nl RV size, no arrhythmia	All
Moderate TR, no significant arrhythmia on ambulatory ECG	IA
Severe	None
Postoperative, if TR mild, nl heart size, no arrhythmia	IA or individualize
Congenital coronary artery anomalies	
Wrong sinus origin	None
>3 months after repair, if no ischemia, arrhythmia, dysfxn at exercise testing	All
Previous MI (individualized, based on resting LV fxn, sxs, arrhythmia, and GXT)	None, or IA, or IA, IIA
Mitral valve prolapse	
No syncope from arrhythmia, sustained/complex arrhythmia, severe MR, LV dysfxn (EF <50%), embolic events, or family hx MVP-related death	All
Any of the above	IA
Systemic hypertension	
pre-hypertension (120/80 mm Hg up to 139/89 mm Hg)	All
Stage 1 htn (140–159 mm Hg/90–99 mm Hg) without target organ damage including LVH or concomitant heart disease	All (monitor BP)
Stage 2 htn (≥160/100 mm Hg)	None (or no IIIA-C) until BP controlled

(continued)

Table 12.5 (*cont.*)

Condition	Sport
Kawasaki disease	
Normal coronary arteries or transient ectasia, convalescent phase, after 6–8 weeks	All
Regressed aneurysms, no exercise ischemia with myocardial perfusion scanning	All
Small to medium isolated aneurysms, no exercise-induced ischemia or arrhythmia; repeat exercise perfusion testing each 1–2 years	IA, IB, IIA, IIB
Large, multiple, or segmented coronary aneurysms with or without obstruction if normal LV fxn, no exercise-induced arrhythmia or ischemia with myocardial perfusion scanning; repeat exercise perfusion testing each 1–2 years	IA, IIA
After MI or revascularization, after ≥6 weeks, nl LV fxn, exercise tolerance, no exercise-induced arrhythmia or ischemia with myocardial perfusion scanning; repeat exercise perfusion testing each 1–2 years	IA, IB
After MI or revascularization, LV EF <40%, exercise intolerance, or exercise-induced ventricular arrhythmia	None
Patients on antithrombotic therapy	Avoid collision sports
Myocarditis	
Full recovery = nl LV fxn, wall motion, and cardiac dimensions; nl ECG; no significant arrhythmia on ambulatory ECG and GXT; serum markers of inflammation and heart failure normalized	None until full recovery (minimum 6 months)
Pericarditis	
Acute phase	None
Full recovery (no evidence active disease, no effusion by echo, and serum markers of inflammation normal)	All
With myocarditis	See myocarditis
Constrictive	None
Inherited arrhythmia syndromes	
Long QT syndrome	None vs. IA
Short QT syndrome	None vs. IA
Ventricular tachycardia, cathecholaminergic polymorphic	None vs. IA
Brugada syndrome	IA
Hypertrophic cardiomyopathy	None vs. IA
Arrhythmogenic right ventricular cardiomyopathy (ARVC)	None vs. IA
Other myocardial diseases (limited data) Dilated cardiomyopathy; primary nonhypertrophied restrictive cardiomyopathy; systemic infiltrative diseases with secondary cardiac involvement such as sarcoidosis; isolated noncompaction of LV myocardium ± systolic dysfunction	None vs. IA

Table 12.5 (*cont.*)

Condition	Sport
Marfan syndrome	
No CV involvement as defined below; reeval 6 months intervals	*IA, *IIA
Aortic root dilation (>40 mm, or z-score > +2), prior aortic root surgery, chronic dissection of aorta or other artery, mod-severe MR; family hx dissection or death in Marfan relative; reeval 6 months intervals	*IA
Aortic insufficiency	see AI (*and, no collision sports)
Ehlers–Danlos syndrome (vascular form)	None

*Some conditions, including repaired tetralogy of Fallot, d-TGV, single ventricle, pulmonary vascular obstructive disease, etc., are associated with a risk of sudden death at rest and during exertion.

Adapted from 36th Bethesda Conference: Eligibility recommendations for competitive athletes with cardiovascular abnormalities. J Am Coll Cardiol 2005;45:1312–1375.

Sports classification is shown in Table 12.4.

Abbreviations: abn, abnormality; AI, aortic insufficiency; AS, aortic stenosis; ASD, atrial septal defect; AVB, atrioventricular nodal block;BD; balloon dilation; BP, blood pressure; CV, cardiovascular; d-TGV, d-transposition of the great vessels; dysfxn, dysfunction; EF, ejection fraction; Elev, elevated; fxn, function;GXT, graded exercise test; htn, hypertension; hx, history; l-TGV, l-transposition of the great vessels; LV, left ventricle or left ventricular; LVE, left ventricular enlargement; LVEDD, left ventricular end-diastolic diameter (echo); LVH, left ventricular hypertrophy; mmHg, millimeters of mercury; MI, myocardial infarct; MR, mitral regurgitation; MVP, mitral valve prolapse; nl, normal; p, pressure; PA, pulmonary artery; PDA, patent ductus arteriosus; PI, pulmonary insufficiency; PS, pulmonary stenosis; pts, patients; PVOD, pulmonary vascular obstructive disease; reeval, reevaluate/reevaluation; R_P, pulmonary vascular resistance; RV, right ventricle or right ventricular; sat, oxygen saturation; sxs, symptoms; TR, tricuspid regurgitation; VO_2 max, maximal oxygen consumption (exercise); VSD, ventricular septal defect.

infants may feed poorly because of dyspnea and tachypnea and may have emesis and/or gastroesophageal reflux because of intestinal edema, thoracic hyperinflation, and esophageal compression from left atrial enlargement. They have greater energy expenditure because of cardiac and respiratory overwork and often require 30–40% more calories than normal infants to achieve minimally acceptable weight gain. If timely surgery is not feasible, alternative feeding methods, such as continuous gastric or transpyloric tube feedings of hypercaloric formula, may be indicated.

Growth and small stature. Children with a cardiac anomaly may be small in stature because of the effect of the condition upon the circulation or because of problems coexisting with the cardiac anomaly (e.g., DiGeorge syndrome). In most children, the latter is true, as evidenced by the observation that growth rates and stature for age often remain unchanged after successful cardiac repair.

Between the ages of 1 and 4 years, the appetite of many children is considered poor by their parents. The parents of healthy children in this age range often complain about their child's eating habits. The rate of weight gain compared with the first year of life markedly decreases at about 1 year of age. Yet many small-statured children with a cardiac problem have a normal rate of growth. Comparison to published "normal" growth curves may help allay parental anxiety.

Each of these factors leads to concern for many parents, and these concerns are increased in the parents of children with a cardiac anomaly who are small statured. They believe that stature would become normal if the child would only eat. This leads to turmoil, unpleasant meal experiences, and frustration. These problems can be reduced by using anticipatory guidance to discuss with the parents what they should expect as their child grows older.

Follow-up medical care

Most children with cardiac anomalies require periodic evaluation. The reasons for the evaluation and the type of information sought depend in large part upon the natural history of the cardiac condition. For instance, in a patient with a large VSD, evidence of the development of pulmonary hypertension or congestive cardiac failure would be sought, whereas in aortic stenosis, evidence of increasing gradient, left ventricular strain, and/or important aortic insufficiency would be looked for. Thus, the frequency of return visits and the type of diagnostic studies performed on the patient's return are dictated by the symptoms and the natural history of the defect.

Usually, infants are evaluated more frequently than older children because changes in circulation take place more rapidly during the first year of life.

Children with cardiac anomalies also require routine pediatric care. In infants with cardiac failure or other major symptoms, physicians can easily overlook or fail to administer routine immunizations, but these are an important component of the child's health care.

Most children with repaired cardiac malformations and many with acquired heart disease are at risk for late complications, such as arrhythmia, endocarditis, progressive obstruction of previously relieved stenosis, and so on. Some patients are at long-term risk for sudden life-threatening events.

Many children with repaired patent ductus arteriosus (PDA), ASD, or VSD are not at great risk for complications and may not require frequent follow-up care by a pediatric cardiologist after they have fully recovered from their cardiac intervention.

Many centers for adults with congenital heart disease have established follow-up programs, which usually include the expertise of pediatric cardiologists.

Insurability and occupational issues
For the young adult with heart disease, insurability and occupational issues remain difficult problems for many patients, especially for those with important physical limitations (e.g., CHF, PVOD, and Marfan syndrome) that severely limit their available employment options to sedentary or light-activity jobs (Table 12.6). Some states have established health insurance pools for patients who are otherwise considered uninsurable (at affordable cost) by commercial insurers because of preexisting conditions.

Infective endocarditis prophylaxis
Endocarditis is a serious life-threatening condition that requires lengthy medical treatment and which in some cases requires surgical treatment. Therefore, prevention is a worthy goal. However, many patients who developed endocarditis had previously received optimal antibiotic treatment and the efficacy of antibiotics given preprocedure appears to be limited.

These issues are addressed in guidelines from the American Heart Association and American Dental Association, published in 2007, and reflect similar recommendations in European and British assessments of endocarditis prevention (Table 12.7 Fig. 12.1). These recommendations represent a considerable departure from the practice of the last several decades, and substantially reduce the number of patients, and the types of conditions, for which endocarditis prophylaxis is recommended.

Children with most forms of congenital cardiac anomalies and those with acquired valvar anomalies are at some degree of increased risk of developing infective endocarditis, but for many lesions this risk is low or similar to that of unaffected patients.

Endocarditis is very rare in repaired and unrepaired ASD, repaired VSD and PDA (after 6 months and with no residual abnormality), and mitral valve prolapse without regurgitation. Children with functional murmurs and those with normal hearts following Kawasaki disease or rheumatic fever are not at risk, either.

Children at high risk are those with prosthetic valves, unrepaired cyanotic lesions, surgically created systemic-to-pulmonary artery shunts, conduits, a past history of endocarditis, patients within 6 months of a repair (surgical or catheter-based), and patients after repair who have residual shunts adjacent to the site of prosthetic material impairing neoendothelialization.

Because the risk of endocarditis also varies with the type of cardiac lesion and also with the type of repair or palliation, antibiotic prophylaxis is indicated for only those with the highest risk if endocarditis is acquired.

Table 12.6 Occupational Guidelines for Adults with Congenital Heart Disease.

Work→	Sedentary	Light	Medium	Heavy	Very Heavy
Peak Lift→	≤10 lb	≤20 lb	≤50 lb	≤100 lb	>100 lb
Frequent Carry→	small objects	≤10 lb	≤25 lb	≤50 lb	≥50lb
Peak Load→	≤ 2.5 cal/min	2.6–4.9 cal/min	5.0–7.5 cal/min		≥ 7.6cal/min
↓ Condition					
AI	—	—	—	—	—
AS	—	severe	moderate	mild	—
ASD	—	severe*	moderate	mild	—
Cardiomyopathy*	—	mod-severe PVOD*	mild-mod PVOD	—	no PVOD
COA	Dilated	Hypertrophic	—	—	—
		—	± op; htn	—	repaired, nl BP rest and exercise
Hypertension	—	—	mod-severe	mild	—
MR	severe (CM and/or AFib)	—	moderate (mild-mod CM)	mild (no CM)	—
MS	severe	moderate	mild	—	—
MVP	—	—	—	—	mild, no sxs
PDA	—	mod-severe PVOD*	mild-mod PVOD	—	no PVOD
PS	—	severe	moderate	—	mild

PA Hypertension (primary)*	PAp ≥ 0.5 systemic	PAp ≤ 0.5 systemic	—	—	—
TOF, post op*	—	mod-severe PVOD* unop or palliated only	RVp > 50 mm Hg mild-mod PVOD post op	RVp < 50 mm Hg no PVOD	—
VSD	—				—
Other Major Defects*	—				—
Arrhythmia	—	VT*	PVC with CHD	AVB; pacemaker†; SVT; VT (nl otherwise)	PAC; PVC (nl heart); WPW*

Wide variation exists among patients with similar diagnoses [Diller G-P, Dimopoulos K, Okonko D, et al. Exercise intolerance in adult congenital heart disease: Comparative severity, correlates, and prognostic implication. Circulation 2005;112(6):828–835.]; recommendations must be individualized. Exercise testing may be advisable for many patients.

Table data adapted from Gutgesell HP, Gessner IH, Vetter VL, Yabek SM, Norton JB. Recreational and occupational recommendations for young patients with heart disease. A Statement for Physicians by the Committee on Congenital Cardiac Defects of the Council on Cardiovascular Disease in the Young, American Heart Association. Circulation 1986;74(5):1195A–1198A.

* Some conditions may be associated with sudden death, even in patients at rest.

† Use of certain equipment (e.g., arc welding) or repetitive shoulder motion may damage pacing system.

AI, aortic insufficiency; AS, aortic stenosis; ASD, atrial septal defect; AVB, atrioventricular block; cal/min, calories/minute; CHD, congenital heart disease; CM, cardiomegaly; COA, coarctation; GXT, graded exercise test; htn, hypertension; lb, pound; mm Hg, millimeters of mercury; MR, mitral regurgitation; MS, mitral stenosis; MVP, mitral valve prolapse; nl, normal; op, operation; PA, pulmonary artery; PAp, pulmonary artery pressure; PDA, patent ductus arteriosus; PS, pulmonary stenosis; PVC, premature ventricular contraction; PVOD, pulmonary vascular obstructive disease; RVp, right ventricular pressure; SVT, supraventricular tachycardia; TOF, tetralogy of Fallot; TR, tricuspid regurgitation; VSD, ventricular septal defect; VT, ventricular tachycardia.

Table 12.7 Primary Reasons for Revision of the IE Prophylaxis Guidelines.

IE is much more likely to result from frequent exposure to random bacteremias associated with daily activities than from bacteremia caused by a dental, GI tract, or GU tract procedure.

Prophylaxis may prevent an exceedingly small number of cases of IE, if any, in individuals who undergo a dental, GI tract, or GU tract procedure.

The risk of antibiotic-associated adverse events exceeds the benefit, if any, from prophylactic antibiotic therapy.

Maintenance of optimal oral health and hygiene may reduce the incidence of bacteremia from daily activities and is more important than prophylactic antibiotics for a dental procedure to reduce the risk of IE.

Reprinted with permission from Wilson W, Taubert KA, Gewitz M, Lockhart PB, Baddour LM, Levison M, Bolger A, Cabell CH, Takahashi M, Baltimore RS, Newburger JW, Strom BL, Tani LY, Gerber M, Bonow RO, Pallasch T, Shulman ST, Rowley AH, Burns JC, Ferrieri P, Gardner T, Goff D, Durack DT. Prevention of infective endocarditis: Guidelines from the American Heart Association: A guideline from the American Heart Association Rheumatic Fever, Endocarditis and Kawasaki Disease Committee, Council on Cardiovascular Disease in the Young, and the Council on Clinical Cardiology, Council on Cardiovascular Surgery and Anesthesia, and the Quality of Care and Outcomes Research Interdisciplinary Working Group. Circulation October 9, 2007;116(15):1736–1754. Epub April 19, 2007. Erratum in: Circulation October 9, 2007;116(15):e376–e377.

Antibiotic prophylaxis (Fig. 12.1) is started within the hour before the procedure and not sooner. Antibiotic administration at this time assures a high blood level of the antibiotic at the time of the bacteremia risk. Beginning antibiotics a day or two before the procedure is unwise; this promotes the development of organisms resistant to the antibiotic being administered. Dental work is the most frequent procedure for which endocarditis prophylaxis is indicated.

In patients receiving continuous antibiotics for prophylaxis of asplenia, rheumatic fever, or urinary tract infection and in patients receiving antibiotics for other acute indications, relatively resistant flora appear in the oropharynx and gut after only a few days of treatment, so an antibiotic of a different class from that currently being taken is indicated for endocarditis prevention.

ADDITIONAL READING AND REFERENCES

General

Kavey RE, Allada V, Daniels SR, et al. Cardiovascular risk reduction in high-risk pediatric patients: A scientific statement from the American Heart Association Expert Panel on Population and Prevention Science; the Councils on Cardiovascular Disease in the Young, Epidemiology and Prevention, Nutrition, Physical Activity and Metabolism, High Blood Pressure Research, Cardiovascular Nursing, and the Kidney in Heart Disease; and the Interdisciplinary Working Group on Quality of Care and Outcomes Research: Endorsed

PREVENTION OF INFECTIVE (BACTERIAL) ENDOCARDITIS
Wallet Card

This wallet card is to be given to patients (or parents) by their physician. Healthcare professionals: Please see back of card for reference to the complete statement.

Name: _____

needs protection from

INFECTIVE (BACTERIAL) ENDOCARDITIS

because of an existing heart condition.

Diagnosis: _____

Prescribed by: _____

Date: _____

You received this wallet card because you are at increased risk for developing adverse outcomes from infective endocarditis (IE), also known as bacterial endocarditis (BE). The guidelines for prevention of IE shown in this card are substantially different from previously published guidelines. This card replaces the previous card that was based on guidelines published in 1997.

The American Heart Association's Endocarditis Committee together with national and international experts on IE extensively reviewed published studies in order to determine whether dental, gastrointestinal (GI), or genitourinary (GU) tract procedures are possible causes of IE. These experts determined that there is no conclusive evidence that links dental, GI, or GU tract procedures with the development of IE.

The current practice of giving patients antibiotics prior to a dental procedure is no longer recommended **EXCEPT** for patients with the highest risk of adverse outcomes resulting from IE (see below on this card). The Committee cannot exclude the possibility that an exceedingly small number of cases, if any, of IE may be prevented by antibiotic prophylaxis prior to a dental procedure. If such benefit from prophylaxis exists, it should be reserved **ONLY** for those patients listed below. The Committee recognizes the importance of good oral and dental health and regular visits to the dentist for patients at risk of IE.

The Committee no longer recommends administering antibiotics solely to prevent IE in patients who undergo a GI or GU tract procedure.

Changes in these guidelines do not change the fact that your cardiac condition puts you at increased risk for developing endocarditis. If you develop signs or symptoms of endocarditis—such as unexplained fever—see your doctor right away. If blood cultures are necessary (to determine if endocarditis is present), it is important for your doctor to obtain these cultures and other relevant tests **BEFORE** antibiotics are started.

Antibiotic prophylaxis with dental procedures is reasonable only for patients with cardiac conditions associated with the highest risk of adverse outcomes from endocarditis, including:

- Prosthetic cardiac valve or prosthetic material used in valve repair

- Previous endocarditis

- Congenital heart disease only in the following categories:

  - Unrepaired cyanotic congenital heart disease, including those with palliative shunts and conduits

  - Completely repaired congenital heart disease with prosthetic material or device, whether placed by surgery or catheter intervention, during the first six months after the procedure*

  - Repaired congenital heart disease with residual defects at the site or adjacent to the site of a prosthetic patch or prosthetic device (which inhibit endothelialization)

- Cardiac transplantation recipients with cardiac valvular disease

*Prophylaxis is reasonable because endothelialization of prosthetic material occurs within six months after the procedure.

Dental procedures for which prophylaxis is reasonable in patients with cardiac conditions listed above.

Figure 12.1 Prevention of infective endocarditis wallet card. Reprinted with Permission www.americanheart.org ©2008, American Heart Association.

All dental procedures that involve manipulation of gingival tissue or the periapical region of teeth, or perforation of the oral mucosa*

*Antibiotic prophylaxis is NOT recommended for the following dental procedures or events: routine anesthetic injections through noninfected tissue; taking dental radiographs; placement of removable prosthodontic or orthodontic appliances; adjustment of orthodontic appliances; placement of orthodontic brackets; and shedding of deciduous teeth and bleeding from trauma to the lips or oral mucosa.

**Antibiotic Prophylactic Regimens
for Dental Procedures**

Situation	Agent	Regimen—Single Dose (30–60 minutes before procedure)	
		Adults	Children
Oral	Amoxicillin	2 g	50 mg/kg
Unable to take oral medication	Ampicillin **OR**	2 g IM or IV*	50 mg/kg IM or IV
	Cefazolin or ceftriaxone	1 g IM or IV	50 mg/kg IM or IV
Allergic to penicillins or ampicillin—Oral regimen	Cephalexin ‡	2 g	50 mg/kg
	OR		
	Clindamycin	600 mg	20 mg/kg
	OR		
	Azithromycin or clarithromycin	500 mg	15 mg/kg
Allergic to penicillins or ampicillin and unable to take oral medication	Cefazolin or ceftriaxone†	1 g IM or IV	50 mg/kg IM or IV
	OR Clindamycin	600 mg IM or IV	20 mg/kg IM or IV

*IM, intramuscular; IV, intravenous.
†Or other first- or second-generation oral cephalosporin in equivalent adult or pediatric dosage.
‡Cephalosporins should not be used in an individual with a history of anaphylaxis, angioedema, or urticaria with penicillins or ampicillin.

Gastrointestinal/Genitourinary Procedures: Antibiotic prophylaxis solely to prevent IE is no longer recommended for patients who undergo a GI or GU tract procedure, including patients with the highest risk of adverse outcomes due to IE.

Other Procedures: Procedures involving the respiratory tract or infected skin, tissues just under the skin, or musculoskeletal tissue for which prophylaxis is reasonable are discussed in the updated document (reference below).

Adapted from *Prevention of Infective Endocarditis: Guidelines From the American Heart Association,* by the Committee on Rheumatic Fever, Endocarditis, and Kawasaki Disease. *Circulation,* 2007; 116: 1736-1754. Accessible at http://circ.ahajournals.org/cgi/reprint/CIRCULATIONAHA.106.183095.

Healthcare Professionals—Please refer to these recommendations for more complete information as to which patients and which procedures need prophylaxis.

American Heart Association. | American Stroke Association.
Learn and Live.

The Council on Scientific Affairs of the American Dental Association has approved this statement as it relates to dentistry.

National Center
7272 Greenville Avenue
Dallas, Texas 75231-4596
americanheart.org

Figure 12.1 *(continued)*

by the American Academy of Pediatrics. Circulation December 12, 2006;114(24):2710–2738.

Diet

Gidding SS, Dennison BA, Birch LL, et al., for American Heart Association; American Academy of Pediatrics. Dietary recommendations for children and adolescents: A guide for practitioners. Pediatrics February 2006;117(2):544–559 and Circulation June 13, 2006;113(23):e857.

Hyperlipidemia

Haney EM, Huffman LH, Bougatsos C, Freeman M, Steiner RD, Nelson HD. Screening and treatment for lipid disorders in children and adolescents: Systematic evidence review for the US Preventive Services Task Force. Pediatrics July 2007;120(1):e189–e214.

Magnussen CG, Raitakari OT, Thomson R, et al. Utility of currently recommended pediatric dyslipidemia classifications in predicting dyslipidemia in adulthood: Evidence from the Childhood Determinants of Adult Health (CDAH) study, Cardiovascular Risk in Young Finns Study, and Bogalusa Heart Study. Circulation January 1, 2008;117(1):32–42.

McCrindle BW, Urbina EM, Dennison BA, et al., for American Heart Association Atherosclerosis, Hypertension, and Obesity in Youth Committee; American Heart Association Council of Cardiovascular Disease in the Young; American Heart Association Council on Cardiovascular Nursing. Drug therapy of high-risk lipid abnormalities in children and adolescents: A scientific statement from the American Heart Association Atherosclerosis, Hypertension, and Obesity in Youth Committee, Council of Cardiovascular Disease in the Young, with the Council on Cardiovascular Nursing. Circulation April 10, 2007;115(14):1948–1967.

Report of the Expert Panel on Blood Cholesterol Levels in Children and Adolescents. Pediatrics 1992;89:525–584.

Third Report of the National Cholesterol Education Program (NCEP) Expert Panel on Detection, Evaluation, and Treatment of High Blood Cholesterol in Adults (Adult Treatment Panel III) final report. Circulation December 17, 2002;106(25):3143–3421.

US Preventive Services Task Force. Screening for lipid disorders in children: US Preventive Services Task Force recommendation statement. Pediatrics 2007;120:e215–e219.

Obesity

Barlow SE, for Expert Committee. Expert committee recommendations regarding the prevention, assessment, and treatment of child and adolescent overweight and obesity: Summary report. Pediatrics December 2007;120(Suppl 4):S164–S192.

Body Mass Index-for-Age. Centers for Disease Control and Prevention; 2000. Including pediatric growth charts. Available from www.cdc.gov/growthcharts/.

Council on Sports Medicine and Fitness; Council on School Health. Active healthy living: Prevention of childhood obesity through increased physical activity. Pediatrics May 2006;117(5):1834–1842.

Tobacco

Fiore MC, Bailey WC, Cohen SJ, et al. Treating Tobacco Use and Dependence. Clinical Practice Guideline. Rockville, MD: U.S. Department of Health and Human Services,

Public Health Service; June 2000. Available from www.surgeongeneral.gov/tobacco/.

The Tobacco Use and Dependence Clinical Practice Guideline Panel, Staff, and Consortium Representatives. A clinical practice guideline for treating tobacco use and dependence: A U.S. Public Health Service report. JAMA 2000;283:3244–3254.

Presports cardiovascular evaluation

Bille K, Figueiras D, Schamasch P, et al. Sudden cardiac death in athletes: The Lausanne recommendations. Eur J Cardiovasc Prev Rehabil December 2006;13(6):859–875. Available from http://multimedia.olympic.org/pdf/en_report_886.pdf.

Corrado D, Pelliccia A, Bjørnstad HH, et al. Cardiovascular pre-participation screening of young competitive athletes for prevention of sudden death: Proposal for a common European protocol. Consensus Statement of the Study Group of Sport Cardiology of the Working Group of Cardiac Rehabilitation and Exercise Physiology and the Working Group of Myocardial and Pericardial Diseases of the European Society of Cardiology. Eur Heart J March 2005;26(5):516–524.

Maron BJ, Chaitman BR, Ackerman MJ, et al. Recommendations for physical activity and recreational sports participation for young patients with genetic cardiovascular diseases. Circulation June 8, 2004;109(22):2807–2816.

Maron BJ, Thompson PD, Ackerman MJ, et al. Recommendations and considerations related to preparticipation screening for cardiovascular abnormalities in competitive athletes: 2007 update: A scientific statement from the American Heart Association Council on Nutrition, Physical Activity, and Metabolism: Endorsed by the American College of Cardiology Foundation. Circulation March 27, 2007;115(12):1643–1655.

Endocarditis prevention

Wilson W, Taubert KA, Gewitz M, et al. Prevention of infective endocarditis: Guidelines from the American Heart Association: A guideline from the American Heart Association Rheumatic Fever, Endocarditis and Kawasaki Disease Committee, Council on Cardiovascular Disease in the Young, and the Council on Clinical Cardiology, Council on Cardiovascular Surgery and Anesthesia, and the Quality of Care and Outcomes Research Interdisciplinary Working Group. Circulation October 9, 2007;116(15):1736–1754. Epub April 19, 2007. Erratum in: Circulation October 9, 2007;116(15):e376–e377.

Adults with congenital heart disease

Gatzoulis MA, Swan L, Therrien J, Pantely GA. Adult Congenital Heart Disease: A Practical Guide. Oxford: Wiley-Blackwell; 2005.

Appendix A
Congestive heart failure – drug therapy

See Chapter 11 for a more complete discussion of CHF management. One or more of the following classes of drugs are employed for management of acute heart failure, with examples of commonly used agents shown. Consult specific drug literature for precautions, contraindications, details of use including maximum doses, etc.

- DIURETICS

Chlorothiazide (Diuril®)			
Age <6 months	2–8 mg/kg/day	bid	IV
	20–40 mg/kg/day	bid	PO
Age >6 months	4 mg/kg/day	qd or bid	IV
	20 mg/kg/day	bid	PO
Adult	100–500 mg/day	qd or bid	IV
	500 mg–2 g/day	qd or bid	PO
Furosemide (Lasix®)	0.5–1 mg/kg/dose	qd or bid	IV
	1–4 mg/kg/day	qd or bid	PO
Spironolactone (Aldactone®)	1–3 mg/kg/day	qd or bid	PO
	Adult CHF 12.5–50 mg/day		PO

- INOTROPES

Digoxin (Lanoxin®)

Load (Total Digitalizing Dose or TDD)   PO (avoid parenteral route)

Premature	20 µg/kg
Term neonates	30–40 µg/kg
Infants–2 years	40–60 µg/kg
Children >2years	30–40 µg/kg

(Give 1/2 of TDD initially, 1/4 of TDD in 6–8 hours, last 1/4 of TDD in 12–16 hours after first dose; reassess clinically before each increment of the TDD is given.)

Maintenance

25% of TDD/day ÷ bid		PO
-or-		
10 μg/kg/day ÷ bid		PO

Dobutamine (Dobutrex®)	1–15 μg/kg/min	IV
Dobutamine (Intropin®)	5–20 μg/kg/min	IV
Epinephrine (Adrenalin®)	0.02–1.0 μg/kg/min	IV
Milrinone (Primacor®)		
bolus	50 μg/kg (over 15 minutes)	IV
infusion (± bolus)	0.25–1.0 μg/kg/min	IV

• AFTERLOAD REDUCING AGENTS

Captopril (Capoten®)	0.25–4 mg/kg/day ÷ tid	PO
	Adult: 12.5–25 mg/dose tid	PO

(No commercially available liquid dose form; captopril rapidly degrades in aqueous solution, mix fresh 1 mg/mL solution each dose, or compound according to Am J Hosp Pharm 1994;51:95–96.)

Enalapril (Vasotec®)	0.1–0.5 mg/kg/day qd or ÷ bid	PO
	Adult: starting 5 mg/day, max 40 mg/day	PO
Enalaprilat (Vasotec®)	Starting 5–10 μg/kg/dose q6h–24 h	IV
	Adult: 0.625–1.25 mg/dose q6h	IV
Nitroglycerin	0.25–20 μg/kg/min	IV
Nitroprusside (Nitropress®)	0.25–20 μg/kg/min	IV

ADDITIONAL READING

FAQ's US Drug Information (with links to International Drug Information sites) US National Library of Medicine. Available from www.nlm.nih.gov/services/drug.html. Accessed March 2008.

Robertson J, Shilkofsky N. (eds.) The Harriet Lane Handbook, 17th ed. Philadelphia: Elsevier-Mosby; 2005.

Taketomo CK, Hodding JH, Kraus DM. (eds.) Pediatric Dosage Handbook, 14th ed. Hudson, OH: Lexi-Comp; 2007.

Appendix B
Management of the cyanotic neonate with congenital heart disease

- Assess and manage ABCs (Airway/Breathing/Circulation) *first*
- Prostaglandin (PGE, Alprostadil®) 0.025–0.1 µg/kg/min IV

  1 vial = 1 mL = 500 µg (micrograms); keep refrigerated until mixed
  Mix options:

  MIX #1 (no calculator needed)

  1 vial in 9 mL NS or D10W = 50 µg/mL
  add 3 mL of this to 47 mL D10W in IV chamber or syringe pump = 3 µg/mL
  infuse at rate (mL/h) equal to neonate's wt in kg for dose delivered of 0.05 µg/kg/min
  double rate for 0.1 µg/kg/min

  -OR- MIX #2

  1 vial in (83/wt in kg) mL of D5W or D10W
  infuse at 1 mL/h for 0.1 µg/kg/min

  -OR- MIX #3

  1 vial in 100 mL
  infuse at (1.25 × wt in kg) mL/h for 0.1 µg/kg/min

  -OR- MIX #4

  (0.6 × wt in kg) mg in 100 mL
  infuse at 1 mL/h for 0.1 µg/kg/min

  Consider intubation, especially before transport
  Side effects   Apnea
                    Hypotension
                    Fever
                    Rash

- *If no PGE available*, Intubate/Paralyze/Anesthetize to minimize oxygen consumption

Appendix C
Management of hypercyanotic (TET) spells from least to most invasive

- Have parent hold and calm child
- Knee/chest position
- AVOID IATROGENIC AGITATION

    limit exam, venipuncture, etc.
    NO INOTROPES (e.g., no digoxin, dopamine, or dobutamine) and NO DIURETICS

- Oxygen (increases R_S, decreases R_P)—Use least aggravating method of delivery.
- Morphine subcutaneous 0.1–0.2 mg/kg (decreases sympathetic tone, decreases oxygen consumption) *or* Ketamine 1–3 mg/kg IM (sedates and increases R_S)
- Fluid bolus (warmed)/Correct anemia/Convert tachyarrhythmia
- Phenylephrine (Neosynephrine®; action: increases R_S)

    bolus: 0.1 mg/kg IM or SC or IV
    start infusion: 0.1–0.5 µg/kg/min IV, titrate to effect (reflex bradycardia indicating raised BP; increased pulse oximeter saturation)

- *or* Methoxamine 0.1 mg/kg IV (action: increases R_S)
- β-Blockers (action: decrease oxygen consumption, may lessen infundibular "spasm")

    esmolol (Breviblock®) load 500 µg/kg × 1 min then, infuse 50–950 µg/kg/min (titrate in 25–50 µg/step)
    or propranolol (Inderal®) 0.05–0.25 mg/kg IV over 5 minutes

- Sodium bicarbonate 1–2 mEq/kg/dose IV
- Intubate/paralyze/anesthetize (reduces oxygen consumption to minimum)
- Surgical shunt, emergently

R_S, systemic vascular resistance
R_P, pulmonary vascular resistance

Appendix D
Acute management of tachyarrhythmia

Patient unstable?

- Cardiovert/defibrillate

Patient stable?

- 12-lead ECG
- ***Run Continuous Rhythm Strip (preferably a three-lead or 12-lead) During Conversion Attempt***
- Vagal Maneuvers

  Valsalva/Gag/Ice to Face

  (Avoid carotid & ocular massage and hypertension-producing drugs)
- Adenosine (Adenocard®, 2 mL/vial × 3 mg/mL = 6 mg/vial) DRUG OF CHOICE
    - Start dose 100 µg/kg IV *push* (fastest bolus possible, follow immediately with saline flush)
    - Increase by 100 µg/kg/dose to "maximum" 500 µg/kg (Theophylline is antagonist; may need ≫ "maximum" dose)
- *Verapamil is absolutely contraindicated* ≤ age 12 months and relatively contraindicated at any age.
- *Digoxin and Verapamil are contraindicated* in WPW
- Obtain 12-lead ECG after conversion

Appendix E
Acute management of bradyarrhythmia

Assess and manage ABCs (Airway, Breathing, Circulation) *first*

Must differentiate *congenital complete AV block* (CCAVB, rare) versus *sinus bradycardia* from noncardiac causes (common).

If CCAVB and

Patient stable?

Obtain 12-lead ECG & rhythm strip and call pediatric cardiologist

-OR-

Patient unstable?

- Isoproterenol (Isuprel®) 0.1–0.5 µg/kg/min IV and/or
- Pace (transcutaneous/transvenous/transgastric)

Appendix F
External direct current (DC) shock

CARDIOVERSION—Electrical termination of any arrhythmia other than ventricular fibrillation

DEFIBRILLATION—Electrical termination of one and only one arrhythmia: ventricular fibrillation

- Use the *largest* paddles that will completely contact skin over their entire surface.
- No dry contacts—Electrolyte pad or paste must completely cover the contact area between paddles and skin. Do not use ultrasound gel.

Dose:

Cardioversion	SVT	1/4–1/2 Joules/kg
	VT	1–2 Joules/kg
Defibrillation	VF	2–4 Joules/kg

Avoid "pilot error":

- *Never SYNC* (synchronize) for ventricular defibrillation
- *Always SYNC* for cardioversion, even for atrial "fibrillation," whenever QRS is distinct
- Connect 3- or 5-lead ECG *cable* for best Sync during cardioversion
- *Power on*
- *Set dose*
- *Charge*
- Call "*Clear!!*" and observe that all personnel are not in contact with the patient
- *Press hard* for good contact (minimal paddle-to-skin electrical resistance)
- Hold *both buttons* depressed for at least 3 seconds (sync takes time, particularly with relatively slow ventricular rates)
- Always record *rhythm strip* during procedure (some machines do this automatically)
- For subsequent cardioversion attempts, push *SYNC* again

Appendix G

ADDITIONAL READING (the following are encyclopedic reference works covering all aspects of pediatric cardiology)

Allen HD, Driscoll DJ, Shaddy RE, Feltes TF. (eds.) Moss and Adams Heart Disease in Infants, Children, and Adolescents Including the Fetus and Young Adult, 7th ed. Philadelphia: Lippincott Williams and Wilkins; 2007.

Anderson RH, Baker EJ, Macartney FJ, Rigby ML, Shinebourne EA, Tynan MJ. (eds.) Paediatric Cardiology, 2nd ed. London: Churchill Livingstone; 2002.

Garson A, Bricker JT, Fisher DJ, et al. (eds.) The Science and Practice of Pediatric Cardiology, 2nd ed. Baltimore: Williams and Wilkins; 1998.

Moller JH, Hoffman JIE. (eds.) Pediatric Cardiovascular Medicine. New York: Churchill Livingstone; 2000.

Index